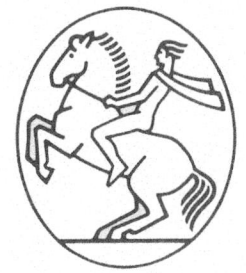

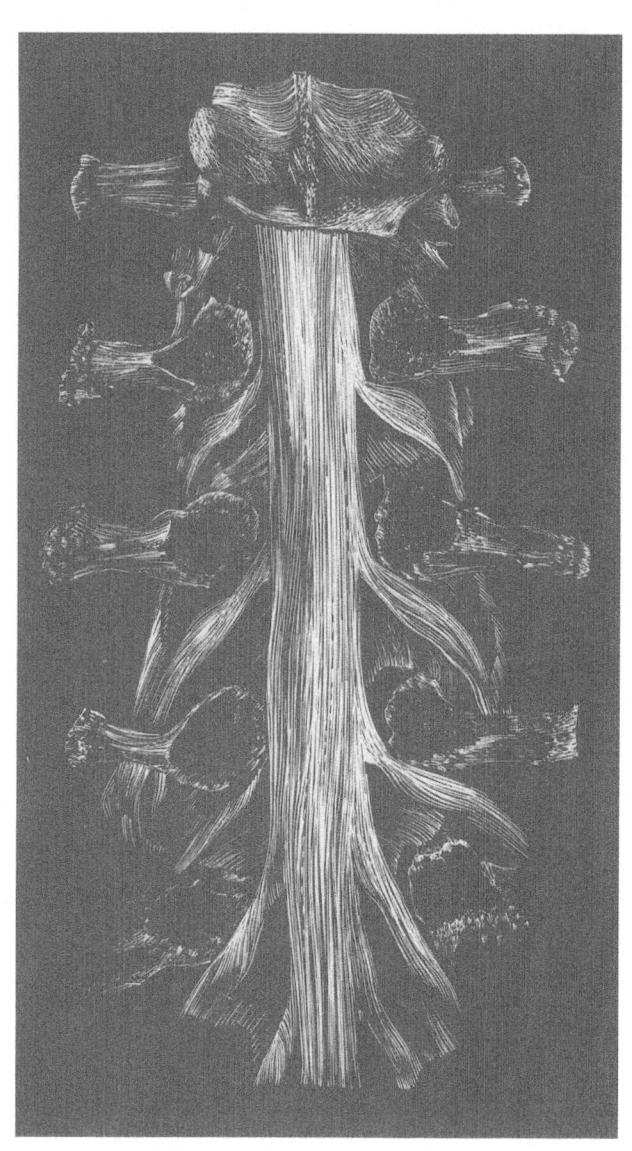

Henry V. Crock

A Short Practice of Spinal Surgery

Second, revised edition

With a Contribution on
Medical Aspects in the Management
of Spinal Surgical Patients
by Bryan P. Galbally

Springer-Verlag Wien GmbH

Henry Vernon Crock, A.O., M.D., M.S., F.R.C.S., F.R.A.C.S.
Consultant Spinal Surgeon, Senior Lecturer, Honorary Consultant,
The Royal Postgraduate Medical School, Hammersmith Hospital and
The Cromwell Hospital, London, U.K.

© 1993 Springer-Verlag Wien
Originally published by Springer-Verlag Wien New York in 1993

Product Liability: The publisher can give no guarantee for information about drug dosage and application thereof contained in this book. In every individual case the respective user must check its accuracy by consulting pharmaceutical literature.

The use of registered names, trademarks, etc. in the publication does not imply, even in the absence of a specific statement, that such names are exempt from the relevant protective laws and regulations and therefore free for general use.

With 278 partly coloured Figures

Frontispiece: From a wood-block by the artist Tate Adams, based on a dissection of the lumbar spine prepared by Dr. Carmel Crock.

ISBN 978-3-211-82351-4   ISBN 978-3-7091-6650-5 (eBook)
DOI 10.1007/978-3-7091-6650-5

Foreword

This volume is a treatise by a master surgeon on the spine. Mr. Crock has already produced classic papers and beautifully illustrated books on the anatomy of the spine and his studies with injection techniques provide new data on the arterial supply and venous drainage of the vertebral bodies, spinal cord and nerve roots. Using this traditional classical method he describes new approaches to spinal surgery, a particularly difficult field. The text is lucidly written and beautifully illustrated with X-rays, injection studies, dissection specimens, CT and MR scans. These are all of the highest quality and many of the techniques used are new and provide information that was previously not available. Mr. Crock divides surgery of the spine into different sections, in most of which he himself has been responsible for adding important new data, especially in nerve root canal stenosis and internal disc disruption. The book covers all aspects of disc disease and spondylolisthesis and there is also a section on surgery of the cervical spine. I feel that this work – the result of personal research, surgical experience and extreme hard work – will be essential reading for all orthopaedic and neurosurgeons who venture to operate around the delicate spinal cord and its major nerve roots.

Sir Roy Calne, F.R.S.

Preface

In the nine years which have passed since the first edition of this book was published many changes have occurred to modify the practice of spinal surgery. There has been an explosive growth of publications including new journals such as Neuro-Orthopaedics, Rachis, The European Spine Journal and hosts of books and monographs on many different topics, scientific and clinical, relating to the human spine in health and disease.

Burgeoning interest in the whole field of spinal disorders has led to the formation of many new spine societies in the 1980's, national and international. Under their influence many of the animosities over the questions of who should treat and operate on patients with spinal problems have begun to break down. Spinal surgery has emerged from the decade as an independent speciality. In this period advances in imaging technology have had the greatest impact on the diagnosis of spinal disorders. The developments in biochemical testing of disc tissues alluded to in the 1983 preface have not had any impact on clinical practice. Hence most practitioners continue to recognise only two forms of disc disease – prolapse or degeneration. Controversy over the treatment of the first persists while the management of the second often remains clouded by uncertainty.

Enthusiasm for the treatment of disc prolapses by chemonucleolysis with chymopapain has waned in the North American continent although work on the use of other enzymes such as collagenase continues. Micro-discectomy and percutaneous discectomy have emerged as the latest methods for dealing with some disc prolapses.

Finally there have been major developments in the design and application of devices for spinal fixation.

I have added important new material while maintaining a rather conservative stand on the use of some of the surgical techniques which have been introduced in the past nine years. I hope that this book will continue to serve as a useful, practical and safe guide to those who care for patients who may require spinal operations.

London 1992   *Henry V. Crock*

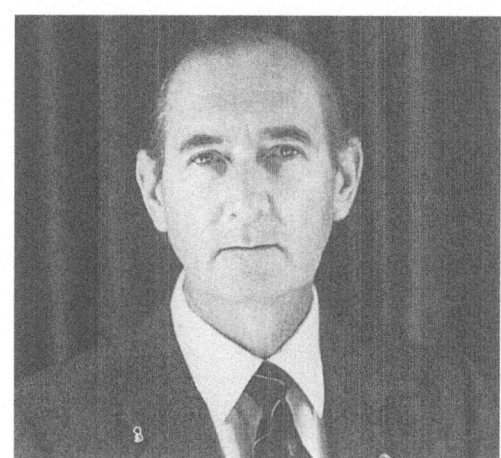

Since 1986 the author has practised in London. He holds the post of Honorary Senior Lecturer and Consultant Spinal Surgeon in the Department of Orthopaedic Surgery at the Royal Postgraduate Medical School, Hammersmith Hospital and is Director of the Spinal Disorders Unit at the Cromwell Hospital, London where he is joined by his wife Dr. M. C. Crock and Dr. B. P. Galbally.

Acknowledgements

The second edition of this book has been produced in England with new material derived from my experience while working in London since 1986. I wish to thank the many colleagues who have given me support since my arrival here, too many to be mentioned individually by name. I am particularly grateful to the British Orthopaedic Association for having elected me to Fellowship. When I first returned to London to commence practice I was given remarkable assistance by Mr. J. P. O'Brien, formerly director of the spinal disorders unit at the Robert Jones and Agnes Hunt Orthopaedic Hospital, Oswestry.

Professor Ruth Bowden (now retired) and Professor C. Sinatamby from the anatomy department at the Royal College of Surgeons of England have both provided me with opportunities to perform dissections which are illustrated in this volume. I have had enormous encouragement from my colleagues in the department of orthopaedic surgery at the Royal Postgraduate Medical School, Hammersmith Hospital where in particular I have worked in Mr. J. Patrick England's unit. Professor Graham Bydder and Professor Robert Steiner of the MRC research unit for magnetic resonance imaging have given me wonderful assistance.

Among my orthopaedic colleagues I am particularly indebted to Peter Baird, John Scott Ferguson, David Sharp, George Raine, and Professor Al Haddad.

At the Cromwell Hospital I have to thank many colleagues but especially Dr. Derek Kingsley and Dr. John Dawson with whom I have worked closely in Neuro-radiology, and Dr. Micheal Espir and Dr. Kevin Zilkha in Neurology. The medical directors, Dr. Nizami and Dr. Hameed have provided excellent facilities for the spinal disorders unit. The nursing staff both on the wards and in the theatres and the physiotherapists Misses Vandana Patel and Amanda Capstick have contributed significantly to the care of many of the patients whose problems are discussed in this book.

I thank also my European colleagues Professor Franco Postachinni from Rome, Dr. Roberto Binazzi from Bologna and Dr. Giuseppe Tabasso from Turin. I have also received enormous encouragement from Professor Peter Schulitz of the University of Düsseldorf, and Professor Sven Olerud of the University of Upsalla.

I am especially indebted to Dr. Joseph Assheuer, one of Germany's leading neuro-radiologists from Cologne, for providing me with the most important MRI images which are reproduced in chapters 3 and 8.

Professor Norbert Gschwend and Dr. Dieter Grob have given me special assistance since my arrival in Europe in 1986.

Shortly before I completed this manuscript my dear friend and collaborator in the first edition of this book died in Perth, Western Australia. Sir George Bedbrook had been a friend to me and to my twin brother since we were medical students in the University of Melbourne in 1949 when we first had contact with him as a teacher of anatomy. Like us he was also an identical twin. I wish to pay a special tribute to his genius and warm humanity.

In addition I wish to record my gratitude to the late Sir Roy Douglas Wright who helped to mould my medical career and that of my twin brother Professor Emeritus Gerard Crock. Pansy Wright wrote the forward to the first edition. He died in 1990.

Sir Roy Calne FRS my friend and colleague since 1957 when we first met as postgraduate students in Oxford has kindly consented to write the Foreword to this edition. I am, as ever, deeply grateful to him.

Many of the new drawings in this edition have been prepared by Miss Lizzie Butler who has worked tirelessly in the past few months on the preparation of all the illustrative material. To her I owe a special debt of gratitude.

My secretaries Misses Andrea Keenan and Linda Wilkinson have prepared this manuscript most skilfully despite their routine heavy workload.

I would also like to thank Dr. Tateru Shiraishi for his remarkable help with the editorial preparation of this manuscript.

Finally I wish to thank the staff of Springer-Verlag, Wien for their continuing support. I have had an excellent working relationship with them now for many years.

Henry V. Crock

Contents

8. Spinal Infections   273

9. The Management of Failed Spinal Operations   291

1

Nerve Root Canal Stenosis

1.1. Isolated Lumbar Disc Resorption

This condition is characterised by gross narrowing of one affected disc space, with sclerosis of the adjacent vertebral bodies. Occurring commonly as an isolated affection in an otherwise normal spine, even late in life, it is seen most commonly at L 5/S1, occasionally at L4/5 and rarely at higher levels in the lumbar spine (Figs. 1.1,2).

Attention was first drawn to the importance of "reduced lumbosacral joint space: its relation to sciatic irritation", by Williams in 1932. The terminology "*isolated disc resorption*" was coined by Crock in 1970, though he was unaware of the existence of Williams' paper at that time.

Isolated disc resorption causes back and leg pain more commonly than does prolapse of an intervertebral disc. This condition therefore assumes great clinical importance and warrants identification as a specific form of disc disease. Knowledge of this entity has increased considerably in the past 8 years due to the wider use of computerised tomography and magnetic resonance imaging in the investigation of spinal disorders. By combining observations on the pathological findings in isolated disc resorption with a sound knowledge of surgical anatomy, different forms of surgical treatment can be planned to suit individual cases. Treated by the standard operation of "laminectomy" used in the management of disc prolapse, results are often poor, whereas they are usually excellent when bilateral nerve root canal and foraminal decompressions are performed. In selected cases, localized spinal fusion is sometimes indicated.

a) Natural History

This condition of narrowing of a single lumbar intervertebral disc space usually progresses slowly over a number of years, the clinical course being punctuated by repeated bouts of acute low back pain lasting 3–4 days which then resolve completely. Following trauma, particularly a fall on to the buttocks, the symptoms may extend to include severe bilateral buttock and leg pains. In some cases buttock and leg pain may be aggravated by standing or sitting and occasionally by walking. The description of nerve root claudication may then be used to describe this particular

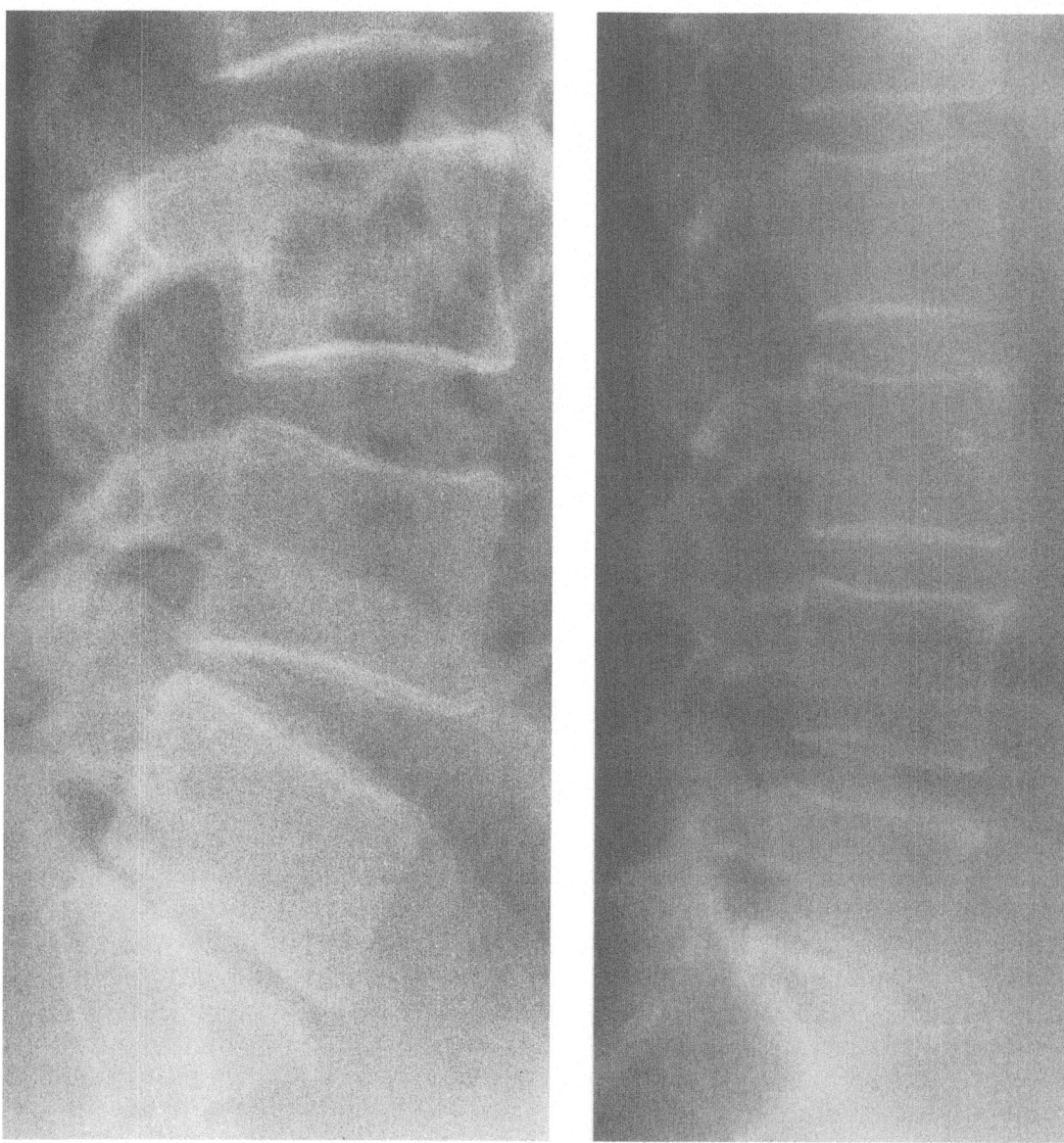

Figure 1.1   **Figure 1.2**

Figure 1.1. A lateral radiograph of the lumbar spine of a 48-year old man showing the classical features of isolated disc resorption at the lumbo-sacral junction

Figure 1.2. A lateral radiograph of the lumbar spine of an 82 year old man presenting with symptoms arising from isolated disc resorption at L5/S1. All the other lumbar discs have maintained a normal height. This patient presented with symptoms of L5/S1 nerve root irritation which were relieved by bilateral foraminal and root canal decompressions at that level

symptom pattern. Characteristically these symptoms may be relieved by postural changes such as stooping to bend forwards or after lying on a bed for a short time. When the L3/4 or L4/5 discs are affected, back pain predominates and may be very severe, preventing any movement. Muscle spasm leads to lumbar tilt – a scoliotic deformity which may persist for hours or weeks. Neurological examination is usually normal in these patients even when symptoms of referred leg pain are severe.

In parallel with the natural history of the symptoms, repeated radiological examination will reveal progressive loss of disc height at the affected level (Figs. 1.3 a–c). In the lower lumbar region in adults, the disc height between adjacent

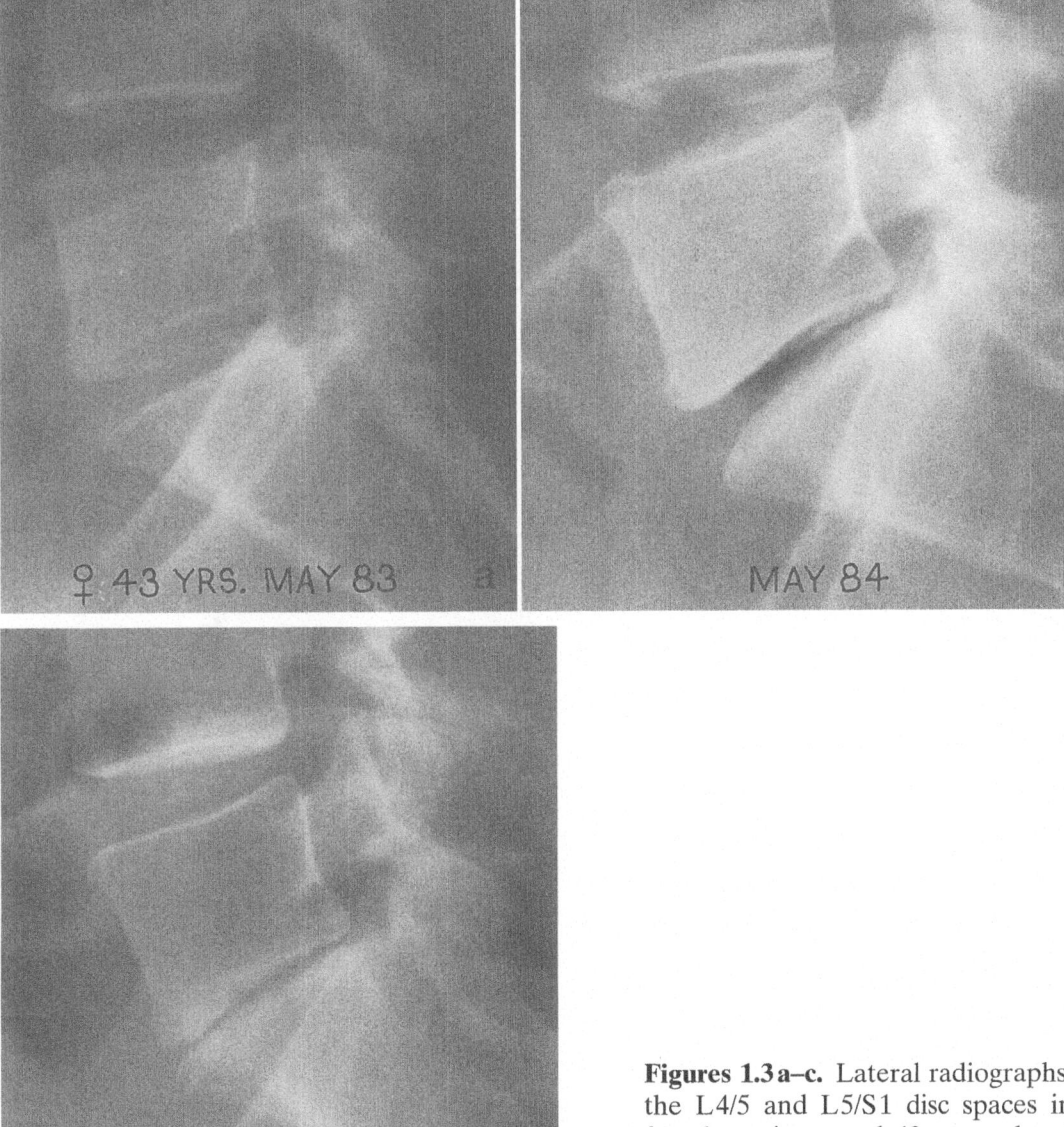

Figures 1.3 a–c. Lateral radiographs of the L4/5 and L5/S1 disc spaces in a female patient aged 43 years showing the rapid evolution of isolated disc resorption at L5/S1. Note the Knuttson vacuum sign in **b**. Vertebral end-plate sclerosis has already appeared in **c**

vertebral end-plates ranges from 10 to 15 mm. In established cases of isolated lumbar disc resorption, the height of the intervertebral disc space may be reduced to 3 mm. The vacuum phenomenon of Knuttson is another prominent radiological feature especially in X-rays taken with the patient standing with the lumbar spine extended. A black gas shadow will then appear in the disc space. Sclerosis of the adjacent vertebral end-plates appears and often extends to involve large areas of the vertebral bodies themselves (Figs. 1.4,5). Marginal osteophyte formation is often minimal but a ridge of bone covered with a thin layer of annular fibre remnants frequently projects into the spinal canal across its whole width. Subluxation of the facet joints related to the resorbed disc is an invariable finding best seen in oblique views of the facets (Figs. 1.6 a,b). This may give rise to retrolisthesis of L5 on S1, further compromising the sizes of the nerve root canals and intervertebral foramina (Fig. 1.5).

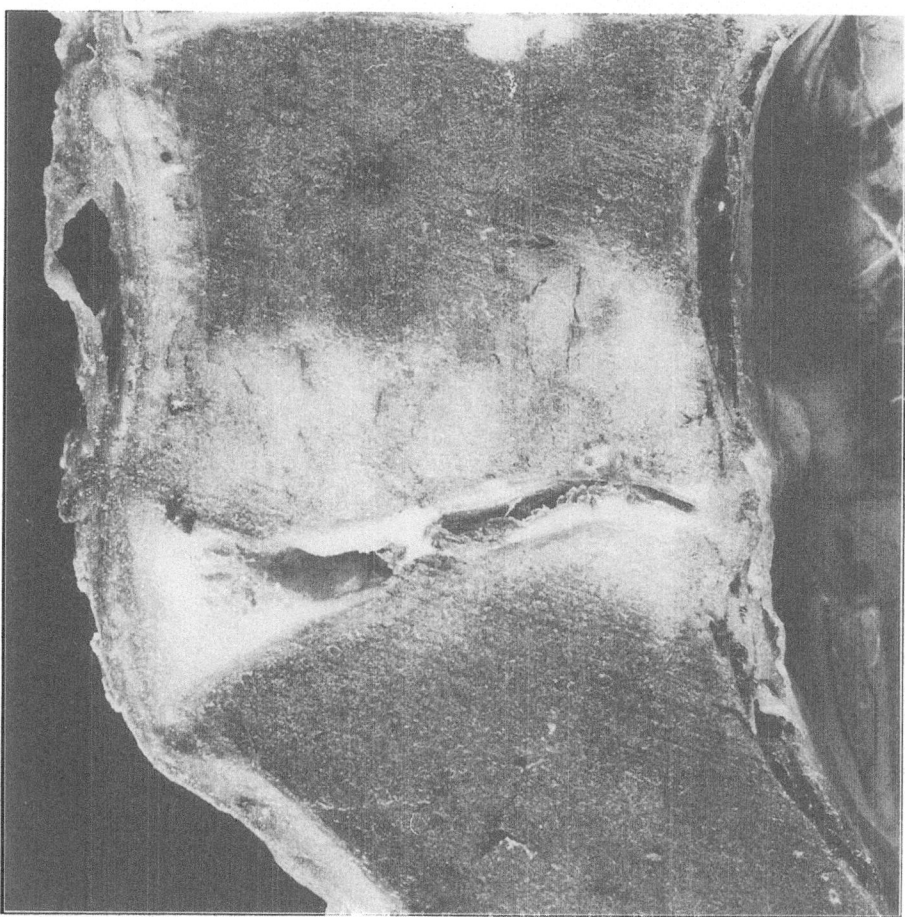

Figure 1.4. A photograph of a mid-line sagittal section of the lumbar spine of a man aged 69 years. The pathological features of isolated disc resorption are well shown, with vertebral end-plate remnants in the posterior two-thirds of the disc space visible on either side of an otherwise empty disc space. Note the marked sclerosis of the vertebral bodies on either side of the disc space

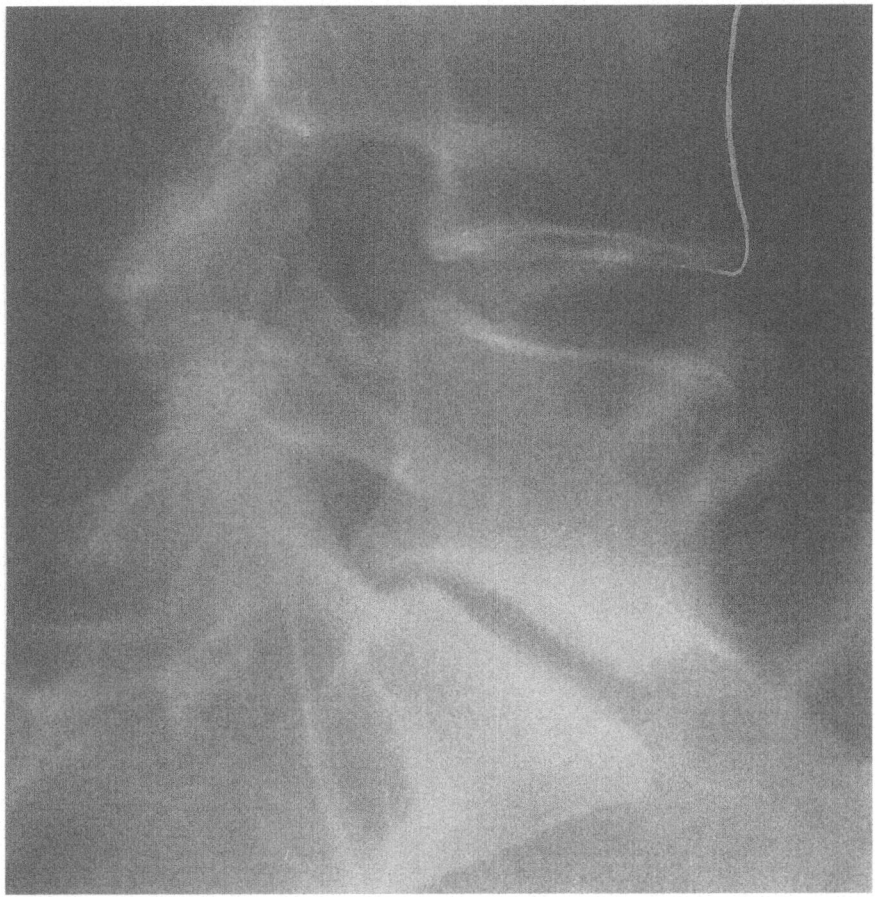

Figure 1.5. A lateral radiograph of the lower lumbar spine showing an example of retro-spondylolisthesis complicating isolated disc resorption at the lumbo-sacral junction. Note the sclerosis which has appeared in the vertebral bodies on either side of the narrowed disc space. The L4/5 disc space is normal

The disc space narrowing which accompanies sacralisation anomalies is not to be confused with that occurring in isolated lumbar disc resorption. Disc resorption at the first mobile segment above a sacralised vertebra is, however, a common finding which often leads to the development of disabling symptoms of isolated disc resorption (Figs. 1.7 a, b).

In established cases where the disc space has become very narrow, with parallel vertebral end-plate settling, symptoms of buttock and leg pain if intractable, are usually bilateral.

Earlier in the course of this disease, a small number of patients may present with unilateral sciatica. These patients may exhibit the classic features of neurological defects in either L5 or S1 roots or both. Usually they will be found to have a seques-trated fragment of vertebral end-plate cartilage impinging on the affected nerve root. At operation in such cases the disc space is virtually empty and clearly recog-nisable necrotic vertebral end-plate cartilage will be found causing the nerve root compression. The volume of sequestrated material is sometimes massive. Clearance

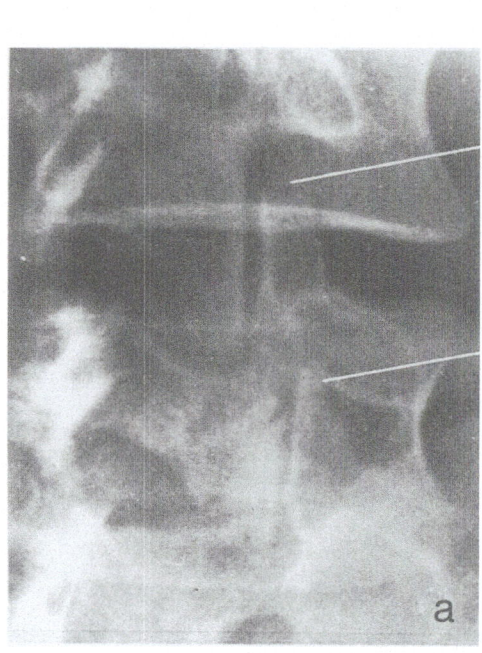

Figures 1.6 a, b

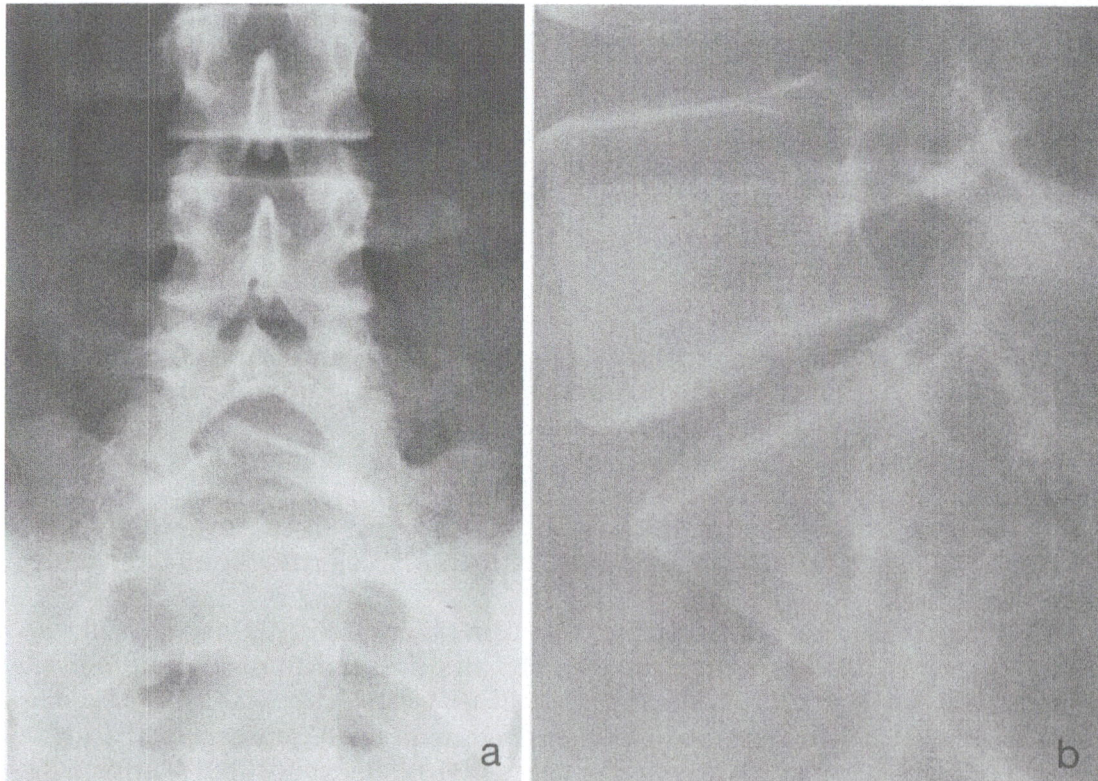

Figures 1.7a, b

of resorbed retained fragments from within the disc space must then be carried out with great care as only fine rongeurs can be used. The danger of these instruments penetrating anterior annular fibres and damaging intra-abdominal contents should be guarded against.

The basic pathology of this condition is still incompletely understood but it is now clear that there is a very active biochemical process leading to degradation of the nuclear and annular portions of the intervertebral disc and eventually to necrosis of the vertebral end-plate cartilages. When vertebral end-plate sclerosis extends into the vertebral bodies, seen best in magnetic resonance imaging and even on plain X-rays, this condition is often mistaken for an infective process (Fig. 1.8).

In some cases the disc space narrowing is associated with punctate defects in opposing vertebral end-plates. These defects are best seen in horizontal CT images while MRI findings both in the sagittal and horizontal planes help to confirm the diagnosis (Figs. 1.9 a–e). Patients with this less common form of isolated disc resorption are often subjected to a wide variety of tests including vertebral biopsy.

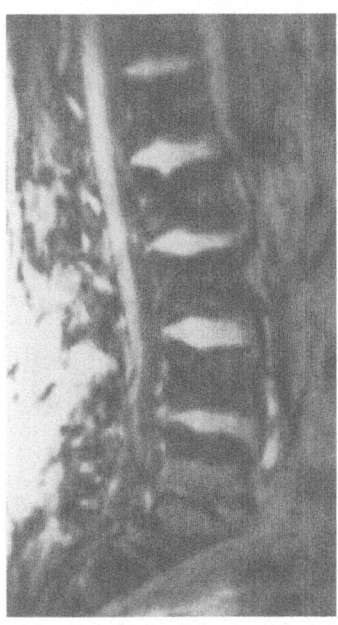

Figure 1.8. A sagittal MR image, T2 weighted sequence, in a male patient aged 35 years showing advanced isolated disc resorption at L5/S1 with extensive signal changes affecting half the vertebral bodies of L5 and S1

Figures 1.6 a, b. An oblique view of the lower lumbar spine showing normal relationships of the facets at the L4/5 level, top marker, and subluxation of S1 up against the pedicle of L5 on the bottom marker, with an explanatory drawing along side

Figures 1.7 a, b. Antero-posterior and lateral radiographs of the lumbar spine of an adult with sacralisation and spina bifida occulta affecting L6 vertebra. In the lateral view of **b** note the isolated disc resorption between L5 and L6

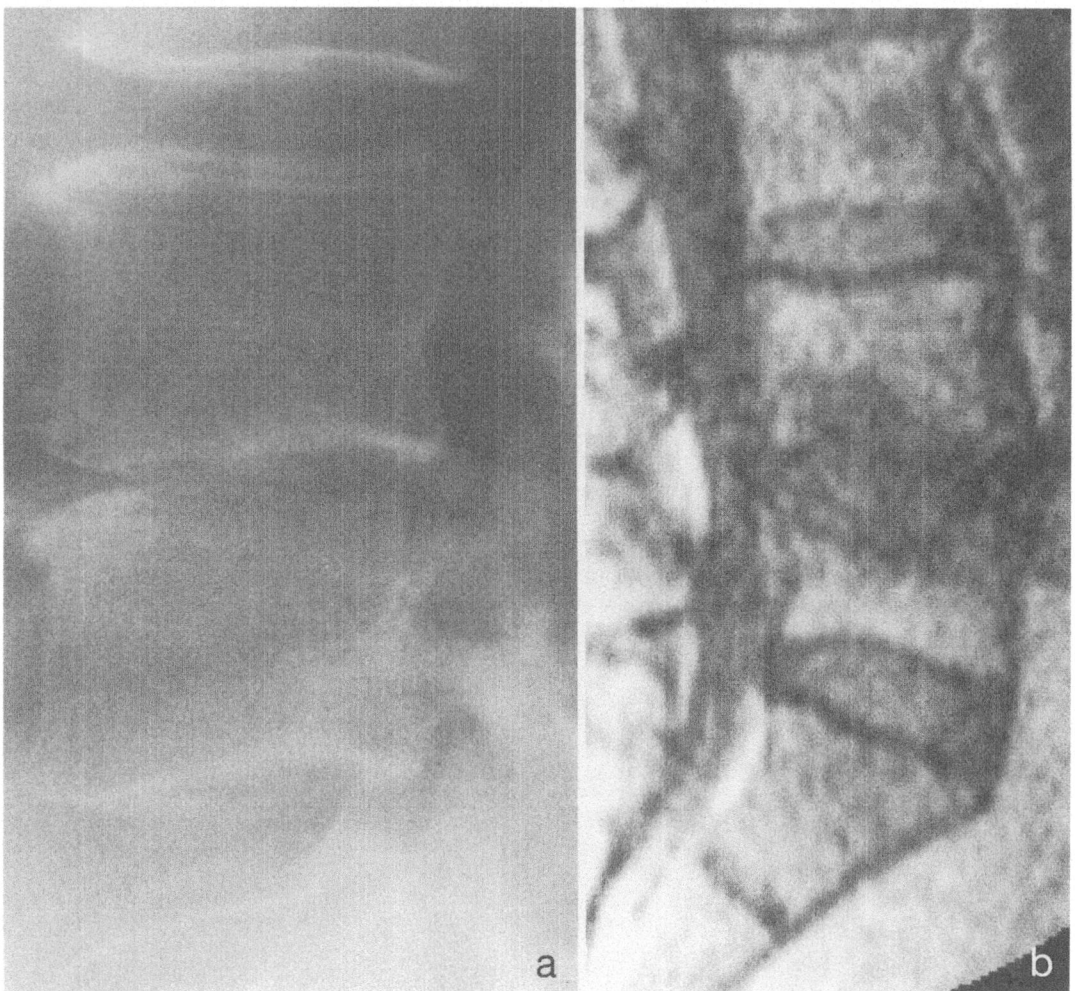

Figures 1.9 a–e. a A lateral radiograph showing isolated disc resorption at L 4/5 in a female patient aged 54 years. **b** A mid-sagittal MR image showing loss of disc height at L 4/5 and changes in the adjacent vertebral bodies consistent with intra-spongeous disc herniation. **c, d** CT images through the vertebral end-plates of L 4 and L 5 showing the classic punctate defects found in this form of isolated disc resorption. This patient had had a negative vertebral biopsy and she had been put on to a course of triple therapy for suspected tuberculous disease despite the fact that there was no evidence of infection on blood tests nor any radiological evidence of para-vertebral abscess formation. She was successfully treated by anterior interbody fusion and histological examinations of tissues removed at operation revealed purely degenerative vertebral end-plate cartilages and disc remnants. **e** A CT image showing the typical punctate defects found in the upper vertebral end-plate of L 5 from a middle aged patient with isolated disc resorption at L 4/L 5

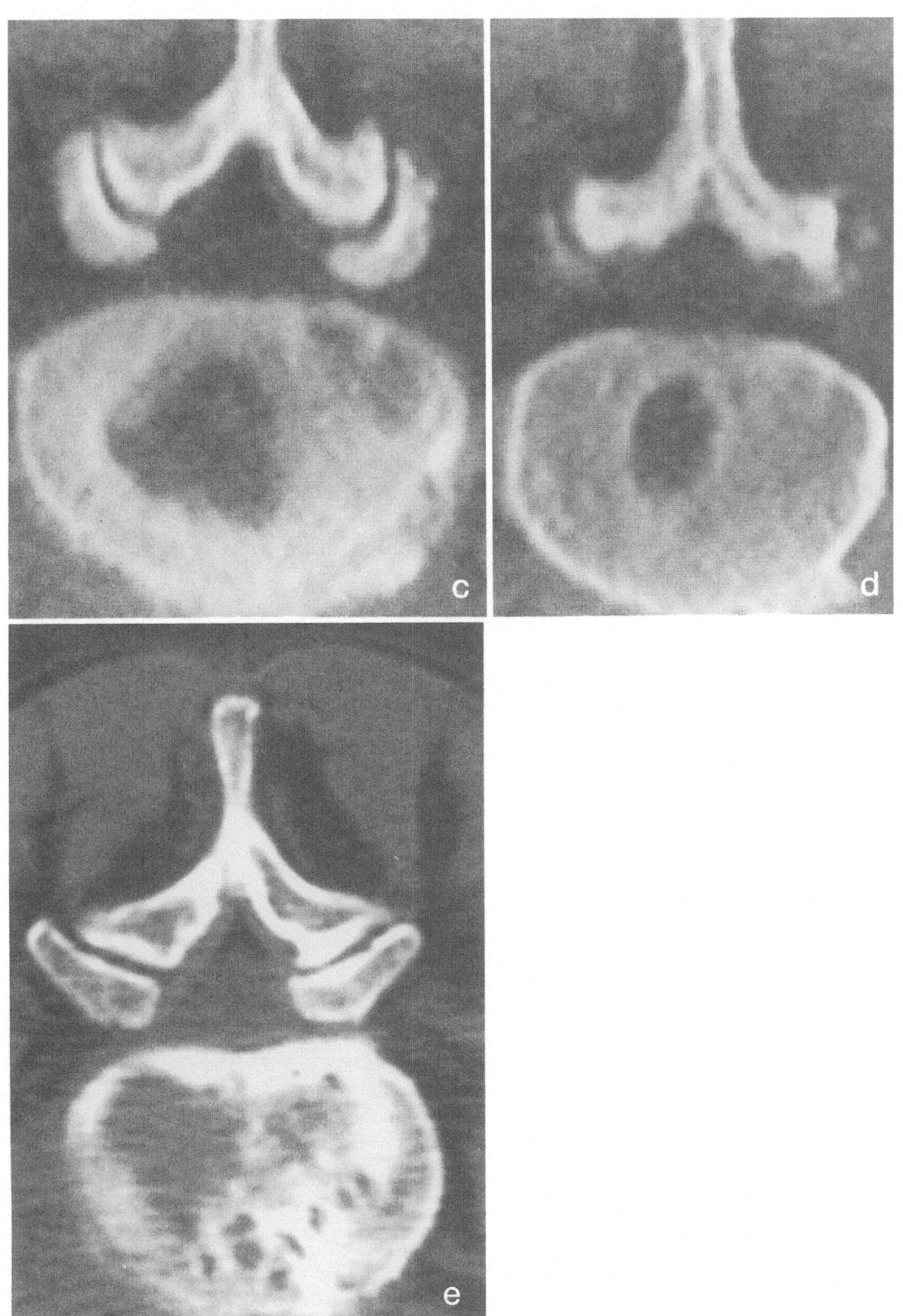

The cause of these lesions remains to be determined. Whether or not they result from a breach in the vertebral end-plate cartilage which allows disc tissue to extend into the adjacent vertebral body or whether the primary lesion is a vascular invasion of a vertebral end-plate defect cannot at this time be confirmed one way or the other (Figs. 1.10 a, b).

The clinical significance of isolated disc resorption is regrettably still not widely appreciated for a number of reasons. The first is that it is regarded by many as an innocuous form of degenerative disease of the spine which is often asymptomatic. While it may give rise to only trivial complaints in the majority of those who are found to have it, on the other hand it is a potent cause of severe disability in a small percentage of patients. Many of these may be denied treatment because they present only with symptoms. Even when their pain is at its worst they may have no abnormal

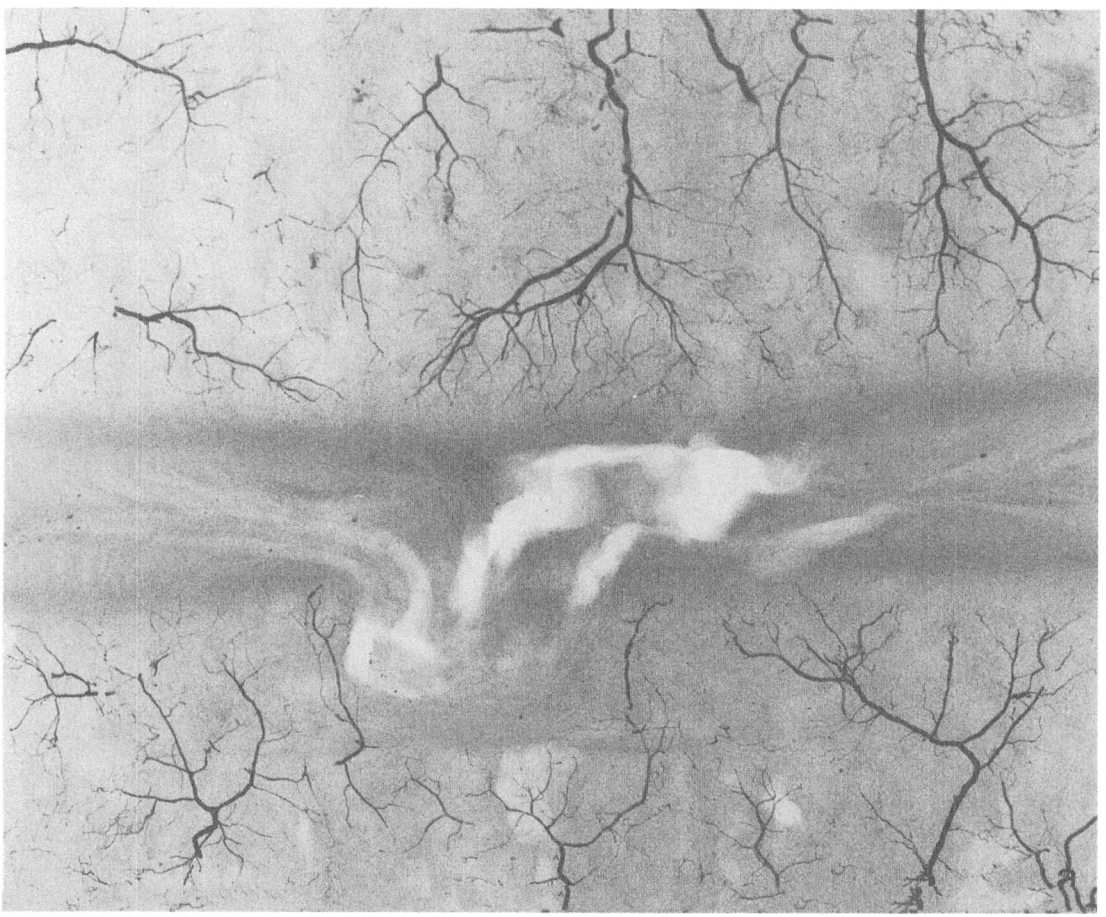

Figure 1.10 a. A thin coronal section obtained at post-mortem from adjacent upper lumbar vertebral bodies following arterial injection of the vertebral vessels. Degenerated nuclear material has herniated into the vertebral body through a defect in the inferior vertebral end-plate. No vascular invasion has occurred into the disc tissues

neurological findings. *The historical account of symptoms is often of more relevance in reaching surgical decisions about treatment than are the physical signs which can be elicited on clinical examination.* Another confusing factor relates to the interpretation of radiculography which is still frequently used in patients with this condition who complain of referred leg pain. Almost invariably the radiculogram is reported as normal and on this basis surgical treatment is frequently denied. Facet subluxation and ligamentum flavum buckling both contribute to venous obstruction in the intervertebral foramina and nerve root canals on either side of the resorbed disc space. This obstructive process may cause remarkable dilatation of the radicular veins leading to oedema of the nerve roots, a finding which is easily overlooked on the radiculograms (Fig. 1.11).

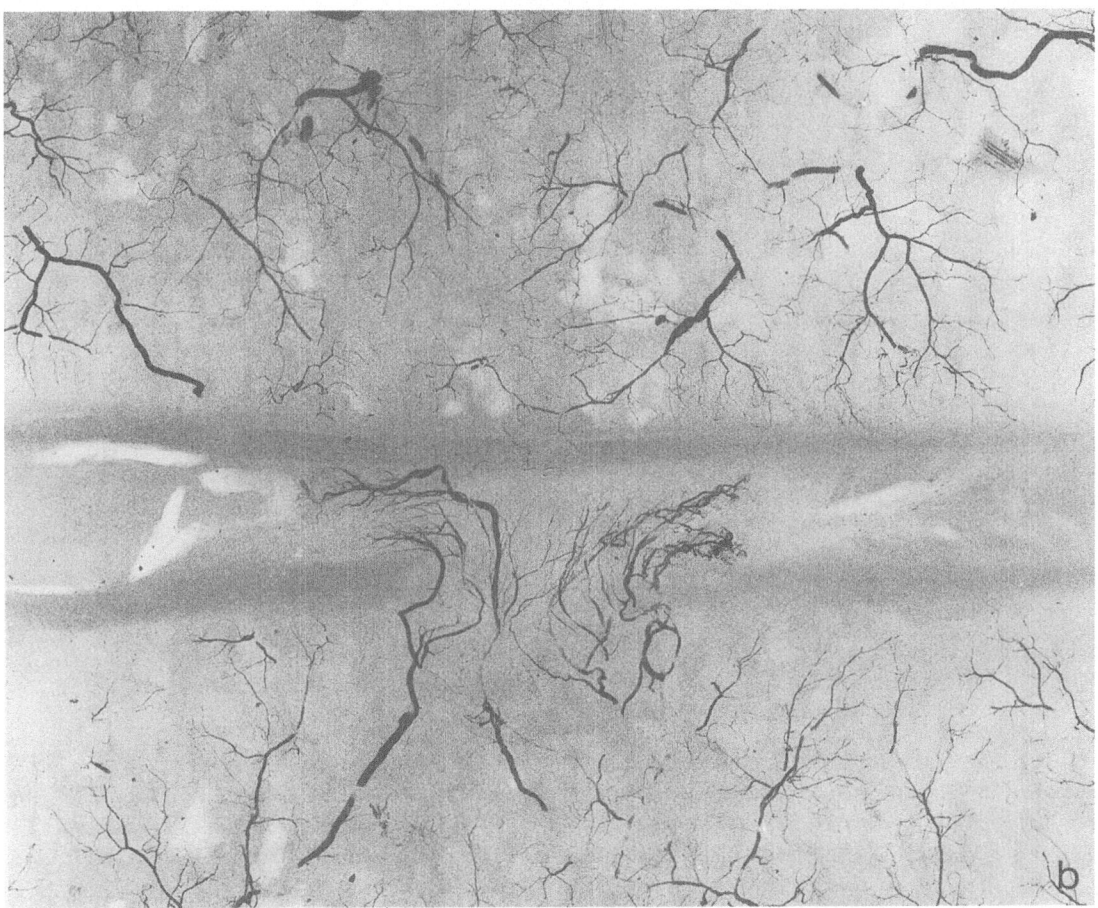

Figure 1.10b. A thin coronal section taken from the upper lumbar region in an adult at post mortem following arterial injection of the vertebral vessels. Note the extensive vascular invasion into the disc space contrasting with the section above

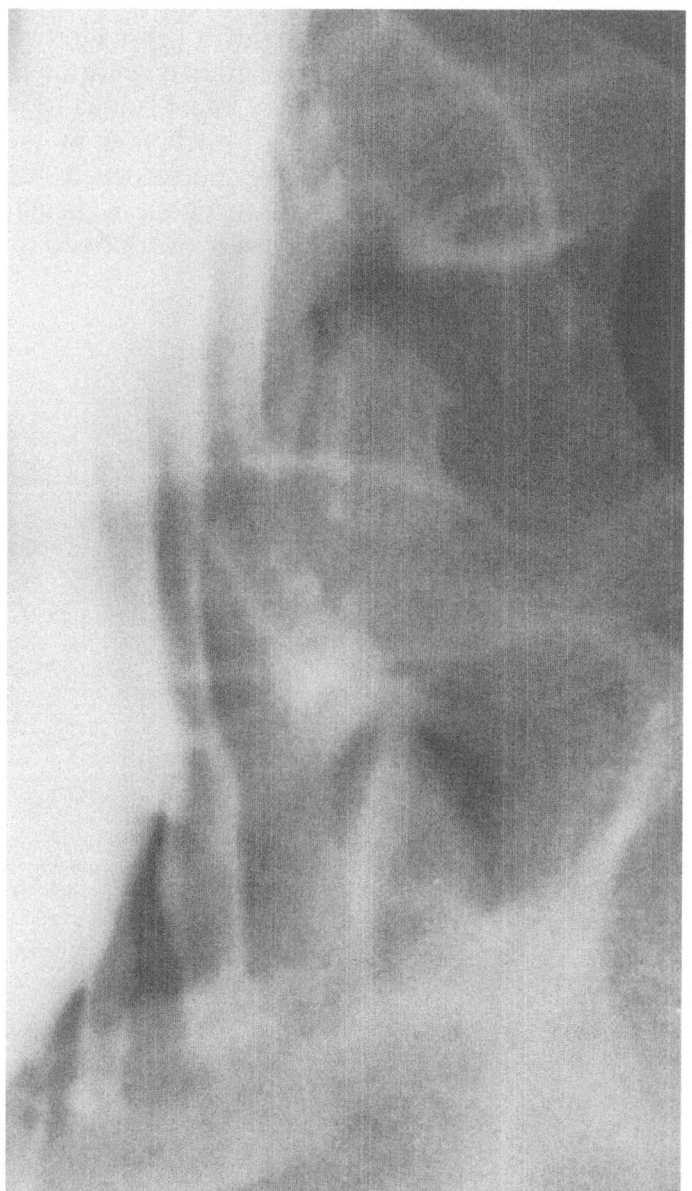

Figure 1.11. A detail from the radiculogram of a patient with isolated disc resorption at L5/S1. Note the approximation of the apex of the superior facet of S1 to the pedicle of L5. Adjacent to the pedicle of L4 a normal nerve root sleeve is outlined. Below that the nerve roots of L5 and S1 are enlarged due to oedema resulting from venous obstruction. The S2 and S3 nerve roots are of normal size. (Reproduced from Spinal Stenosis Edited by J. E. Nixon from Chapter 2 Principles of Anatomy Applied to the Surgery of Lumbar Spinal Stenosis H. V. Crock Page 32, Edward Arnold 1991 by kind permission of John E. Nixon)

b) Anatomy of the Nerve Root Canals and Intervertebral Foramina

i) Normal

The understanding of the genesis of the symptoms and signs which may occur in cases of isolated disc resorption depends largely on knowledge of the normal and pathological anatomy of the lumbar nerve root canals and intervertebral foramina.

The lumbar nerves run obliquely downwards and laterally from the lateral aspects of the dural sac, emerging at their respective intervertebral foramina and lying inferior to the lumbar pedicle in the upper part of each foramen (Fig. 1.12).

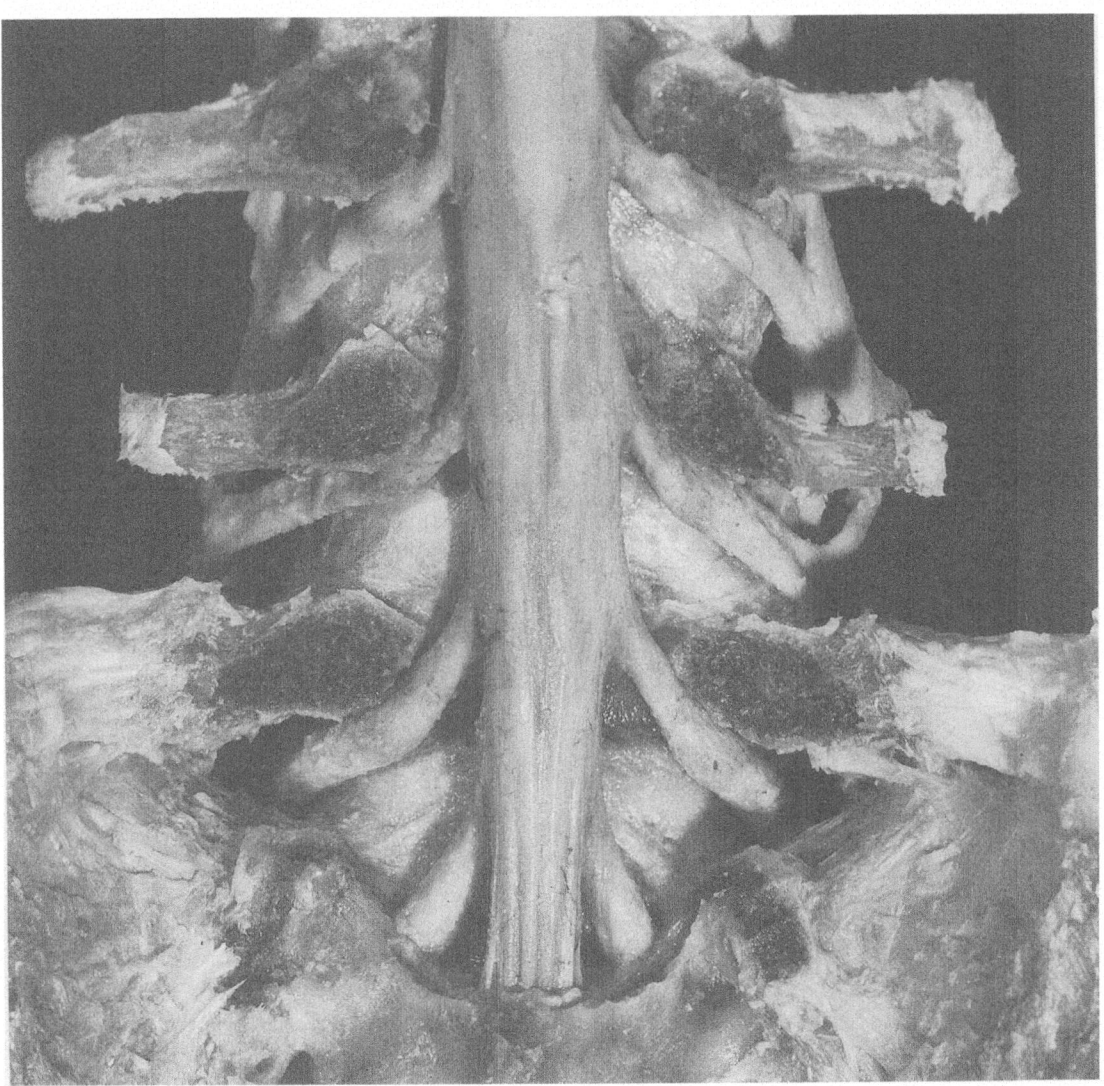

Figure 1.12. A photograph of a dissection of the lower lumbar spine in an adult to show some of the relations of the lumbar nerve roots. Note especially the origins of the nerve root sleeves from the dural sac and the courses of the nerve roots in relation to the pedicles (dissected by Dr. M. C. Crock)

Anomalies excluded, each nerve root is intimately related to the medial and inferior aspects of the adjacent vertebral pedicle.

The intervertebral foramen has fixed boundaries, though its dimensions vary depending on the height of the individual disc space and on the size of the related facet joints and thickness of the ligamentum flavum (Figs. 1.13 a,b). Bounded above and below by the vertebral pedicles, the floor from above downwards is formed by the postero-inferior margin of the upper vertebral body, the intervertebral disc and the postero-superior margin of the lower vertebral body (Fig. 1.14). The roof is formed by the ligamentum flavum, terminating at its outer free edge, and posterior to this structure lies the pars interarticularis and the apophyseal joint formed between the adjacent inferior and superior vertebral facets (Fig. 1.15). The intervertebral foramen is analogous to the doorway at the end of a passage, its vertical height being determined by the vertical height of the corresponding intervertebral disc space.

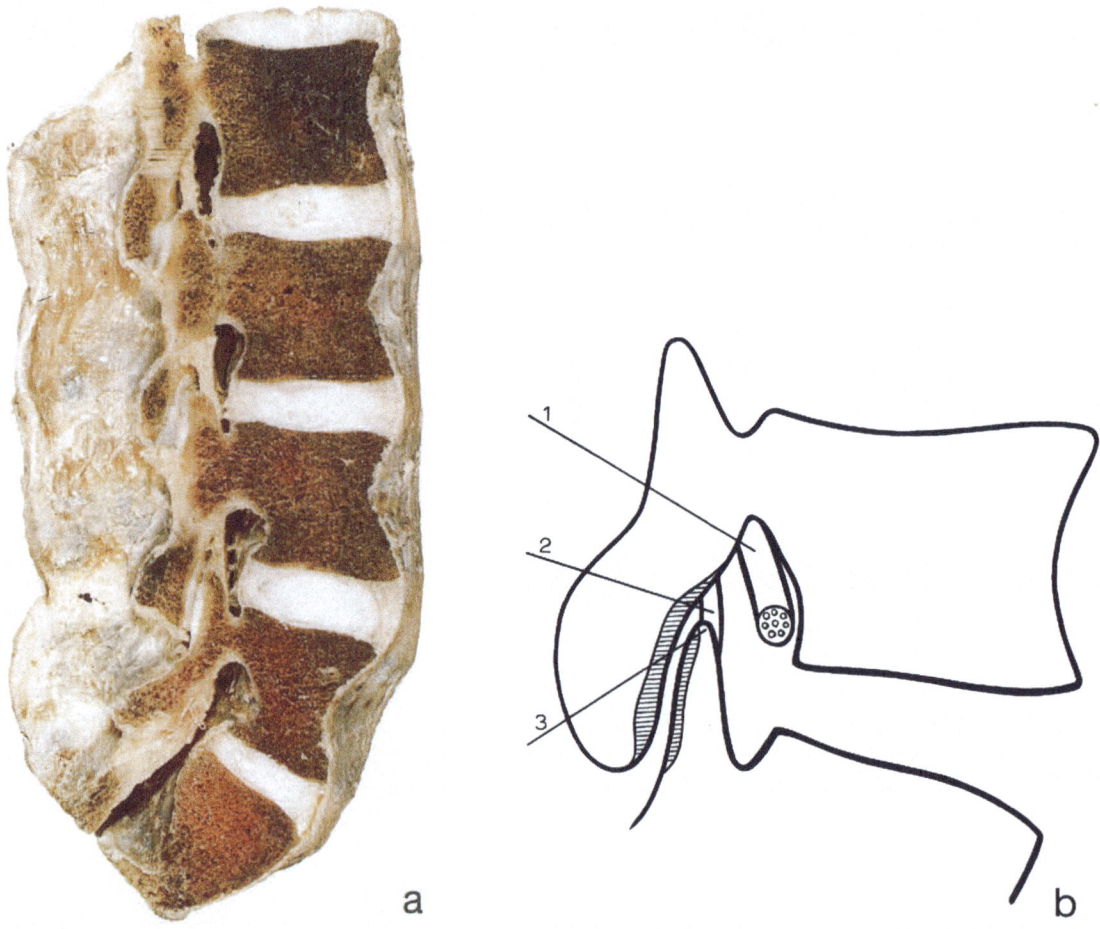

a   b

Figures 1.13 a,b. a A sagittal section through the level of the pedicles of a normal lumbar vertebral spine of an 18 year old male to show the boundaries and major structural relations of the intervertebral foramina. The structure and relations of the ligamentum flavum are best seen at L4/5 in this specimen. **b** A line drawing to show the principal relations of the L5 nerve root at the L5/S1 intervertebral foramen. *1* the nerve root; *2* the ligamentum flavum; and *3* the apex of the superior facet of S1

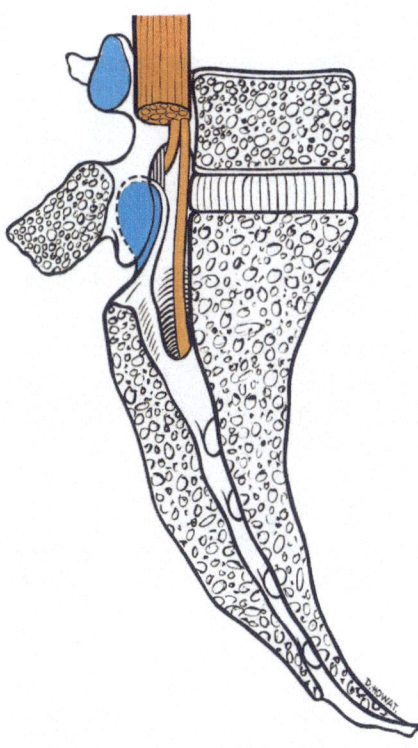

Figure 1.14. A drawing showing the relations of the S1 spinal nerve root canal viewed from within the spinal canal. The L5/S1 disc is of normal height

A nerve root canal, by contrast, is a tubular canal of variable length, arising from the lateral aspect of the dural sac. Viewed from within the sac, the hiatus through which the component motor and sensory nerve roots pass to the spinal nerve has the shape of a funnel. Viewed from without, the dural sheath clothes the spinal nerve on all sides as it courses obliquely downwards and laterally towards the intervertebral foramen (Fig. 1.16). The upper lumbar nerve roots are often orientated almost at right angles to the dural sac and their intraspinal portions are, therefore, very short. The nerve root canal in such cases becomes, in effect, a useless concept, as the dural sac lies against the medial wall of the upper lumbar pedicle. The emerging lumbar spinal nerve passes at once into the intervertebral foramen at its upper boundary immediately below the pedicle.

The shape of the dural sac changes from a rounded tubular outline, tapering progressively from the level of L3 downwards. Contrasting with the upper two lumbar spinal nerves, the lower lumbar nerves are longer and come off at more acute angles from the sides of the dural sac. The concept of a nerve root canal is of greatest significance in relation to the two lower-most lumbar and first sacral nerves.

In Fig. 1.16, the origin of the S1 nerve from the dural sac is shown just below the level of the inferior margin of the fifth lumbar pedicle. Medially at its origin it is related to the lateral aspect of the dural sac. The nerve courses downwards and obliquely as it passes laterally, lying first medial to the fifth lumbar nerve root and

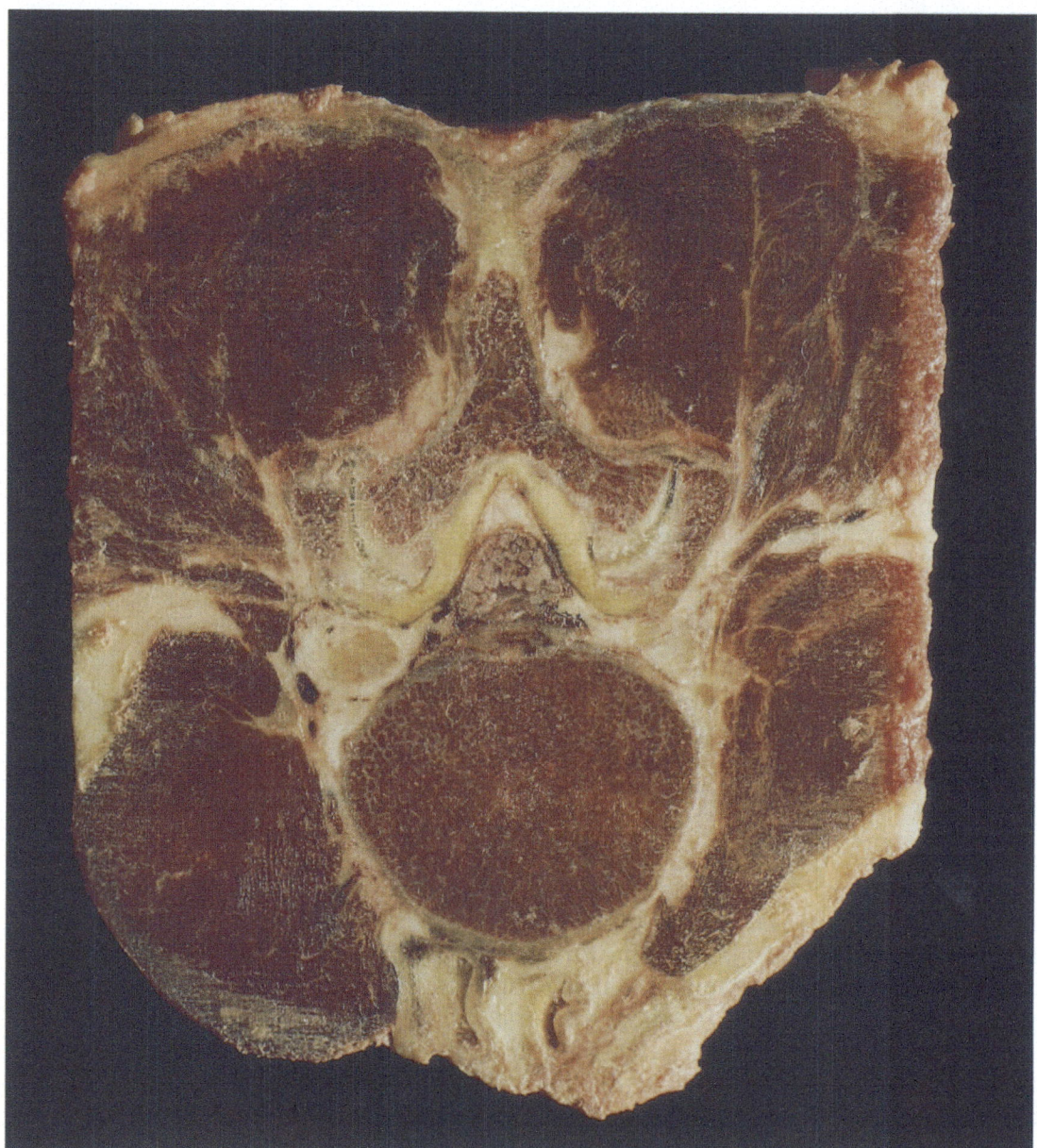

Figure 1.15. A transverse section through the lower lumbar spine at the level of the intervertebral foramen, the section passing through the vertebral body. On the left of the specimen note the posterior relations of the nerve root. In the midline, the cauda equina can be clearly seen with a triangle of epidural fat lying posteriorly. On the right side of the specimen the relations of the ligamentum flavum to the facet joint are shown with its free outer edge in the roof of the intervertebral foramen

below that, medial to the L5/S1 intervertebral foramen; it then lies adjacent to the medial aspect of the pedicle of S1. At the lower border of this pedicle it enters the first sacral intervertebral foramen (Figs. 1.14, 1.16).

The anterior relations of the S1 nerve root canal from above downwards are: the posterior aspect of the body of L5, the intervertebral disc, the posterior aspect of the body of S1. These constitute the floor of the canal when viewed from behind (Figs. 1.14, 16).

The posterior relations vary considerably depending on the length of the individual nerve root and on the orientation of the lamina of L5, which will vary with the lumbo-sacral angle. From above downwards, the uppermost posterior relation of the root canal at its origin is the bony ridge raised on the anterior aspect of the lamina of L5 by the superior attachment of the ligamentum flavum (Fig. 1.17). The nerve root is then covered by the antero-medial aspect of the S1 facet (Fig. 1.16).

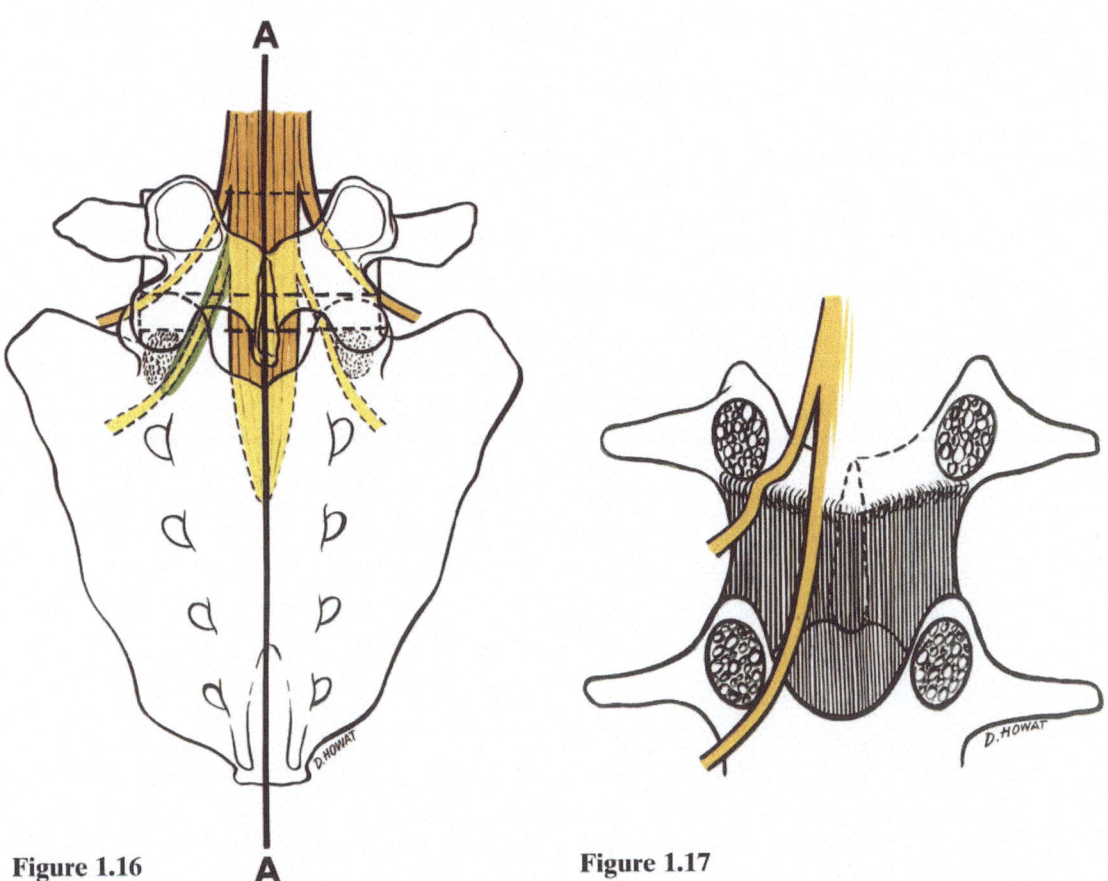

Figure 1.16   **A**   **Figure 1.17**

Figure 1.16. A drawing of the normal lumbo-sacral junction. Note the spinal nerve root canal of S1 outlined in green on the left side of the diagram. The line marked AA represents the plane of section for drawings illustrated in Figs. 1.14, 1.21 and 1.25

Figure 1.17. A drawing of two lumbar laminae viewed from within the spinal canal, showing the bony ridge of the upper attachment of the ligamentum flavum to the superior lamina of the intervertebral space. The L5 nerve root on the left side is shown kinked forward by this ridge at the level of the upper attachment of the ligamentum flavum. The S1 nerve root may be similarly deformed from behind in some cases

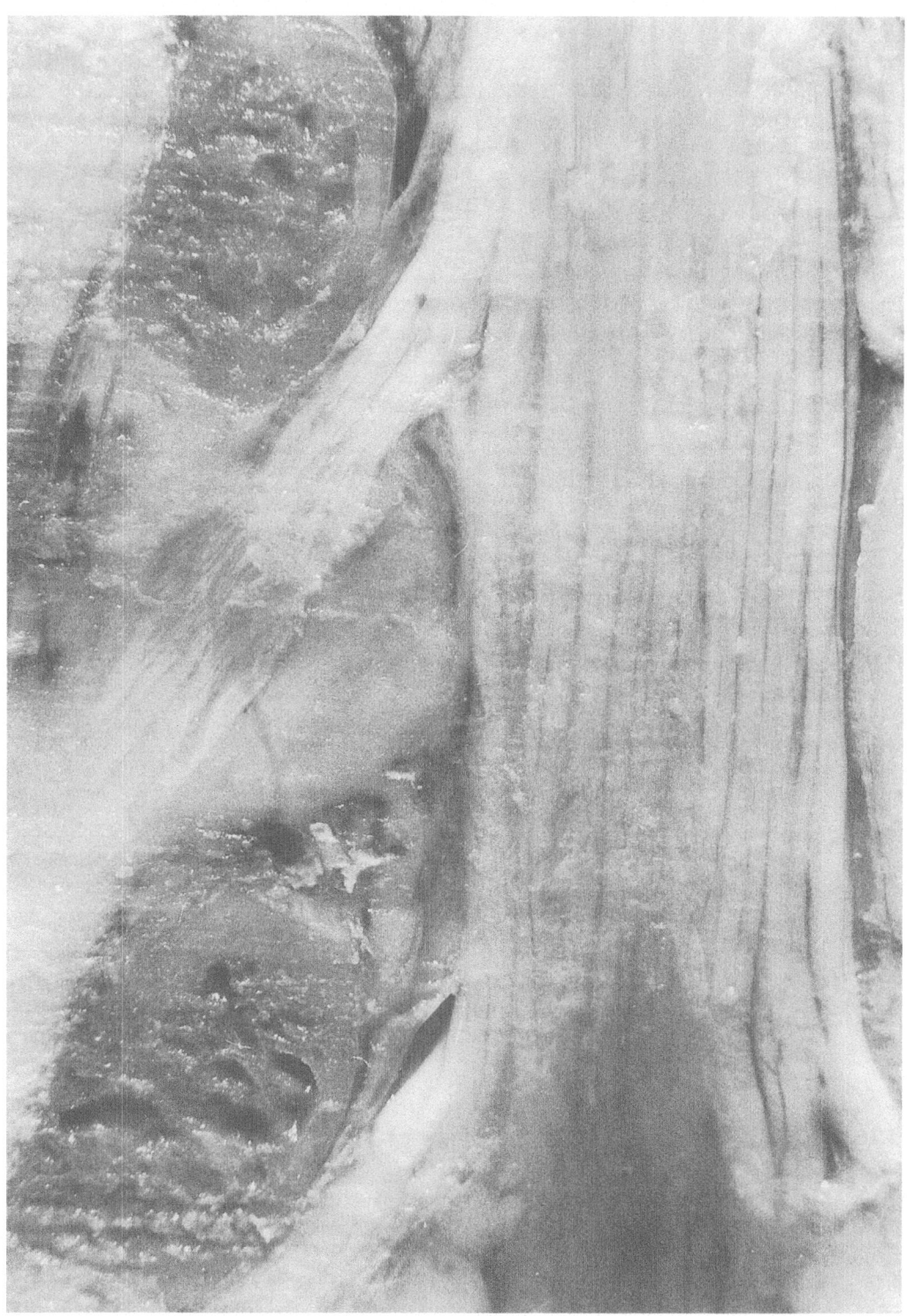

Figure 1.18. A coronal section from the mid-lumbar region of an adult, showing the cauda equina and two lumbar nerve roots on the left, each related to a vertebral pedicle. Note the epidural fat pads surrounding the upper of the two nerve roots

Epidural fat surrounds the spinal nerve root throughout its course to the intervertebral foramen (Fig. 1.18).

The arterial and venous relations of the spinal nerve roots are of great importance.

Knowledge of the anatomy of these veins helps the surgeon to protect them during spinal exploration, avoiding venous haemorrhage which may lead to faulty technique in nerve root canal and foraminal decompressions simply because the fine structures cannot be identified in the pool of blood in the depth of the dissection. *Venous obstruction is a cause of symptoms in nerve root canal stenosis and the task of relieving it is made easy by a knowledge of this local vascular anatomy.*

Relations of the nerve root arteries assume practical significance during difficult spinal canal operations. These vessels should be protected when spinal nerves are being manipulated. Diathermy of their branches should be kept to a minimum, thereby minimizing the risk of iatrogenic nerve root injury which may be permanent.

Detailed descriptions of these vessels have been given by Crock and Yoshizawa (1977). The salient features of this anatomy are seen in the accompanying illustrations on pp. 19 and 20 (Figs. 1.19 a, b, 1.20).

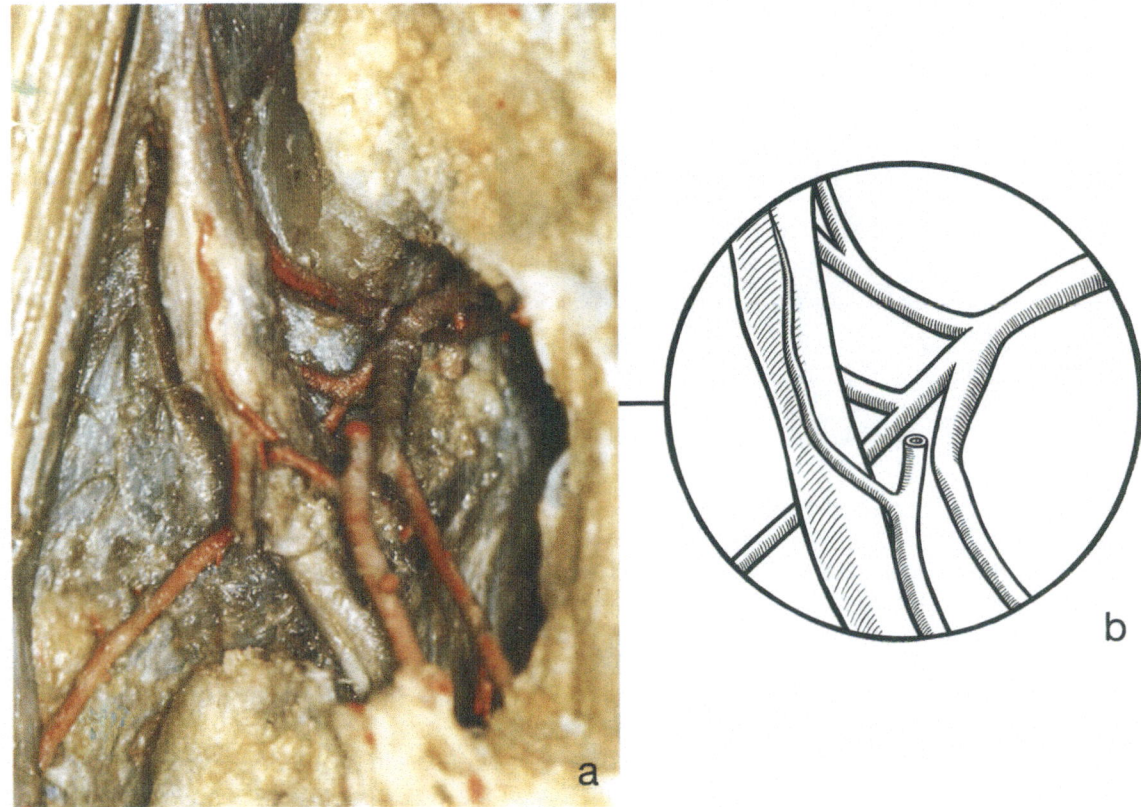

Figures 1.19 a, b. A detailed photograph to show the anterior spinal canal branches of the lumbar artery lying anterior to the emerging lumbar nerve root in the middle of the floor of the intervertebral foramen. Just above those branches related immediately to the infero-medial margin of the pedicle and passing on to the side of the dural sheath, the anterior and posterior radicular arteries can be seen. The single artery on the front of the nerve root ganglion is destined to supply it. The arteries have been injected with red latex rubber. The specimen is from a female aged 18 years

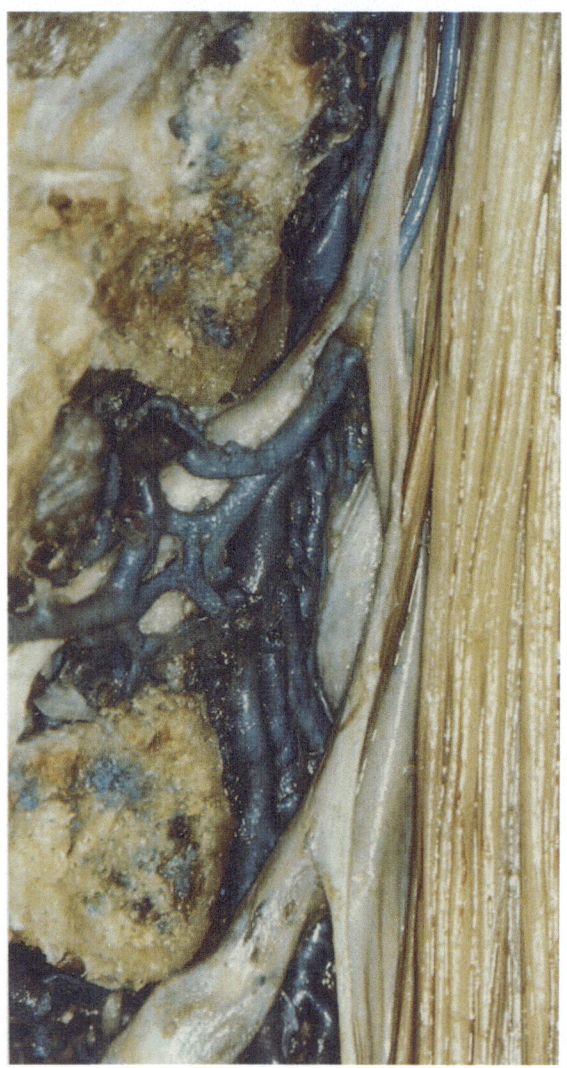

Figure 1.20. A photograph of a dissection showing details of the internal vertebral venous plexus from a male aged 71 years. The plexus was injected with blue latex rubber. The dorsal aspect of the dural sac has been removed to expose the cauda equina.

Radicles of the internal vertebral venous plexus surround emerging nerve roots from their origins at the dural sac and along their courses to the intervertebral foramina. The anterior and posterior component channels are of equal dimensions. This fact is not widely appreciated as the veins which form the dorsal internal vertebral venous plexus readily contract in spasm following the introduction of instruments into the spinal canal.

Radicular veins drain into the internal vertebral venous plexus in the axilla between the medial dural margin of the nerve root sheath and the lateral edge of the dural sac. In this specimen a *radicular vein* (top right) can be seen inside the dural sac, from which it emerges in the axilla between the medial border of the nerve root sheath and the outer margin of the lumbar dural sac. The intradural diameter of this *radicular vein* is approximately 50% smaller than the radicle of the posterior internal vertebral venous plexus into which it drains. Suh and Alexander (1939) have described valve-like structures in the veins at this site.

Damage to the dorsal internal vertebral venous plexus may obstruct the venous drainage of the cauda equina. The axilla of the nerve root sheath is therefore a critical area. The use of diathermy in this zone is potentially dangerous

ii) Pathological

When the vertical height of the lumbo-sacral disc space is greatly reduced, changes occur in the floor and roof of the S1 nerve root canal and also in the L5/S1 intervertebral foramen (Fig. 1.21). A narrow transverse bulging ridge formed by posterior fibres of the remaining annulus fibrosus and posterior longitudinal ligament protrudes into the floor of the S1 nerve root canal. Coupled with the movement upwards of the S1 facet towards the pedicle of L5, the anterior and medial edges of the S1 facet come to lie very close to this ridge and occasionally even to the postero-inferior surface of the fifth lumbar vertebral body. In consequence, mechanical obstruction of the S1 nerve root develops.

In some cases, in addition to the infolding of ligamentum flavum, hypertrophy of the bony ridge for its upper attachment may occur, further contributing to stenosis of both the S1 nerve root canal at its origin and, immediately lateral to it, to stenosis of the L5 nerve root canal just medial to the L5 pedicle (Fig. 1.17).

Appreciating these various contributing factors in the stenosis which may affect the S1 nerve root canal and the L5 nerve root at the L5/S1 intervertebral foramen, the planning of an effective surgical decompression can be logically organized (Figs. 1.22–25).

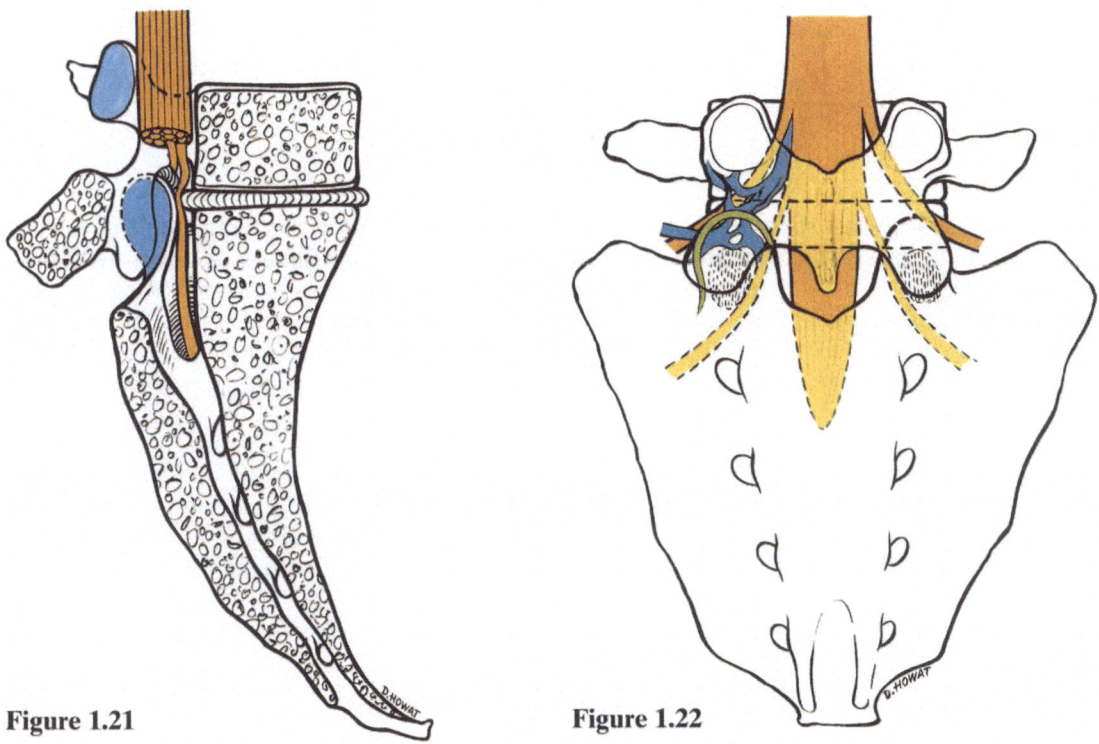

Figure 1.21   **Figure 1.22**

Figure 1.21. A drawing showing the pathological changes which accompany L5/S1 disc resorption. Note the buckling of the ligamentum flavum into the intervertebral foramen, compressing the L5 nerve root. The S1 nerve root is distorted along its course in the "nerve root canal" where it is compressed between the disc in front and the medial border of the S1 facet behind

Figure 1.22. A drawing showing the normal neural and venous vascular relations at the L5/S1 level. The outline of the upper border of the S1 facet is shown in green

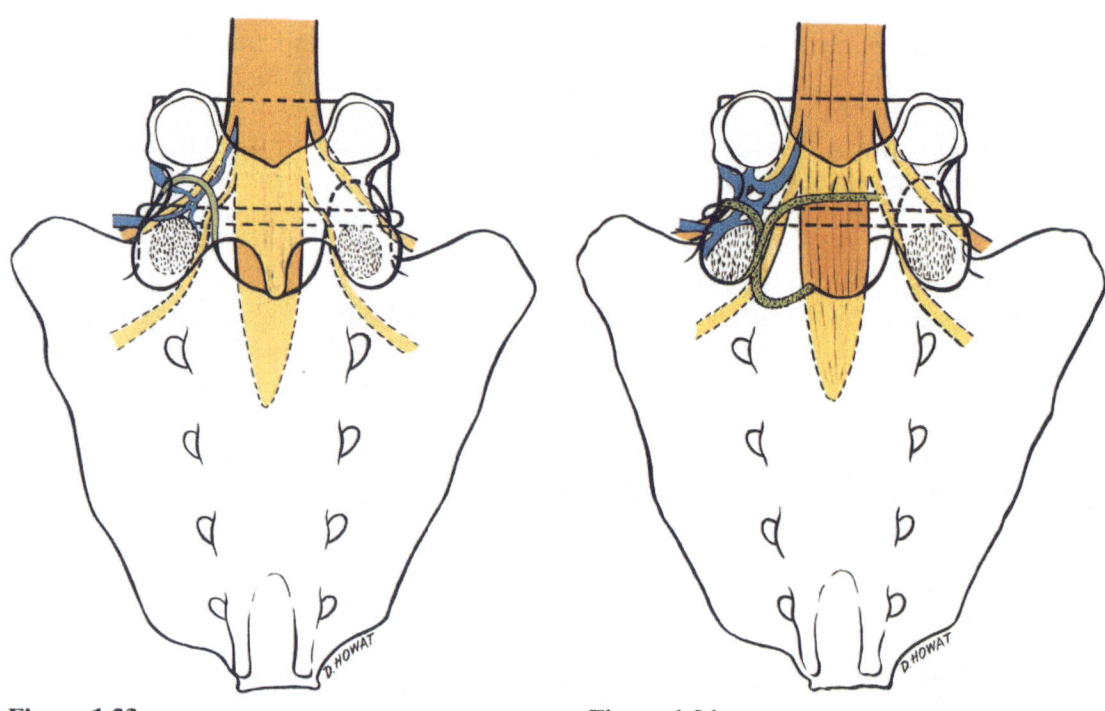

Figure 1.23   **Figure 1.24**

Figure 1.23. A drawing showing distortion of the S1 nerve root canal and of the L5/S1 intervertebral foramen due to subluxation upward of the S1 facet in isolated disc resorption of the lumbar L5/S1 disc. Note particularly the obstructed veins around the nerve roots. The outline of the medial and apical portions of the S1 facet is shown in green. Venous obstruction of this degree may lead to oedema of the L5 and S1 nerve roots as the centrifugal flow in their respective radicular veins is blocked. *This diagram shows only the site of the venous obstruction*

Figure 1.24. A drawing showing the restoration of normal neuro-venous-vascular relations after decompression of the S1 nerve root canal and the L5/S1 intervertebral foramen on the left side at L5/S1. The central portion of the neural arch of L5 is preserved. The outline of the cut surfaces of bone is shown in stippled green and black. The spinous processes of L5 and S1 should be preserved along with the interspinous and supraspinous ligaments

c) *Venous Obstruction*

While the mechanical obstruction to the S1 nerve root in its canal can be readily appreciated in the condition of isolated disc resorption, the finding of venous obstruction is less widely known. The occlusion of veins that is found in advanced cases of isolated disc resorption is demonstrated in Fig. 1.23. These veins are shown refilled after the operative procedure which is designed to relieve symptoms in this condition (Figs. 1.24, 1.25).

The deep seated buttock and thigh pain in these patients which comes on after standing or sitting is a form of *nerve root claudication due to this venous obstruction.*

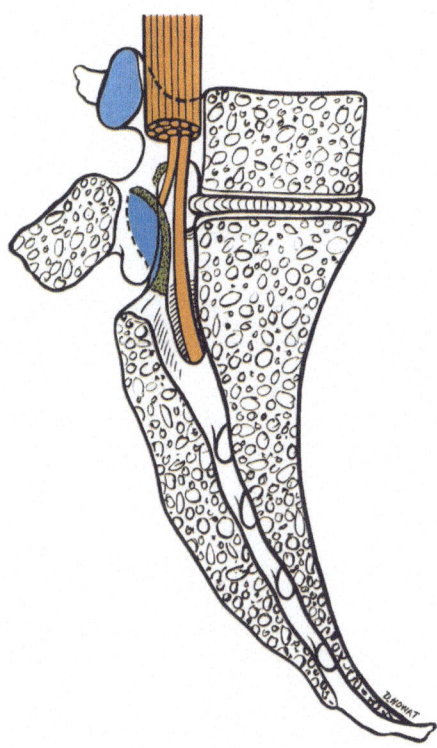

Figure 1.25. A drawing depicting the view from within the spinal canal after foraminal and nerve root canal decompressions. The ligamentum flavum has been totally excised. A stippled green and black outline indicates the extent of bony excision of the superior facet of S1 and of the bony ridge on the anterior aspect of the lamina of L5 at the level of the upper attachment of the ligamentum flavum. The L5 spinal nerve is shown emerging unimpeded through the intervertebral foramen. Dissection of the upper attachment of the ligamentum flavum and bony bar to which it is attached on the anterior aspect of the lamina of L5 is facilitated by the use of 45 degree forward angled rongeurs with a 300 mm long shaft. (Manufactured by Link – English Representatives: New Splint Ltd., Hawley House, Hawley Road, Blackwater, Camberley, Surrey GU17 9ES)

d) Clinical Studies

Venner and Crock (1981) published an analysis of the symptoms and signs in a group of 50 patients suffering from isolated disc resorption at the L5/S1 level. 94% of these patients complained of low lumbar pain and 48% noted radiation of pain to one or both buttocks. 76% had pain in one or both legs, and 50% complained of paraesthesiae. Only 8% reported exacerbation of their pain on coughing, but 18% gave a history of increasing leg pain or paraesthesiae on walking distances up to 500 yards (root claudication). Some patients had weakness and occasional dragging of the feet or difficulty in standing, but these symptoms settled on resting, usually by sitting. 94% had lumbar tenderness, but only 8 patients had reduced lumbar movement as defined by Moll and Wright (1976).

Signs of root irritation, evidenced by limited straight leg raising, painful bow-string test or sciatic nerve tenderness were detected in only 6%; and reduced nerve conduction indicated by wasting, motor weakness, sensory abnormality or reflex depression in 16%. One or both ankle jerks were absent in 10%.

In Table 1.1, measurements of the height of the L5/S1 intervertebral disc space in these 50 patients are recorded.

Table 1.1. Height of the L5/S1 intervertebral disc (50 patients)

	Anterior height			Posterior height	
	>10 mm*	10–5 mm	<5 mm	>5 mm	<5 mm
Male	7	20	3	5	25
Female	3	14	3	4	16
Totals	10	34	6	9	41

*In only one patient was the height more than 15 millimetres.

e) Investigations

Plain X-rays and magnetic resonance images together can provide comprehensive information on isolated disc resorption.

i) Plain X-Rays

Typical findings are: gross disc space narrowing, vertebral body sclerosis especially close to the vertebral end-plates, the Knuttson vacuum sign on the lateral extension film, minimal evidence of osteophyte formation and facet joint subluxation. This intrusion of the superior facet of the lower vertebra into the intervertebral foramina at the affected level is best seen in oblique views of the spine.

ii) Radiculography

Disc prolapse is an infrequent occurrence in established cases of isolated disc resorption, so that lumbar radiculography is unnecessary except in special circumstances; for example, when the patient has severe unilateral leg pain. Disc prolapse at another level may be found, or vertebral end-plate sequestration at the level of the disc resorption may be confirmed. The radiculogram in a typical case is often reported as normal (Fig. 1.11). This could influence a surgeon who is not fully aware of the nature of this condition to advise against the surgery that should be indicated.

iii) Magnetic Resonance Imaging

This investigation is emerging as the most useful single test in establishing the diagnosis of isolated disc resorption and in studying its evolution. Loss of signal on the T2 weighted image of the peripheral portions of the nucleus pulposus appears to be one of the earliest changes associated with the decrease in height between vertebral end-plates (Fig. 1.26). These changes are associated with a uniform bulging of the posterior annular fibres into the spinal canal seen in the sagittal images. As the

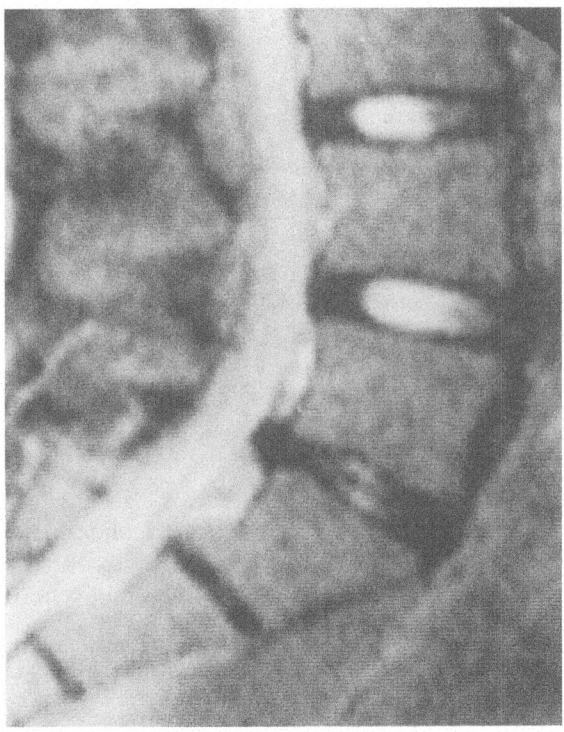

Figure 1.26. A mid-sagittal MR image, T2 weighted sequence, from a female patient aged 37 years showing a loss of signal from the peripheral portion of the nucleus pulposus, decreased disc height and peripheral bulging of the posterior annulus into the spinal canal. This does not represent a disc prolapse but rather a "flat tyre" effect due to bulging posterior annular fibres across the width of the floor of the spinal canal

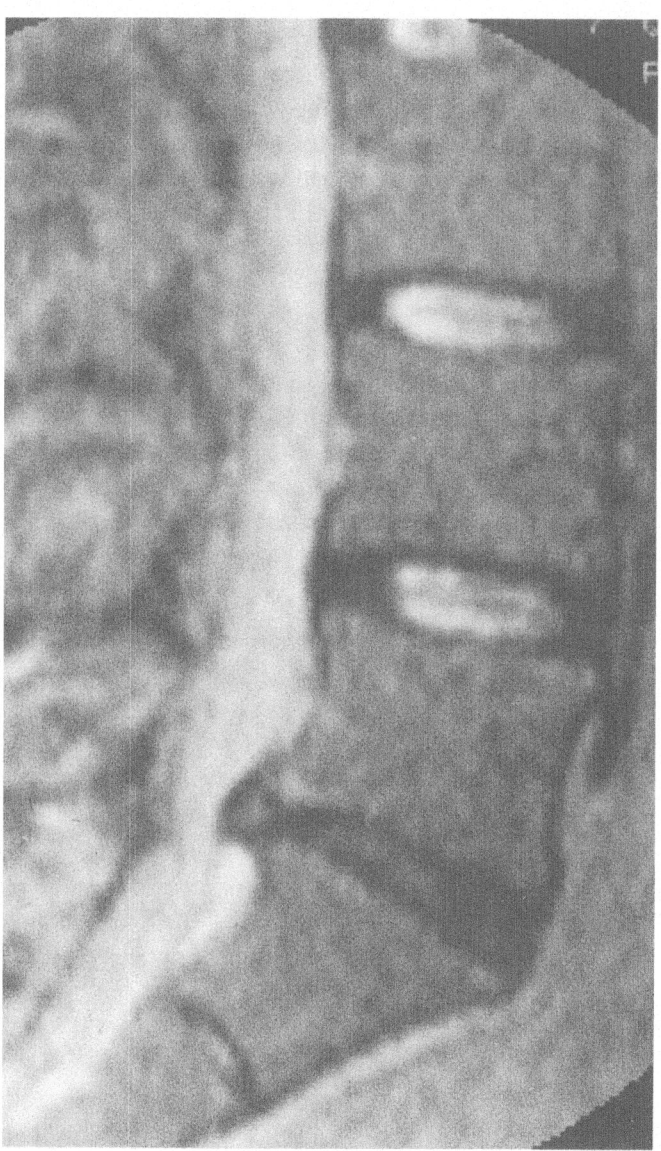

Figure 1.27. A mid-sagittal MR image of the lumbar spine of a male aged 43. Isolated disc resorption is well established at L5/S1 with loss of disc height, almost complete loss of the nuclear signal and heightened signal appearing in the vertebral bodies of L5 and S1 adjacent to the vertebral end-plates. The dural sheath is compressed by the bulging rim of the posterior annular fibres. *This is not a disc prolapse* and it should not be disturbed at operation

process continues, signal changes begin to appear in the vertebral bodies adjacent to the vertebral end-plates and these extend in some cases to extensive changes involving almost half of the vertebral bodies on either side of the narrowed disc space (Figs. 1.8, 1.27). In cases with unilateral sciatica due to prolapse of disc remnants the size of the lesion is best assessed by using gadolinium enhancement (Asseheuer 1991).

iv) Lumbar Discography

This investigation, valuable in other forms of disc disease, has no place in the investigation of isolated disc resorption.

v) Computerised Axial Tomography

Reconstructed CT scanning is useful in confirming the foraminal and nerve root canal stenosis that occurs in this condition. However, transverse scanning at the lumbosacral junction is difficult to interpret in relation to the demonstration of root canal stenosis. It is particularly valuable, however, in demonstrating the punctate vertebral end-plate lesions which are sometimes found in isolated disc resorption (Fig. 9 c–e). Rarely these defects may coalesce and disc remnants herniate into the adjacent vertebral bodies causing severe intractable low back pain. Spinal infection may be suspected but can be excluded if blood examinations are normal and the psoas shadows are not distorted.

vi) Epidural Venography

Obstruction of the intervertebral veins can be demonstrated satisfactorily with this special investigation. However, its demonstration is of theoretical interest as the venous obstruction is a concomitant pathological finding in established cases of isolated disc resorption with facet joint subluxation, facet intrusion into the intervertebral foramen and ligamentum flavum buckling.

f) Operations

i) Types

The treatment of choice in cases with bilateral buttock and leg pain is bilateral nerve root canal and foraminal decompressions. The technique of this operation will be outlined below and is described in detail on pp. 30–35.

In cases where there is an associated unilateral sciatica, a sequestrum of necrotic vertebral end-plate cartilage attached to remnants of annular fibres will usually be present. The protruding fragment is often adherent to the nerve root and its exposure can be difficult, requiring careful dissection of the nerve root sheath. Venous bleeding should be controlled with a sucker and pattie. When the disc fragment has been clearly defined it should be withdrawn with a fine straight pituitary rongeur.

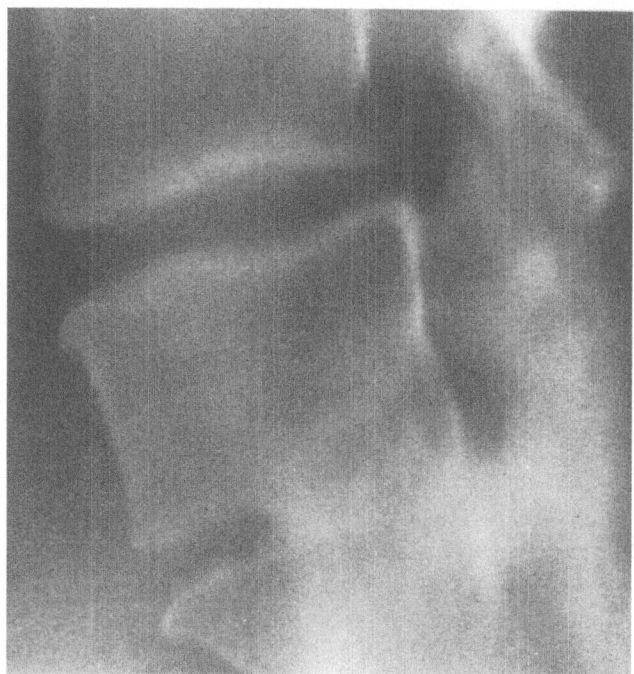

Figure 1.28. A lateral tomogram of the lower lumbar spine in a 31 year old airline pilot treated by posterior interbody fusion for isolated disc resorption at the lumbo-sacral junction. This film was taken 5 years after operation

The intervertebral space is usually too small to admit any but fine instruments. However, it is essential to remove any loose disc remnants from within the disc space, remembering the real danger of instruments slipping unexpectedly forward to penetrate into the abdominal cavity in this type of disc disease. At the same time, bilateral foraminal and nerve root canal decompressions should be performed.

If, at the time of nerve root canal decompression, marked vertebral instability is noted at the site and the patient's symptoms have included the complaint of intractable back pain, then spinal fusion should be carried out. Inter-transverse-alar sacral fusion is recommended. Theoretically, in this circumstance, the ideal procedure is posterior interbody fusion using either the Cloward or Wiltberger techniques, because the grafts fit accurately between the vertebral bodies, producing a strictly localised spinal fusion (Fig. 1.28).

When low back pain is the dominant symptom, primary anterior interbody fusion at the affected level may be indicated (Fig. 1.29).

The cause of the back pain in these cases is not related to nerve root canal and foraminal stenosis. It emanates from either the vertebral bodies, or the arthritic subluxed facet joints which are stressed by degrees of rotatory vertebral body instability, particularly with disc resorption at L4/L5 or L3/L4.

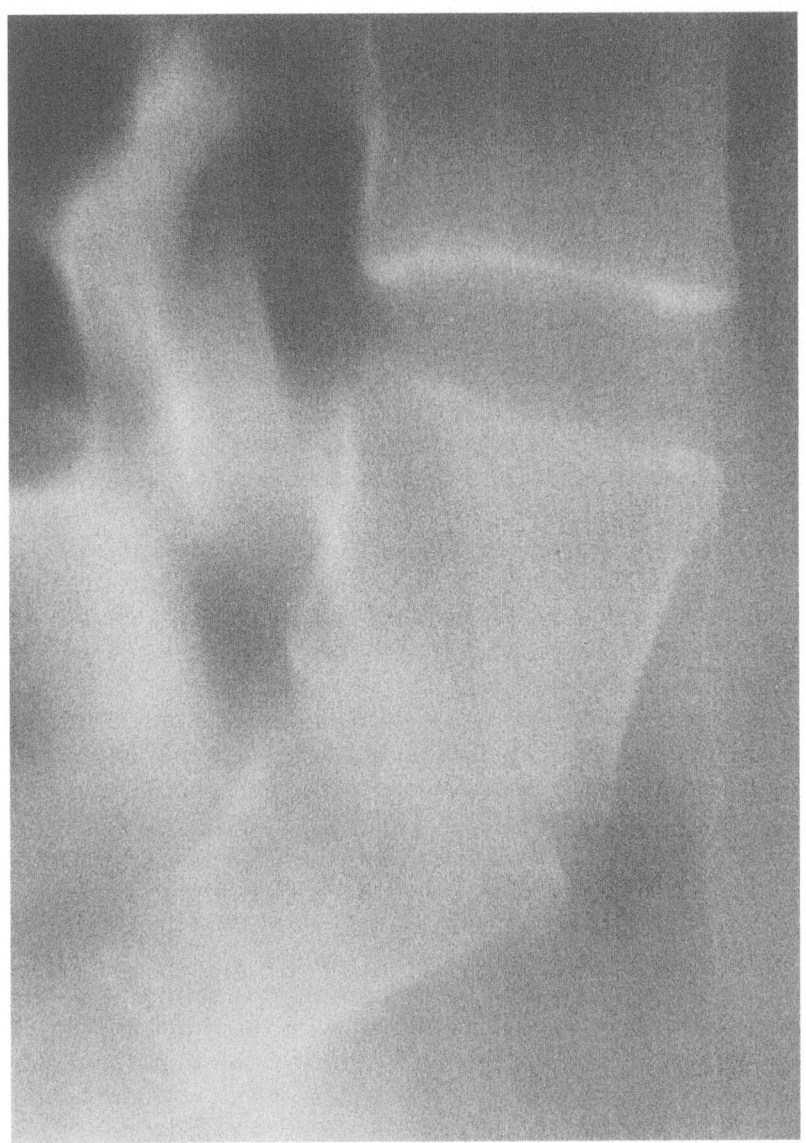

Figure 1.29. A lateral tomogram showing interbody fusion following anterior disc excision and autogenous bone grafting in a female aged 37 years with isolated disc resorption at the lumbo-sacral junction

ii) Technique of Lumbar Nerve Root Canal and Foraminal Decompressions at L5/S1 Level

The surgical approach to the L5/S1 interspace is described on pp. 127–138. Details of the decompression technique via the spinal canal are set out below:

At the outset of this description consider that the ligamentum flavum has already been removed laterally to the level of the medial margin of the S1 facet. In the process of its excision a few millimetres of bone will have been removed from the upper margin of the inferior lamina on each side of the spinous process and interspinous ligament.

Depending on the dimensions of the S1 facet between its medial margin and the inner margin of the S1 pedicle, the S1 nerve root sheath may or may not be visible. The dural sac with overlying epidural fat can be seen. The curved end of a Watson-Cheyne dissector should be introduced *gently* into the spinal canal to identify the medial and superior margins of the S1 pedicle. As it is passed laterally and upwards beneath the S1 facet, the S1 nerve root and its surrounding blood vessels are separated from the roof of the nerve root canal. The underlying ridge of the resorbing disc should then be identified.

If the probe is manipulated vigorously, especially in the region of the upper edge of the S1 pedicle, or far laterally beneath the superior facet of S1, profuse venous haemorrhage may ensue. Performed carefully, this examination allows an accurate assessment to be made of the degree of S1 nerve root canal stenosis, first on one side of the spinal canal, then on the other.

Many individual local variations of pathological anatomy may be encountered. In general terms only three problems need to be addressed; the first a tight mechanical obstruction affecting the S1 nerve root as it traverses the nerve root canal, compressed between the bulging rim of the resorbed disc in the floor of the canal and the antero-medial margin of the S1 facet in its roof; the second, obstruction of the vertebral venous plexus in the intervertebral foramen; and the third compression of the fifth lumbar nerve root and its surrounding veins in the intervertebral foramen and distal end of its nerve root canal beneath the fifth lumbar lamina.

The goal of foraminal and nerve root canal decompression is achieved at this level by trimming the medial margin of the S1 facet flush with the inner margin of the S1 pedicle. Then the S1 facet apex and all remnants of the ligamentum flavum in the intervertebral foramen are removed along with the uppermost attachment of the ligamentum flavum to the bony ridge on the anterior surface of the L5 lamina.

A wide range of instruments should be available as indicated in the illustrations prepared for this chapter (Figs. 1.30–33). Good lighting is essential and the use of low magnification loops is sometimes useful.

Figure 1.30. A photograph of a Watson-Cheyne dissector. The curved tip on the right hand side is pointed and the left-hand end is a blunt probe. These instruments should be available in varying sizes and lengths

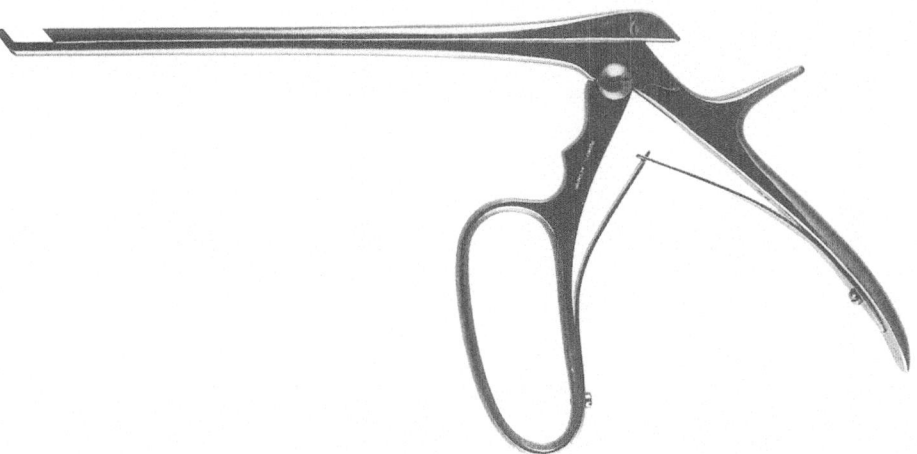

Figure 1.31. A photograph of a 45 degree forward angled oblique punch. A range of these punches should be available with cup sizes varying from 1 mm up to 4 or 5 mm. Some instrument manufacturers are now providing these instruments with long shafts. They are ideally suited for operations designed to decompress the spinal canal, nerve root canals and intervertebral foramina with preservation of the laminal arch and spinous processes. Because of the added length, the handles of the instrument can be lowered even between the buttocks allowing for the insertion of the cutting tip of the instrument high up under a lamina. In addition they can be safely manipulated beneath the interspinous ligaments from one side of the spinal canal to the other so that the apices of superior facets and ligamentum flavum remnants can be removed safely

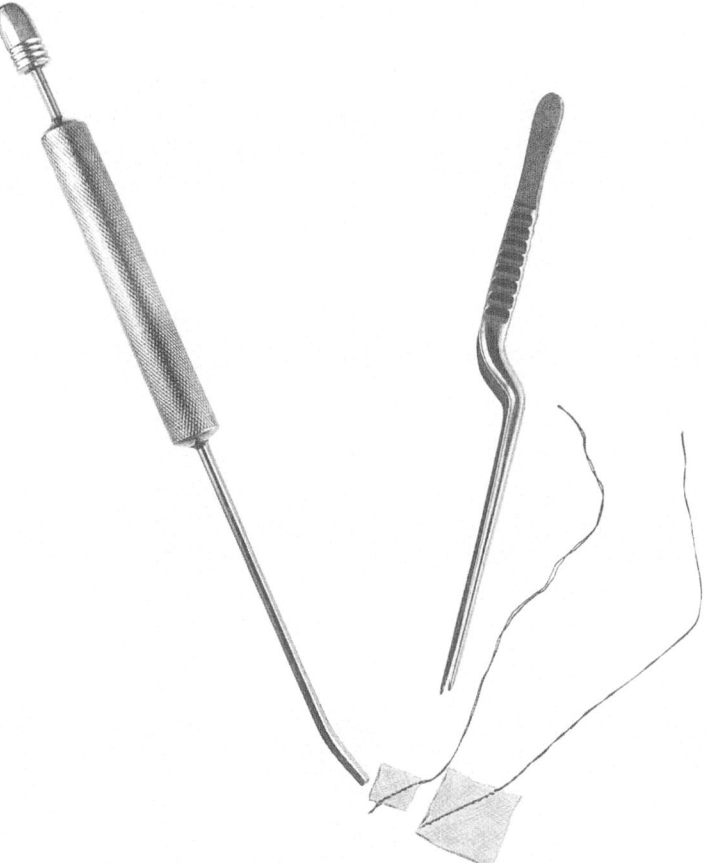

Figure 1.32. A photograph showing sucker and bayonet forceps with patties of different sizes. These are important implements for use in spinal canal explorations

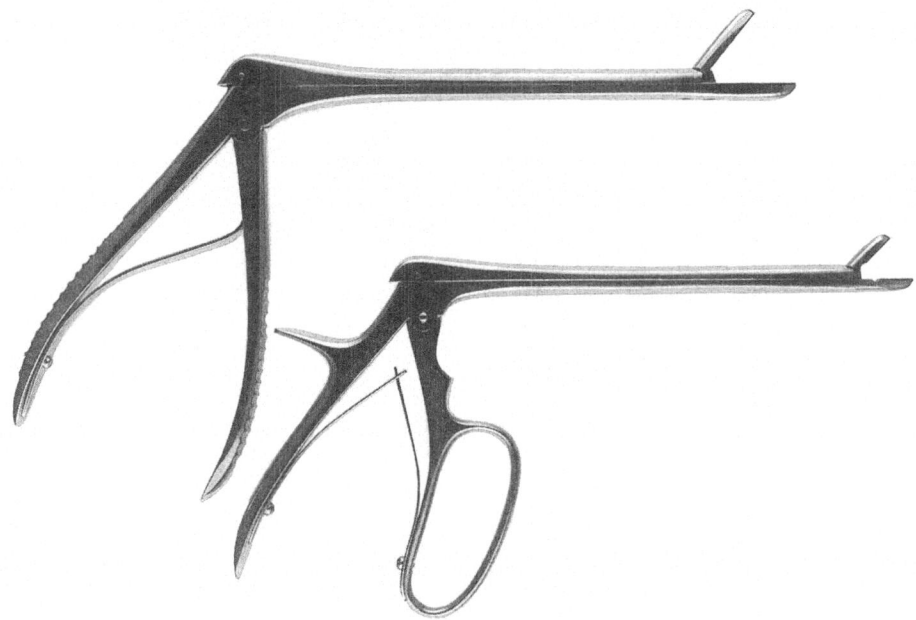

Figure 1.33. A photograph showing straight pituitary rongeurs of varying sizes. A range of these should be available for use during spinal canal decompressions, cup sizes varying again between 1 and 5 mm with straight and forward and backward angled tips

Recent advances in technique now dictate the preservation of spinous processes and interspinous ligaments so that the lumbo-dorsal fascia can be re-attached to the supraspinous and interspinous ligaments at the conclusion of the operation, Crock and Crock (1988).

The surgeon should move freely from one side of the operating table to the other as the opposing nerve root canals and foramina are decompressed, the right sided structures being decompressed from the left side of the table and vice versa. While the right sided decompression is being performed the table should be rolled towards the left and the light adjusted to facilitate the surgical approach. The most difficult manoeuvres are those involving removal of the upper attachment of the ligamentum flavum and the apex of the S1 facet. Use of a 45 degree forward angled 2 mm curette or of an oblique laminal punch with a 300 mm long shaft facilitate this dissection which involves looking obliquely upwards from below, manipulating a sucker with a pattie on its tip in one hand and a long rongeur in the other. In order to remove the apex of the S1 facet it may be necessary to pass the sucker and a fine forward angled laminal punch beneath the interspinous ligament from one side of the spinal canal to the other (Fig. 1.34). *It is not practical to attempt bilateral foraminal and nerve root canal decompressions with the use of an operating microscope.*

The most striking finding at operation following relief of the stenosis is the dramatic refilling of the vertebral venous plexus that ensues. Haemorrhage from these vessels in the spinal canal can always be controlled with gelfoam and light packing with moistened patties. *Diathermy, even with bipolar coagulation, should be avoided* (Figs. 1.35 a, b).

The accompanying diagrams depict alternative methods of relieving stenotic lesions, so minimizing risks of nerve root, dural or vascular damage in particular situations (Figs. 1.36 a–d).

In some instances excision of the bony ridge and upper attachment of the ligamentum flavum can be achieved only after excision of the central arch of the lamina of L5. When this becomes necessary, care is taken to preserve the partes interarticulares of this lamina on both sides, leaving the cut bony surfaces smooth and coating them with bone wax; excision of the apex of the S1 facet, together with the lateral edge of the ligamentum flavum is then facilitated.

Rarely is it necessary to interfere with the floor of the S1 spinal nerve root canal in cases of isolated lumbar disc resorption. Occasionally a sub-rhizal vertebral end-plate sequestrum will be found in this location; it should be removed from beneath the S1 nerve root.

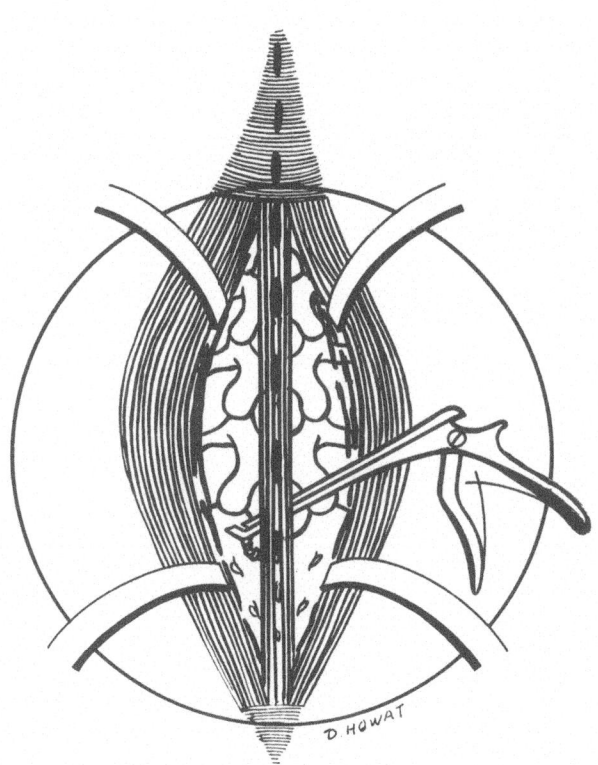

Figure 1.34. A drawing depicting manipulation of a 45 degree forward angled rongeur as it is passed underneath the supraspinous and interspinous ligaments from the right hand side of the lumbar vertebral column at the lumbo-sacral junction, to allow removal of the medial and apical portions of the left superior facet of S1. With practice these manoeuvres can be carried out swiftly on either side of the mid-line, so that adequate decompression of the spinal canal and of the nerve root canals and intervertebral foramina can be achieved

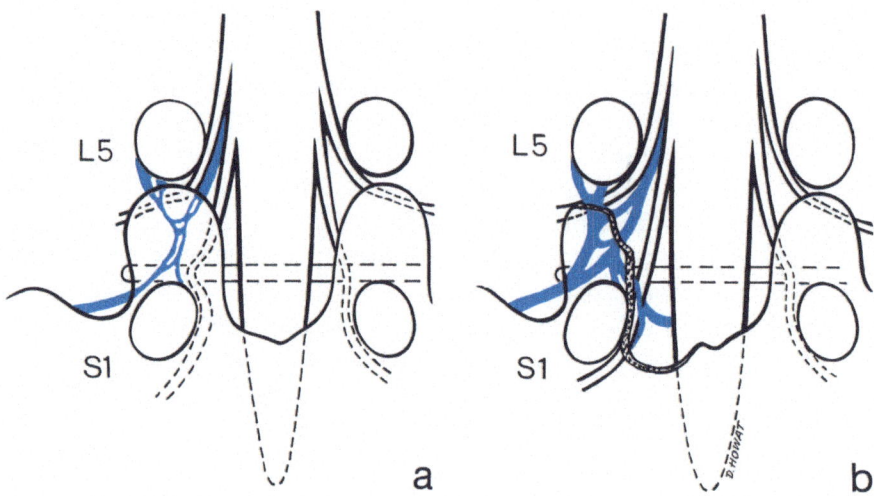

Figure 1.35 a, b. a A drawing to highlight the feature of venous obstruction which is a concomitant of foraminal and nerve root canal stenosis at L5/S1 in a case of isolated disc resorption. Note the distension of the radicular vein proximal to the apical and medial margins of the S1 facet. This may result in swelling of the nerve root sheath as seen in radiculograms (Fig. 1.11). **b** On the right following decompression by excising the apical and medial portions of the S1 facet and the ligamentum flavum, note that the mechanical obstruction of the nerve roots is relieved and the venous drainage re-established. Refilling of these veins at operation is dramatic. Haemorrhage from the radicles should be controlled with gelfoam and patties. The use of diathermy within the spinal canal for the control of haemorrhage should be avoided, particularly in the region of the axilla between the inner margin of the dural root sleeve and the outer edge of the dural sac

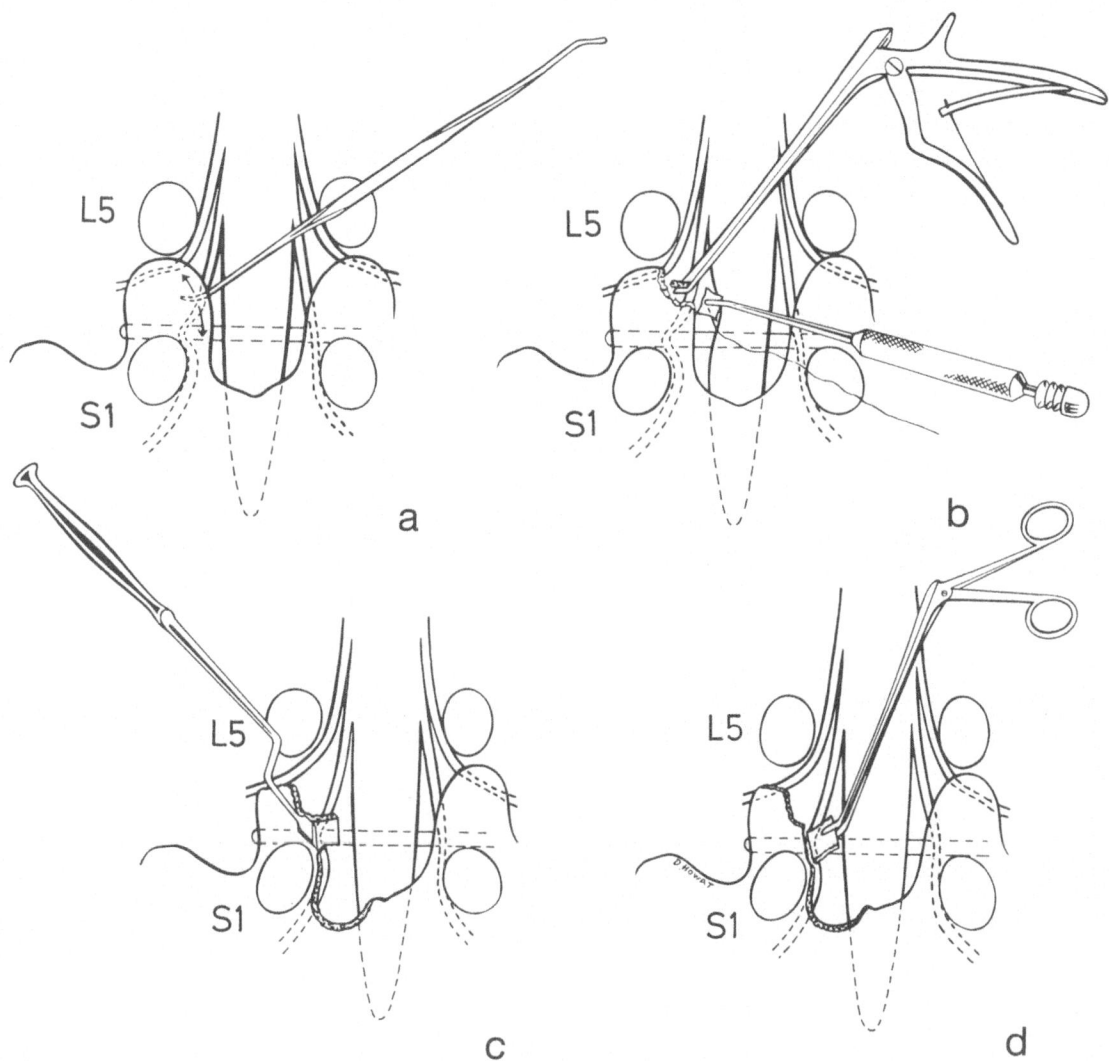

Figure 1.36 a–d. a A diagrammatic representation of the findings of S1 nerve root canal stenosis at the L5/S1 level in isolated disc resorption. Note the use of the curved pointed end of the Watson-Cheyne dissector being used to free the soft tissues anterior to the medial edge of the S1 facet. **b** Note the disposition of the sucker and pattie and the use of a 45 degree forward angled fine cup pituitary punch to excise the apical portion of the facet of S1. This manoeuvre can be carried out as depicted in this drawing from the left side of the laminal interspace or from below and on the right, the tip of the instrument passing beneath the interspinous ligament from the right to the left side of the spinal canal posterior to the dural sac. **c** A drawing depicting the use of a fine chisel to split off the remnants of the medial aspect of the S1 facet where the S1 nerve root canal is most tightly constricted. **d** A drawing depicting the removal of a segment of the S1 facet to complete the decompression of the S1 nerve root canal at the level of the medial margin of the sacral pedicle. A fine pointed forward angled pituitary rongeur is used for this purpose

Results

Symptoms arising from isolated lumbar disc resorption have been shown to be severely disabling. The study published by Venner and Crock in 1981 suggests that nerve root canal decompression in isolated disc resorption is a useful addition to the surgical armamentarium for the treatment of pain in the back and leg. In a series of 45 patients with isolated disc resorption independently reviewed on an average of 45 months after surgical decompression of the S1 or lower lumbar nerve roots complete success was achieved in 62% of the patients and partial success in 24%.

Table 1.2. Success rate of the operation for isolated disc resorption based on six criteria (45 patients)

Criteria	Success rate for each individual criterion (per cent)	Overall success rate of operation (per cent)	
Operation considered by the patients to be "worthwhile"	84	Complete success (6 criteria)	62
Functional disability reduced	71		
Return to work	78	Partial success (3–5 criteria)	24
Relief of backache	84		
Relief of pain in the legs	91	Failure (<3 criteria)	14
Independent observer's assessment: Dr. R. M. Venner	71	Good	71

1.2. Miscellaneous Causes of Nerve Root Canal Stenosis

a) Congenital Abnormalities

Some congenital abnormalities of the lumbar spine may easily go unnoticed. Congenital hypertrophy of facets is an important cause of nerve root canal stenosis which may be overlooked, particularly if the intervertebral disc spaces are of normal height (Figs. 1.37 a–c).

Congenital deficiencies of facets are less common and the defects are sometimes unilateral. The "missing" facet is usually replaced by a bulky soft tissue mass that can cause both foraminal and root canal stenosis (Figs. 1.38 a–c).

b) Space Occupying Lesions

Occasionally, in an otherwise normal spinal canal, space-occupying lesions related to abnormalities in the dura or arachnoid may occur. Extra-dural arachnoid cysts of the Schreiber type or peri-neural cysts of the Tarlov type may produce symptoms of nerve root canal stenosis (Figs. 1.39 a, b) (Gimeno, 1978). These lesions may be large and lead to bony erosions requiring either simple decompression or occasionally, formal excision (Figs. 1.40 a, b, c).

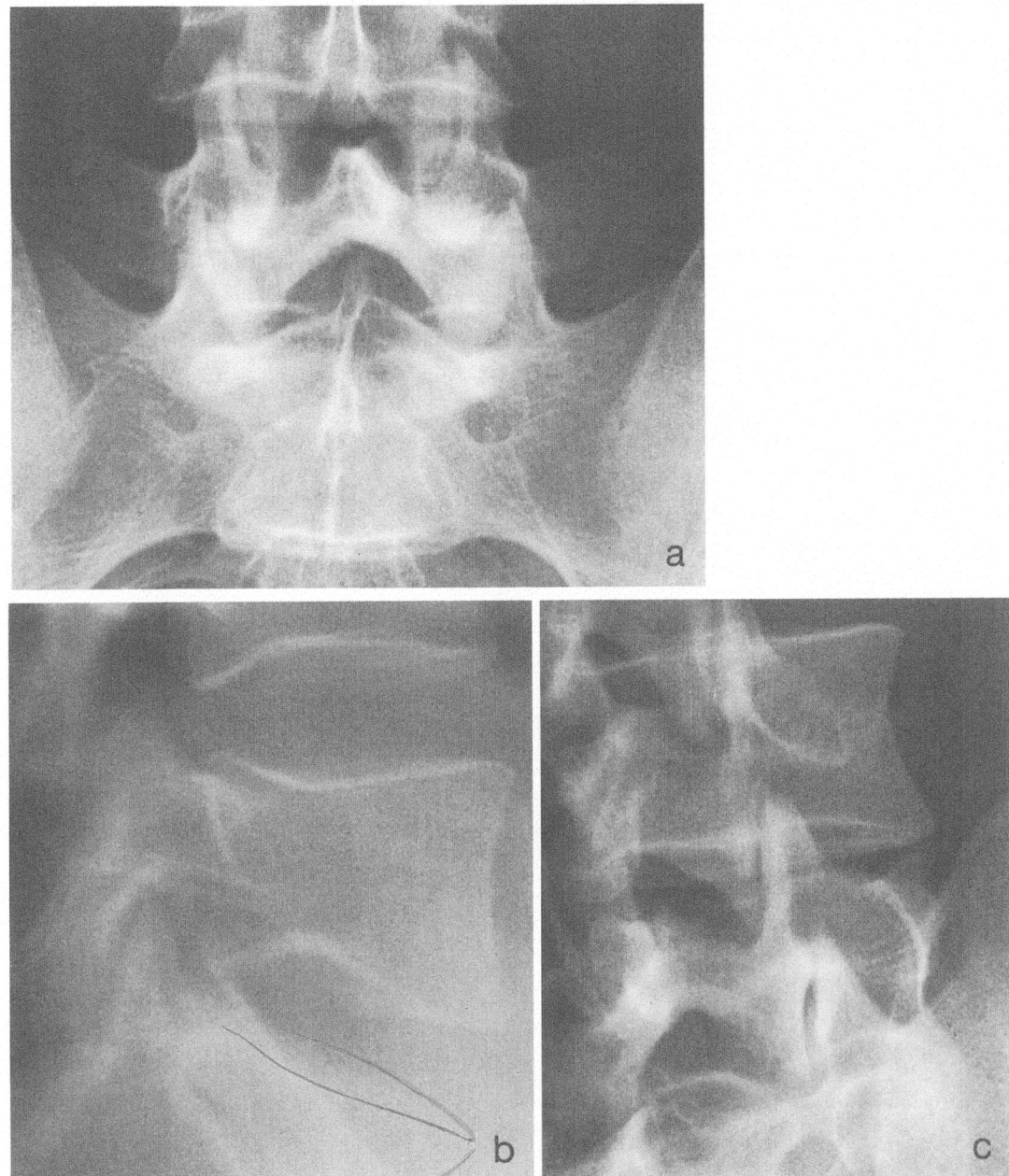

Figure 1.37a–c. a An antero-posterior radiograph of the lower lumbar spine in a man aged 38 years presenting with symptoms of bilateral buttock and thigh pain extending to the back of the knee, aggravated by standing, sitting or walking. Note the orientation of the facets at L5/S1 with the apices of the S1 facet visible on the AP view in close proximity to the inferior borders of the pedicles of L5. **b** A lateral radiograph of the spine in the same patient showing normal discs at L4/5 and L5/S1. Note the congenital large S1 facets projecting upwards into the intervertebral foramen at L5/S1, the apex of the facet being visible close to the inferior surface of the pedicle of L5. **c** An oblique view of the same spine showing the hypertrophic S1 facet, the apex of which lies close to the inferior border of the pedicle of L5. The relationships of the apex of the superior facet of L5 and the pedicle of L4 provide a marked contrast to the findings at the lower level

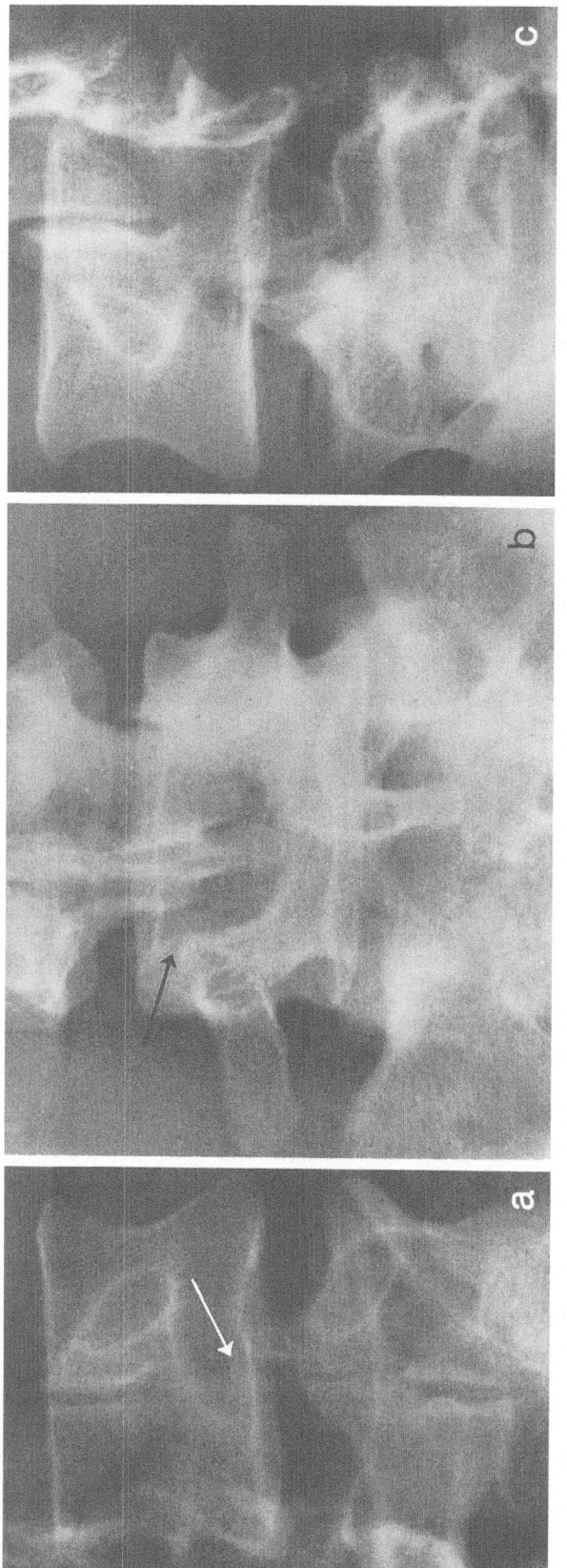

Figure 1.38a–c. a An oblique view of the lower lumbar spine of a woman aged 34 who presented with unilateral buttock and leg pain aggravated by standing and walking. The arrow points to the congenital abnormality at the pars interarticularis with absence of the inferior facet of L4. **b** An antero-posterior radiograph of the same spine showing the unilateral congenital abnormality with absence of the inferior facet of L4 on one side. In the area indicated at the tip of the arrow, there was a bulky mass of soft tissue found at operation, semi-cartilaginous in consistency, causing foraminal and nerve root canal stenosis. **c** An oblique view of the opposite side of the spine showing the normal laminal arrangement and intact inferior facet

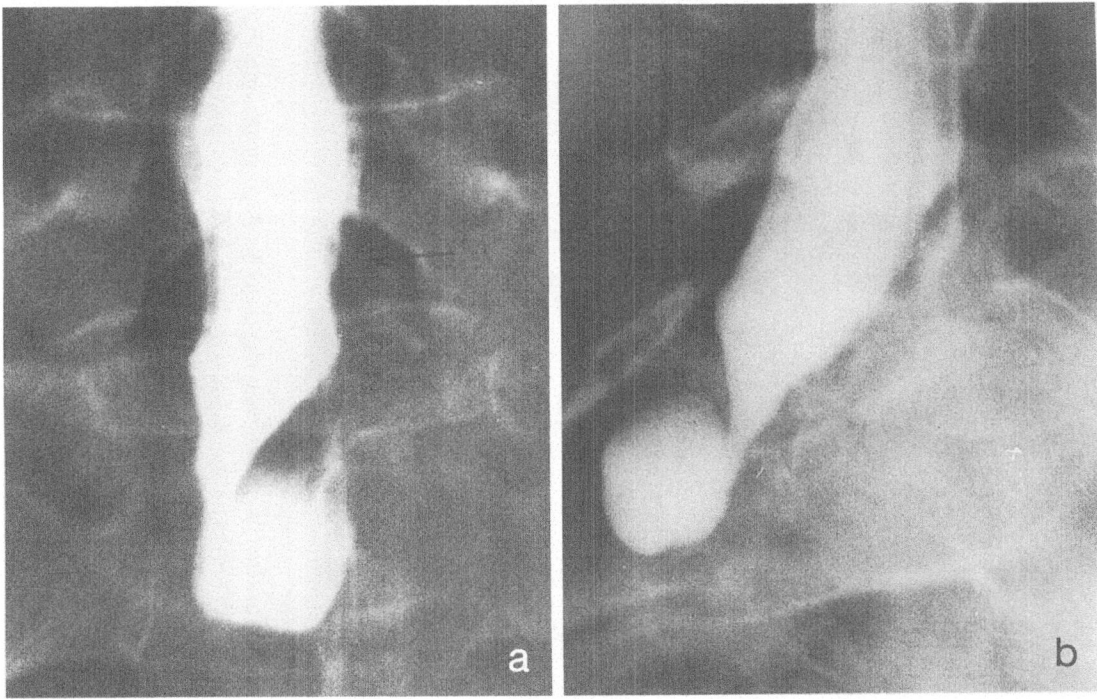

Figure 1.39a,b. a An antero-posterior radiograph of the lower lumbar and upper sacral area showing a myelographic defect produced by an extra-dural arachnoid cyst of the Tarlov type. **b** A lateral radiograph of the myelogram in the same spine, showing the deformation of the lower end of the lumbosacral dural sac produced by a large extra-dural arachnoid cyst, acting as a space occupying lesion in the nerve root canal in this area, there being no associated abnormality of the disc or vertebral column. These lesions are very well shown in magnetic resonance images

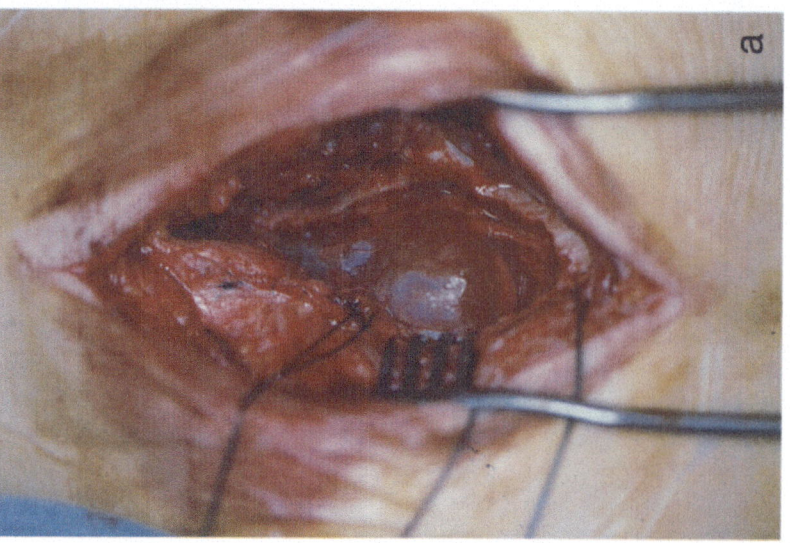

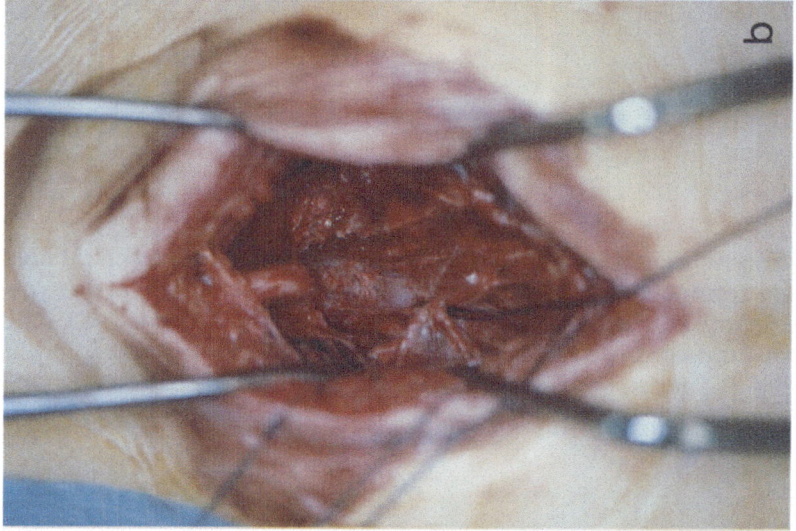

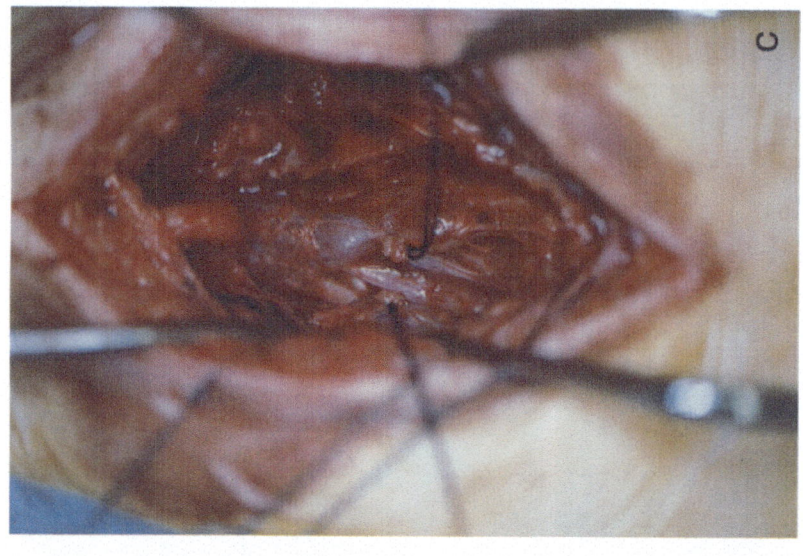

Figures 1.40a–c. a An operative photograph showing a large arachnoid cyst related to the S 4 nerve root, exposed by decompressing the upper three segments of the sacrum. This cyst was producing erosion of the sacral laminae and bodies of the sacral vertebrae. **b** An operative photograph showing the passage of a suture around the base of the neck of the arachnoid cyst after expressing the cerebrospinal fluid from it, back into the dural sac. **c** Showing the decompressed area in the region of the termination of the sacral dural sac with three sacral nerve roots visible on the left

c) Localized Degeneration

More common causes of nerve root canal stenosis are seen in localized degenerative disorders. For example,

   i) In isolated disc resorption, retrolisthesis of L5 on S1 may occur, aggravating the tendency for the development of spinal nerve root canal stenosis which occurs commonly in this condition (Fig. 1.5).

   ii) Retrolisthesis of one lumbar vertebra on another often occurs in association with disc resorptive changes in the first mobile segment above sacralization anomalies in the lower lumbar spine (Figs. 1.7 a,b).

   iii) Unilateral facet osteoarthritis may occur at a single level, most commonly at the lumbo-sacral junction, where it can produce unilateral sciatica (Figs. 1.41 a,b). The use of myelography in the diagnosis of these problems is recommended and typical changes, with gross local deformity, can be seen in a number of the miscellaneous causes referred to in this text (Figs. 1.42 a,b). However, it is very important to recall that the myelogram may be reported as normal in many of these cases especially if root oedema has not been identified. The surgeon must then fall back on his clinical assessment of the patient, aided by plain X-ray findings, while deciding whether or not to recommend surgical treatment in a particular case.

Accuracy of diagnosis has been enhanced since the advent of C.T. scanning and MRI though it must be remembered that these expensive instruments are not universally available. In addition, unless the computer facilities can produce high resolution reconstructions in three planes, the value of images in a single plane in the diagnosis of these particular problems is seriously restricted. Problems in the nerve root canal are not readily appreciated throughout its length by studies of transverse sections alone. Unless this is appreciated, together with the fact that myelography may not define the anatomy of the nerve root canals completely in particular cases, the surgeon presented with apparently normal myelography and normal C.T. scanning in the transverse plane alone, may be disinclined to believe that the patient is seriously disabled and so deny him or her the surgical treatment which would relieve the symptoms.

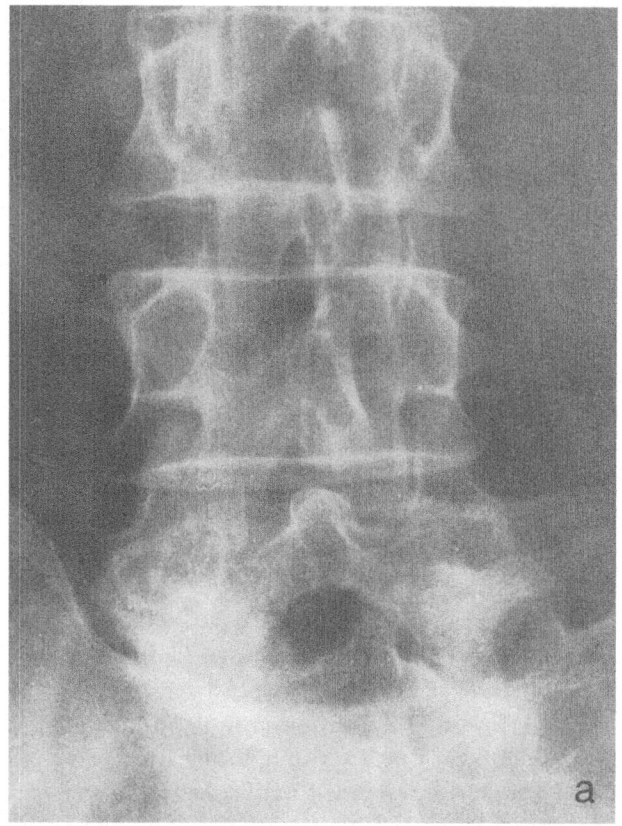

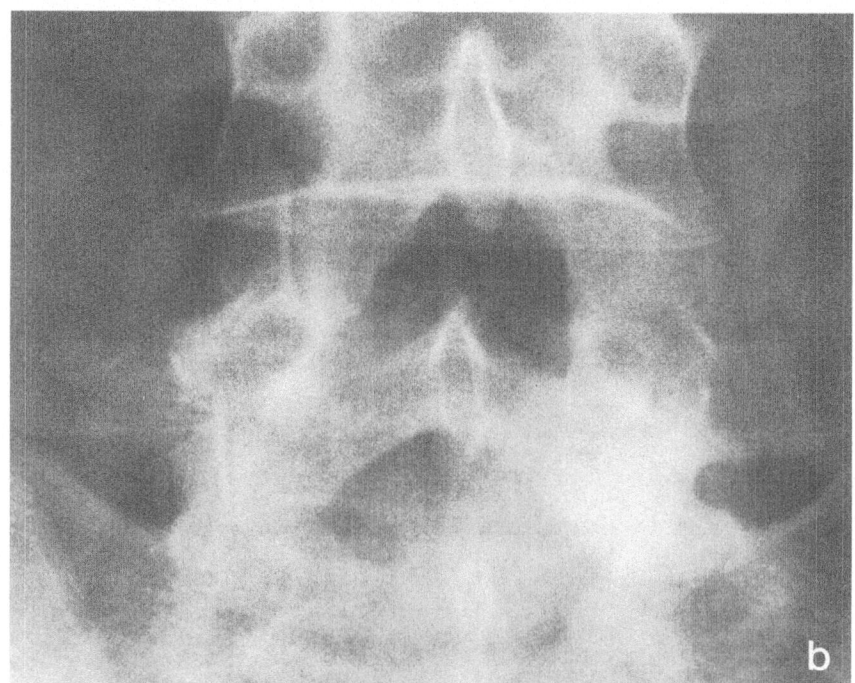

Figure 1.41

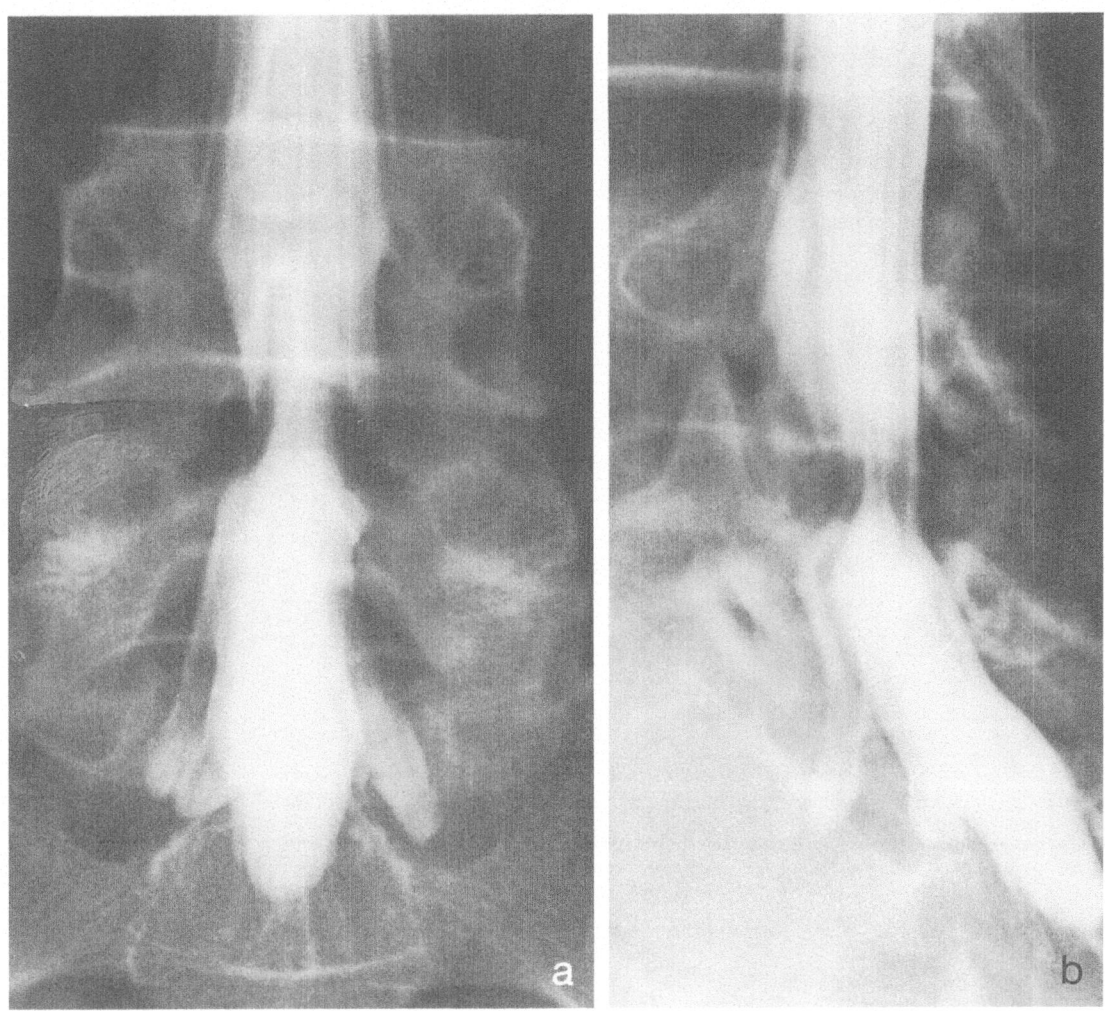

Figure 1.42a,b. **a** An antero-posterior radiograph of the lower lumbar spine to show a myelographic defect (metrizamide radiculogram) with partial spindling of the main column produced by bilateral facet hypertrophy of the inferior facets of L4. This deformity is often reported erroneously as being due to a large central disc prolapse, whereas it results from facet joint and ligamentum flavum hypertrophy. **b** An oblique view highlighting the relationship of the deformity in the column of dye to the medial border of the inferior facet of L4. Although there is an element of central spinal canal stenosis the principal defect is due to bilateral stenoses of the nerve root canals and intervertebral foramina, confirmed at operation

Figure 1.41a,b. **a** A radiograph of the lower lumbar spine in a woman aged 49 years showing unilateral facet hypertrophy due to osteoarthritis, leading to unilateral nerve root canal stenosis. **b** An antero-posterior radiograph of the lower lumbar spine of a man aged 30 with unilateral osteoarthritis of a facet at L5/S1 producing root canal stenosis

2

Internal Disc Disruption

This term was introduced in a paper titled: "A reappraisal of intervertebral disc lesions", published in the Medical Journal of Australia (Crock, 1970).

The condition is common and should be readily identified clinically, though magnetic resonance images or CT discography are essential investigations for its confirmation.

The clinical syndrome which may be associated with this type of disc disorder usually follows severe trauma inflicted on the disc, for example, by sudden unexpected weight lifting, or by forces transmitted through the disc or discs during high speed accidents. Meat industry workers, miners and foundry workers and building labourers are prone to single or repeated episodes of trauma which may give rise to this syndrome. It is also commonly seen among nurses whose work frequently involves moving heavy or disabled patients.

2.1. Clinical Features

a) Symptoms

Patients affected by severe grades of internal disc disruption present with an array of symptoms which should arouse the clinician's suspicion early in the course of management, especially if the history of the mechanism of injury is placed in its proper perspective. Back pain is prominent, having the character of a deep-seated dull ache. It is aggravated by physical activity, physical therapy and spinal manipulation. It is often sufficiently severe to disturb sleep at night. The patient with limb pain due to internal disc disruption always finds difficulty in describing it as the limb pain differs remarkably from that described by patients with impingement neuralgia due to disc prolapse. Usually these limb pains are widespread and described as being deep inside it, having an intolerable aching character.

When these patients first present for treatment, one may be unimpressed with their description of symptoms and struck by the complete absence of abnormal physical signs in many of them. Observation over two or three months will reveal their low tolerance for physical activity. Their symptoms may become widespread with severe occipital headache, intractable spinal pain, nausea and weight loss.

There has been a tendency to label as "functional" or "psychological" many of the symptoms described by patients with lumbar disc disruption including those of headache and temperature dysaesthesia in the legs (Hakelius *et al.*, 1969).

b) Spinal Movements

When standing, many have difficulty in rising from a flexed position. They usually assist themselves by placing the palms of their hands on the anterior aspects of their thighs, literally climbing up from the stooped position using the hands as props. Similarly, when attempting to sit up from a lying position, they may find it impossible without placing both hands flat on the bed behind them and exerting pressure on the upper limbs to raise themselves to a sitting position. At other times they may turn on to one side and get up into a sitting position by rolling their legs over the side of the bed and then levering themselves up slowly and awkwardly, obviously in pain. Spasm of the paraspinal muscles, as seen in cases with disc prolapse or in some with isolated disc resorption, is very uncommon in this condition.

c) Body Weight Loss

In patients who are clearly constitutionally ill as a result of internal disc disruption, *weight loss may be profound* over the course of a few months, ranging from 6–18 kg. Surprisingly features of weight loss and loss of energy are often over-looked even after these patients have been seen by a number of specialists. Conversely, some actually gain weight, due to their enforced physical inactivity.

d) Neurological Signs

Abnormal neurological signs in the limbs are uncommon, though complaints of weakness, clumsiness, and sympathetic nervous system disturbances as described above, are often made.

e) Psychiatric Disturbances

The psychological responses to this form of disc injury are partly predictable. These patients are usually incapacitated for many months before the diagnosis is established. They soon realise that their symptoms are a mystery not only to themselves but often to their doctors also. They feel that their problems are being taken too lightly. Financial worries soon begin to plague them and shortly the whole fabric of their lives begins to disintegrate, leading to an acute anxiety state. The view is often expressed that these problems and others, glibly described as litigation neurosis, will not loom as major obstructions to recovery if treatment is undertaken quickly (Macnab, 1969). Iatrogenically induced neurosis is often seen in these patients, especially if they have been under treatment for more than nine months without relief of symptoms.

There is a range of psychiatric disturbances seen in this group which is distinct from the simpler psychological disturbances seen in patients with disc prolapse requiring surgery.

Following total disc excision and interbody fusion for internal disc disruption, a significant, but small percentage of them, develop an acute psychiatric illness within a few days. They may become disorientated and violent. This phenomenon is rarely seen following any other orthopaedic operation. One is tempted to relate such disturbances to some biochemical abnormality in the damaged disc tissue, postulating that the psychiatric upset is caused by the sudden release of a sensitizing substance into the general circulation at the time of operation.

In managing patients with this type of disc disorder, it is desirable to work closely with a psychiatrist who has a special interest in these matters. The following comments come from the pen of such a consultant psychiatrist, H. G. Stevenson, writing in 1970, pp. 47–48:

"Psychiatric problems following disc disease appear to be labelled functional by the surgeon whose treatment has failed to relieve symptoms, and iatrogenic by his colleagues in the profession who have been fortunate not to be involved in the actual surgical onslaught. Neither of these labels appears to be justifiable in the vast majority of cases.

i) Acute Psychotic Reaction

Two major patterns of disturbance are seen. Firstly, an acute psychotic reaction occurring shortly after operation on either the cervical or lumbar spine varying from a manic type of reaction to one which appears to be schizophrenic in type. The nearest parallel to these are the puerperal psychoses which are accepted as being due to a sudden alteration in biochemical function of the individual following the major physiological alterations of birth, and considered to occur only in patients with a covert psychosis.

In those who react in this way to spinal surgery, there is probably an underlying covert psychotic make-up which may otherwise never have become apparent without the operation. The acute reaction is usually short-lived, responds to conservative anti-psychotic treatment readily and seldom needs intensive psychiatric or physical treatment.

Given that patients suffering from this syndrome are probably prone individuals of whom there is no dearth in the normal community, it could be fairly said that even with a mild whiplash injury to the neck, a state of depression follows.

ii) Reaction to Prolonged Disease

With more serious disc disease, particularly of the cervical spine, one finds the second typical syndrome, characterized by irritability, intolerance to noise, periods of severe depression, headaches starting at the back of the head, going over the front of the head and often causing blurring of vision, a gross degree of introspection which is again probably a factor of a true depressive illness, reduced sexual function, in both male and female and extending particularly in the male to the state of complete impotence, dizziness often postural in type and frequently directly related to the intensity of the headache; pain in the limbs not corresponding to the anatomical areas of sensory supply but notably consistent over a great number of patients, a poor memory and reduced concentration. The overall syndrome responds poorly to anti-depressive medication and the added anxiety of litigation increases the failure of therapy. However, even without litigation this typical syndrome is seen and the "cure" appears to be more an adjustment to an altered way and principle of living than a return to "normal". Whether the cause is biochemical, or due to alteration in the blood supply to the base of the brain, or affection of the sympathetic nervous system is questionable, but this in turn appears to be in parallel with the disc injury rather than a result of the prolonged symptoms or the failure of orthopaedic treatment. Physical strain patterns following damage to the head and neck suggest that the centre of stress is in the region of the hypothalamus, which area has been the focus of attention in most research on depressive states, and this in itself could bring about an alteration in the biochemical balance, particularly in relation to the 5-hydroxytryptamine and plasma cortisol levels.

Follow-up studies on these patients suggest that the depressive state persists for a considerable time, that it tends to recur, perhaps in that the patient has learned a depressive form of reaction to stress and this then becomes his normal pattern to stress in the future. The alteration in the personality adjustment in at least some cases appears to be permanent. The relationship of strain from lower back disease affecting the upper regions of the spine and a typical depressive state occurring in parallel is also seen. Most attention has been centred on the medico-legal aspects, and efforts by Cole (1970), Stevenson (1970) and Parker (1972) have thrown some doubt on Miller's (1961) article on accident neuroses, so that more accurate psychiatric diagnosis in these post-traumatic spinal conditions is gaining acceptance".

When internal disc disruption goes unrecognised on the clinical features described above, the patients drift from doctor to doctor, often seeing as many as ten, including family doctors, rheumatologists, "pain specialists", general surgeons, neurologists, neurosurgeons, orthopaedic surgeons and psychiatrists. Many also seek relief with osteopaths or chiropractors.

2.2. *Pathology*

a) *Macroscopic Changes*

The primary defects appear to lie in the field of histochemical pathology and probably also in alterations to the mechanism of disc nutrition.

Macroscopically, disrupted disc tissue is soft, often slightly yellow in colour but otherwise indistinguishable from disc tissue in the early phases of degeneration.

Circumferential tears between adjacent rings of the annulus fibrosus or radial tears in these fibres, short of complete extension to the outer annular layers, can be demonstrated radiographically by CT discography (Fig. 2.1). After many years of clinical observation, the conclusion is inescapable that in certain individuals these changes in the discs are associated with biological dynamics which lead to a disabling syndrome, precipitated by trauma and further aggravated by repeated minor trauma. The relationships observed in these patients between the degree of their physical activity and the onset of their pain with profound fatigue and lassitude are striking. The greater their activity the worse their symptoms become both in severity and duration. Their tolerance for physical therapy is limited. Good physical therapists will stop treatment, recognizing that they are simply aggravating their patients' problems by continuing exercises. On purely clinical grounds it seems reasonable to conclude that there must be an increase in "noxious fluid exchanges" across the vertebral end-plates in these patients, varying with degrees of their physical activity.

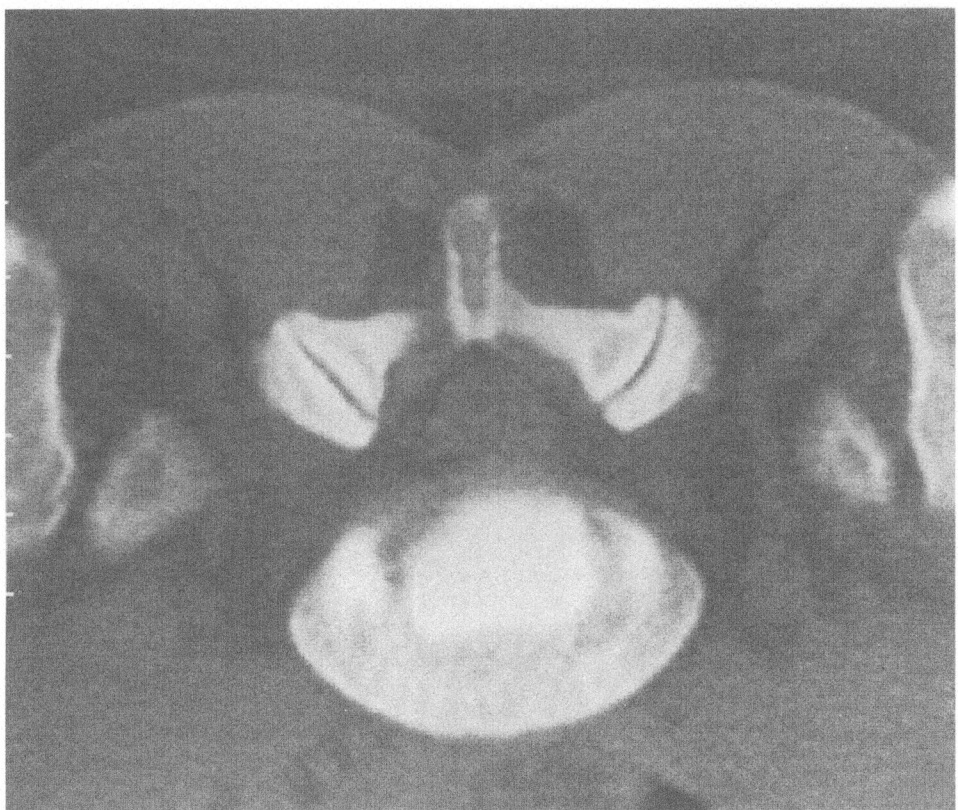

Figure 2.1. CT discogram from a female patient aged 18 years showing internal disc disruption at L5/S1

Studies of fluid exchanges within the intervertebral disc and across the vertebral end-plates have, to date, failed to raise awareness of their potential clinical significance, Ghosh (1988). *Despite rising interest in the biochemistry of the disc, the principal focus of attention in clinical practice, both at the investigative and therapeutic levels, remains set on disc prolapse and the elusive entity of vertebral instability.*

That some dynamic pathological process is active gains further support in observations made during vertebral interbody fusion operations for this condition. For example, the lumbar sympathetic trunk may be found matted to such an affected disc and the adjacent paravertebral lymph nodes seen to be enlarged. In addition, the vascularity of the vertebral bodies adjacent to such a disc appears to be increased and their bony densities somewhat reduced.

The significance of these findings relates to observations made during experiments on auto-immunity in the intervertebral discs of rabbits, reported by Bobechko and Hirsch (1965). Credit for first drawing attention to the possible auto-immune basis to the development of biochemical changes in disc prolapse should be given to Naylor (1962). With added knowledge of the anatomy of the circulation in the region of the vertebral end-plates, Crock and Yoshizawa (1977), Crock and Goldwasser (1983), (Figs. 2.2–10), and with further evidence on the movement of radio-opaque dyes from disc tissues into the veins of the vertebral bodies (Figs. 2.11, 2.12), it seems

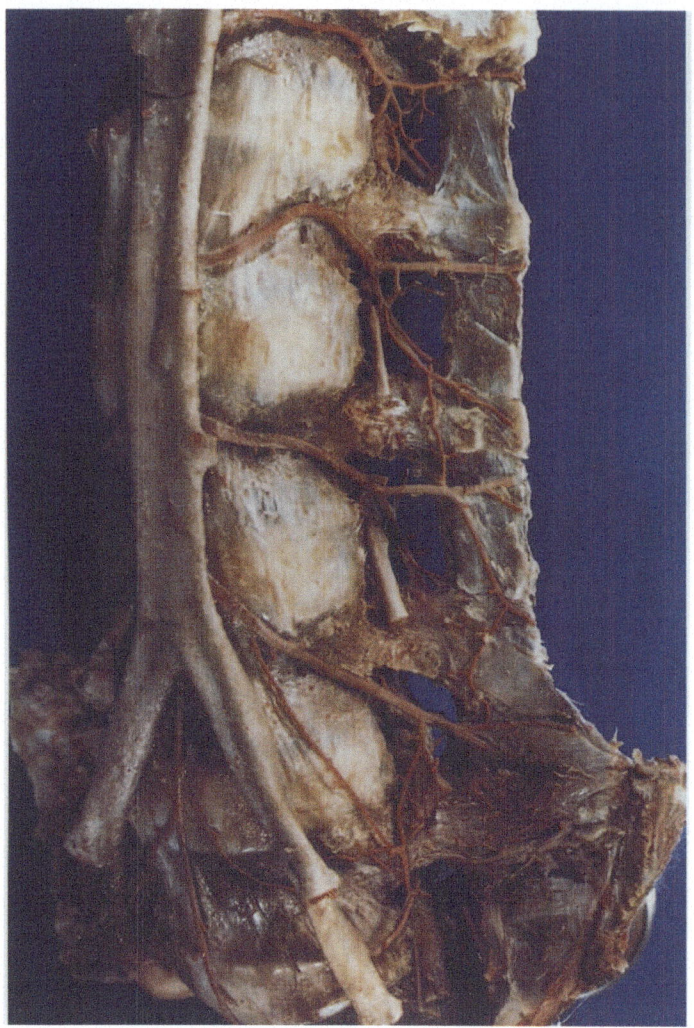

Figure 2.2. A photograph of a dissection of the lumbar vertebral column in an adult viewed from the left side, showing the origins and distribution of the lumbar arteries from the aorta. The median sacral artery is also clearly shown. The psoas muscle has been removed

likely that auto-immunity may play an important role in the development of the severe disabilities that afflict patients with the syndrome of internal disc disruption. Up to the present time despite approaches to workers in various departments of biochemistry and immunology, both in Australia and in Great Britain, fruitful inter-professional liaisons have not yet been successfully established. Selby (1991) has recently instigated a multi-centre clinical study in North America on *internal disc disruption.*

Familiarity with the vascular anatomy of the vertebral bodies and with spinal circulation in general is central, on the one hand, to the understanding of the theoretical bases of many spinal pathological processes, including internal disc disruption, and, on the other hand, vital as a guide to safe surgical practice. For these

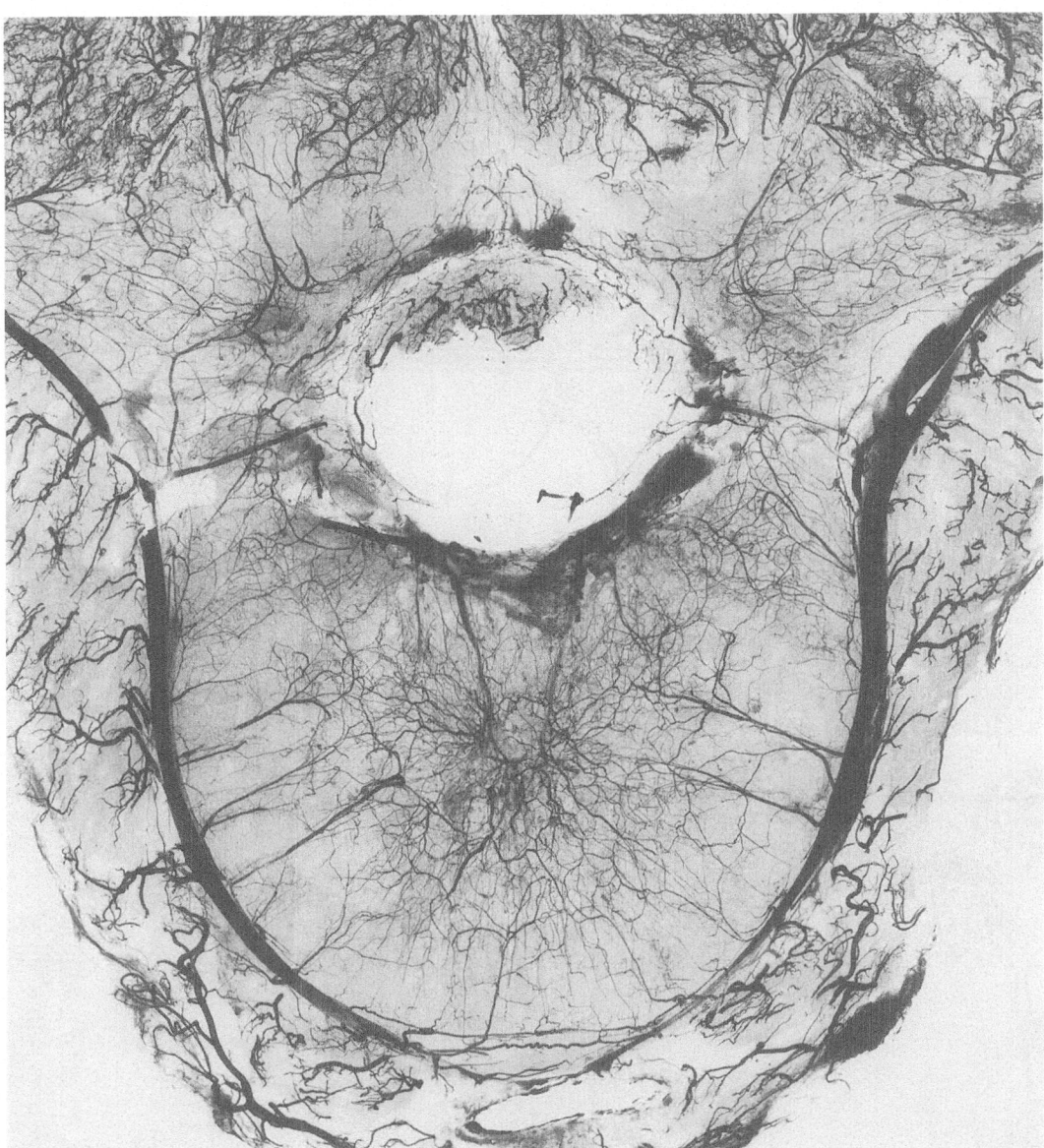

Figure 2.3. A transverse section through the lumbar vertebral body of a child aged 13 years. The radiate distribution of the centrum branches arising from the inner surface of the lumbar arteries on each side has been shown. Note the muscular branches passing directly into the muscles from the outer side of the main trunk of each lumbar artery. [Reproduced by courtesy of J. B. Lippincott and Company from: Clin. Orthop. Rel. Res., No. 115 (1976)]

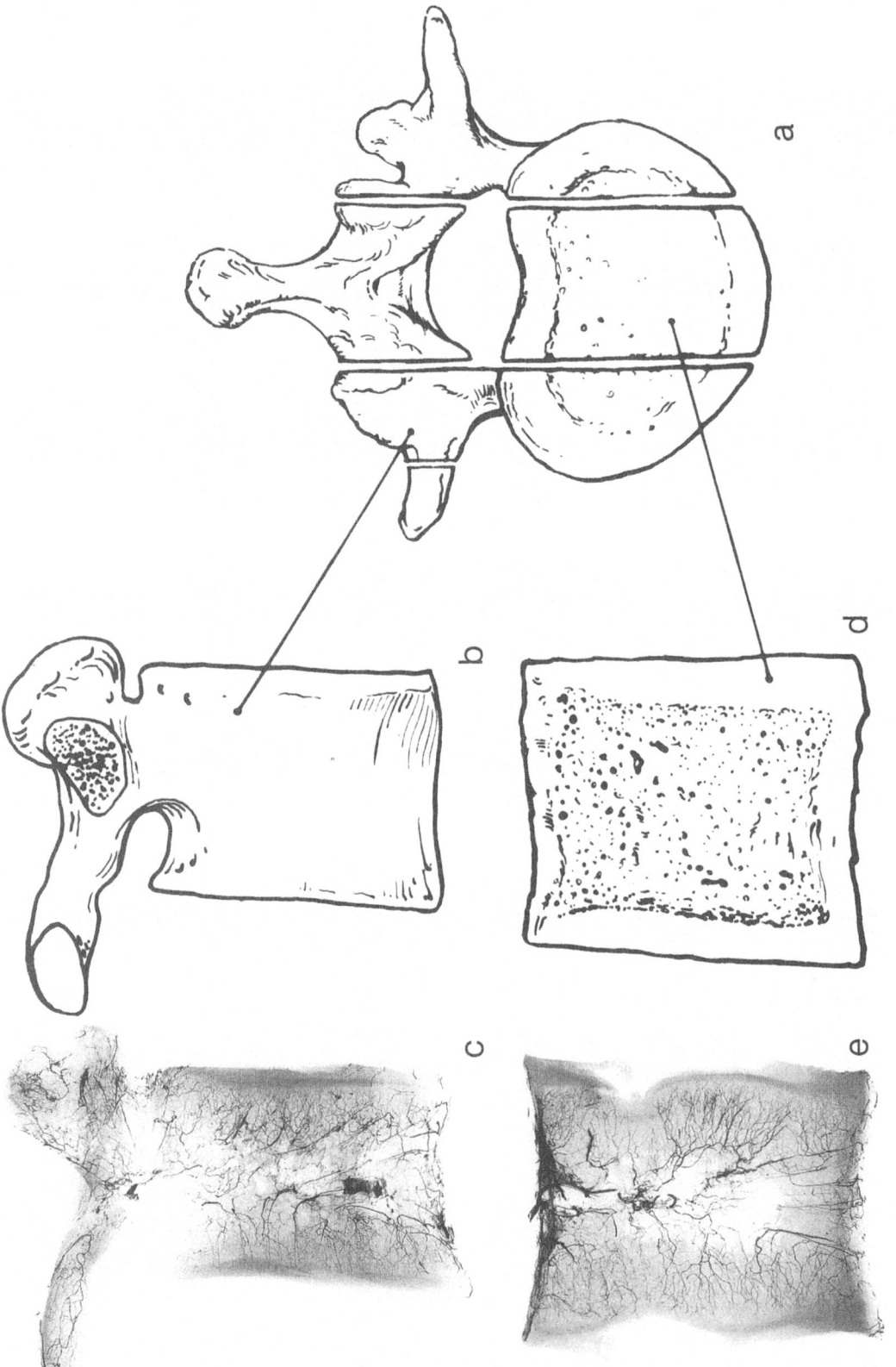

Figures 2.4a–e. Line drawings **a, b, d** indicating the division of a lumbar vertebra into sagittal sections. Sections **c** and **e** of the specimen alongside show the distribution of arteries within the vertebral body from a male aged 30 years. The feeding branches to the centrum grid can be seen in both sections. [Reproduced by courtesy of J. B. Lippincott and Company from: Clin. Orthop. Rel. Res., No. 115 (1976)]

reasons details of the vertebral circulation relative to the arterial supply and venous drainage of vertebral bodies and, in particular, of their vertebral end-plate zones, are illustrated, with descriptive legends in Figs. 2.2–10, while aspects of the gross anatomy of the major vessels related to the lumbar spine will be found, serving as a guide to safe surgical exposures of its antero-lateral surfaces in Figs. 2.29–32a,b.

Sites of Lesions

Post-traumatic internal disc disruption may occur at any level in the spine. In the neck it often follows high speed injuries (see Chapter 7). It is rarely seen in the thoracic spine though, if suspected on the basis of loss of nuclear signal on T2 weighed sequences in MRI, its diagnosis can be confirmed by CT discography (Figs. 2.13 a–c).

In the lumbar spine, the lower discs are most commonly affected. As with disc prolapses, it is rarely found in the upper lumbar discs.

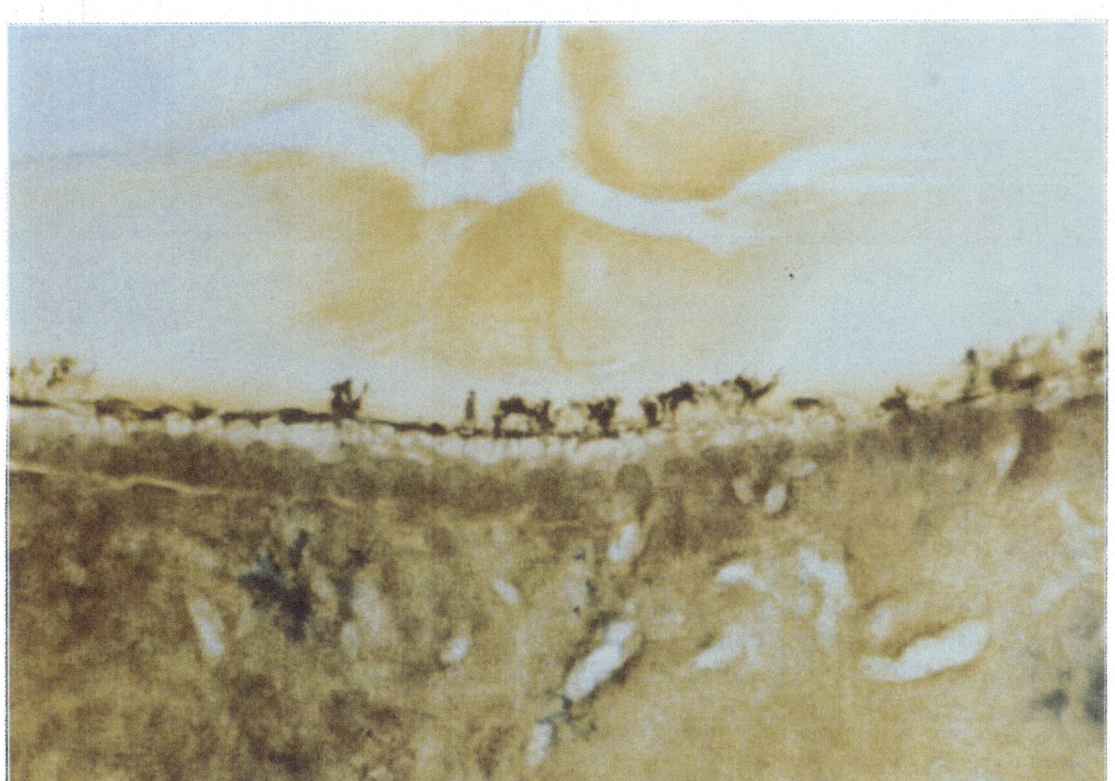

Figure 2.5. A detailed photograph taken from the central area of the disc and vertebral body (500 μm thick) from a woman of 30 years. Spalteholz-cleared specimen (approximately × 20). The demarcation line between the intervertebral disc and vertebral end-plate cartilage is clearly visible. The vertebral end-plate cartilage capillary bed is shown, with vertical tributaries draining to the sub-chondral post-capillary venous network orientated parallel to the vertebral end-plate

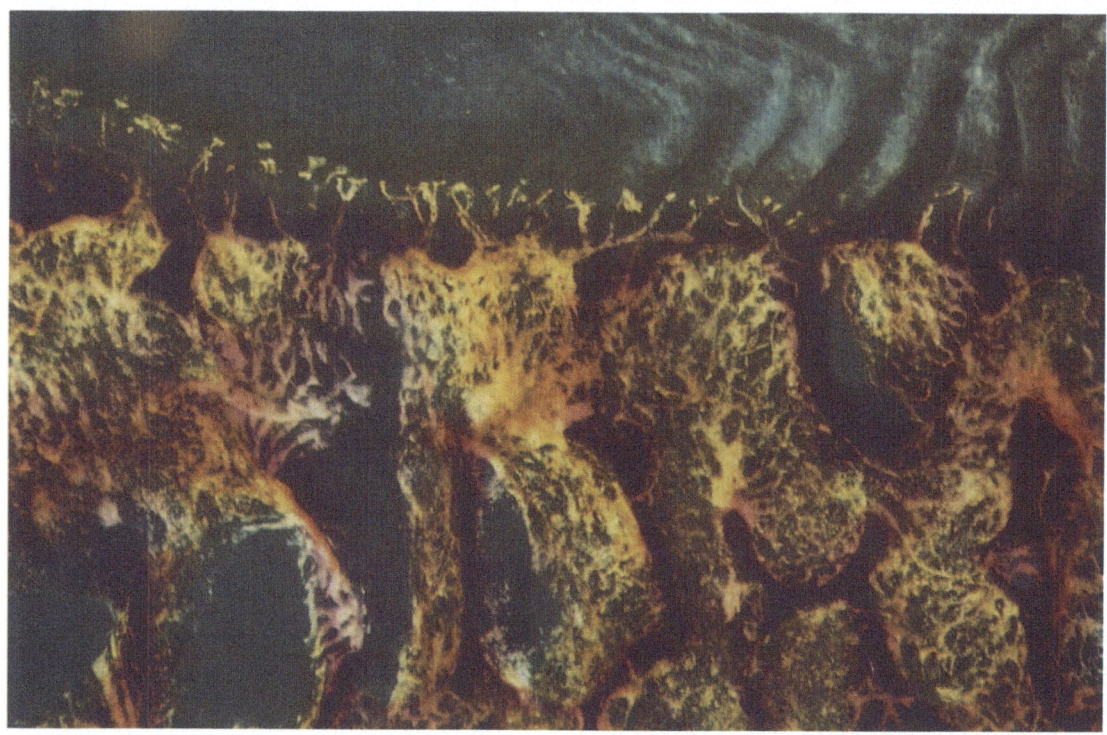

Figure 2.6. A micro-photograph (× 60 approximately) showing the capillary bed in the vertebral end-plate cartilage in the lower lumbar region in an adult dog. Note the drainage of these capillaries directly into the marrow spaces of the vertebral bodies. This is almost certainly the pathway for the passage of substances from a damaged "avascular" disc into the patient's immune system. (Prepared by Drs. H. V. Crock and M. Goldwasser)

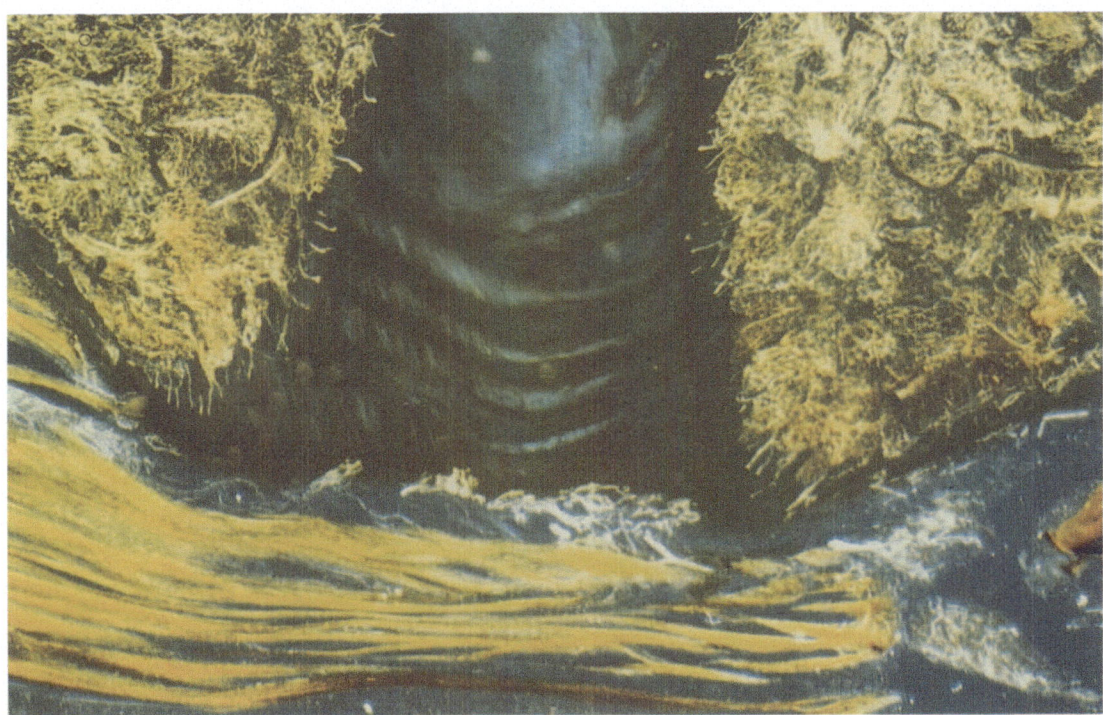

Figure 2.7. A photo-micrograph (× 20 approximately) to show the distribution of capillaries in the vertebral end-plate cartilages at the anterior disc margin in the lower lumbar disc of an adult dog. (Prepared by Drs. H. V. Crock and M. Goldwasser)

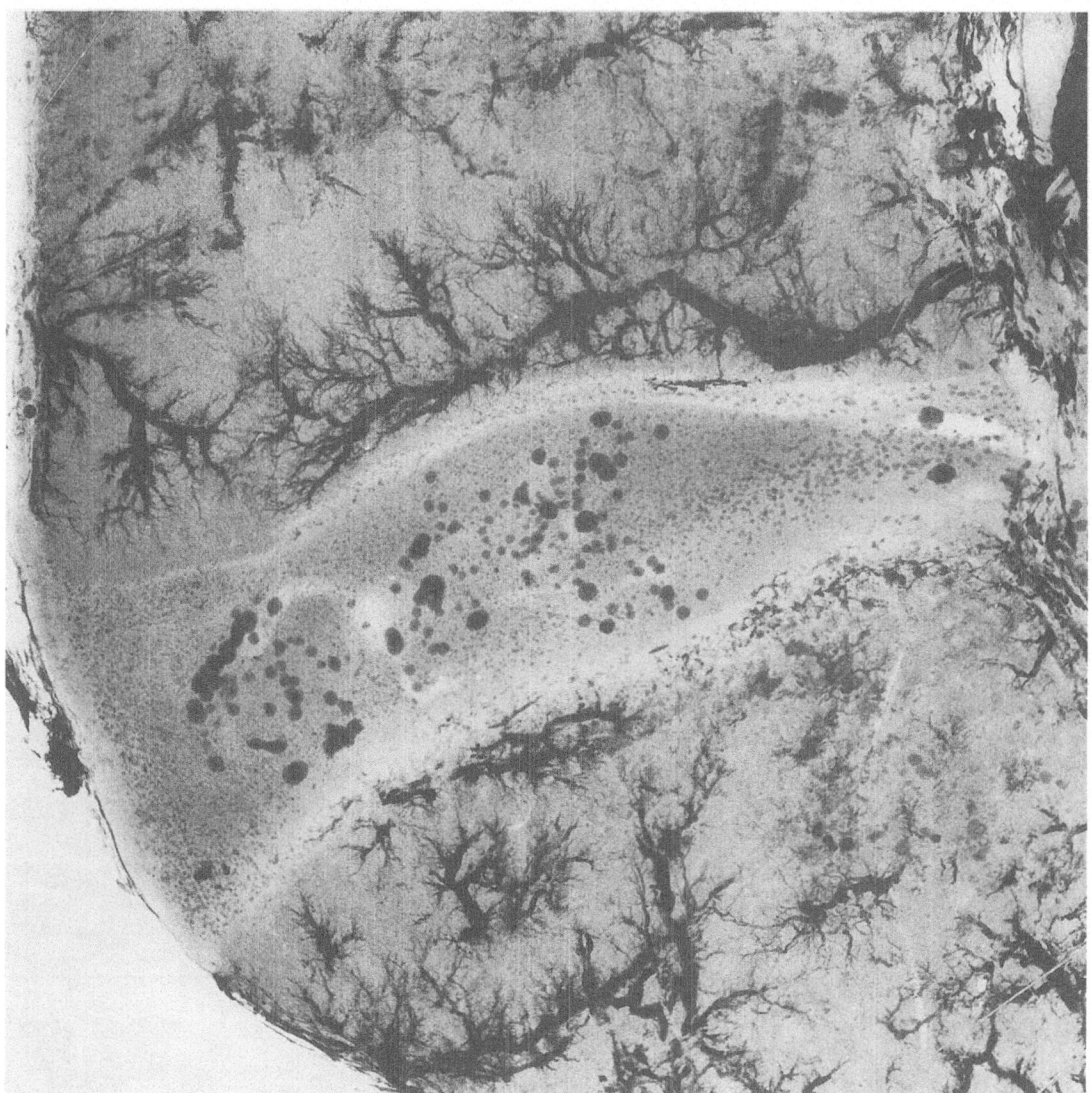

Figure 2.8. A radiograph of a thin sagittal section cut laterally near the vertebral pedicle from the lumbo-sacral junction of a woman aged 67 years. Some fragments of barium sulphate debris have adhered to the cut surface of the disc. The horizontal sub-articular collecting vein system of the vertebral body can be seen running parallel to the vertebral end-plate area on the lower surface of the 5th lumbar vertebra. Nearer the disc, of smaller calibre, running parallel to the vertebral end-plate cartilage, the sub-chondral post-capillary venous network can be seen. It is only partly filled. This system drains by vertical stems through perforations in the vertebral end-plate into the larger horizontal sub-articular collecting vein system. In this specimen only one such stem can be seen joining these two venous channels. [Reproduced by courtesy of the Editor, J. Bone Joint Surg. *55b* (1973), and J. B. Lippincott and Company from: Clin. Orthop. Rel. Res., No. 115 (1976)]

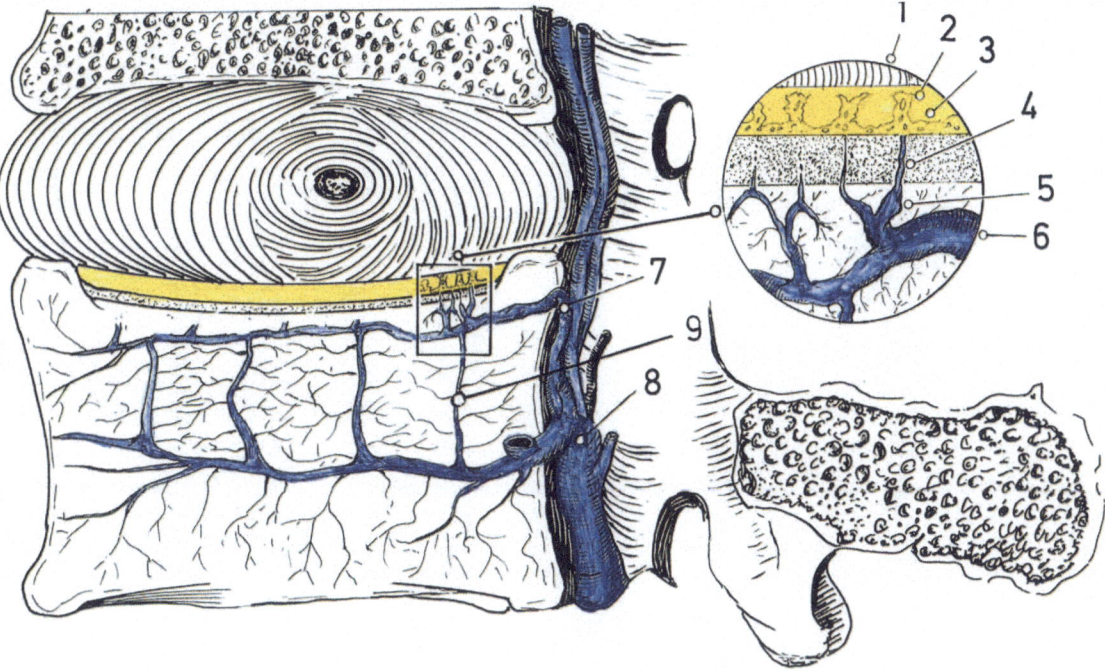

Figure 2.9. A schematic drawing to show the spatial relationships of the veins of a typical vertebral body. *1* intervertebral disc; *2* capillary bed in vertebral end-plate cartilage; *3* sub-chondral post-capillary venous network on the vertebral end-plate; *4* vertebral end-plate perforated by short vertical venous tributaries; *5* vertical tributaries from the sub-chondral post-capillary venous network, draining to the horizontal sub-articular collecting vein; *6* horizontal sub-articular collecting vein; *7* horizontal sub-articular collecting vein joining the anterior internal vertebral venous plexus; *8* basi-vertebral vein joining the anterior internal venous plexus; *9* vertical tributary of the basi-vertebral system of veins

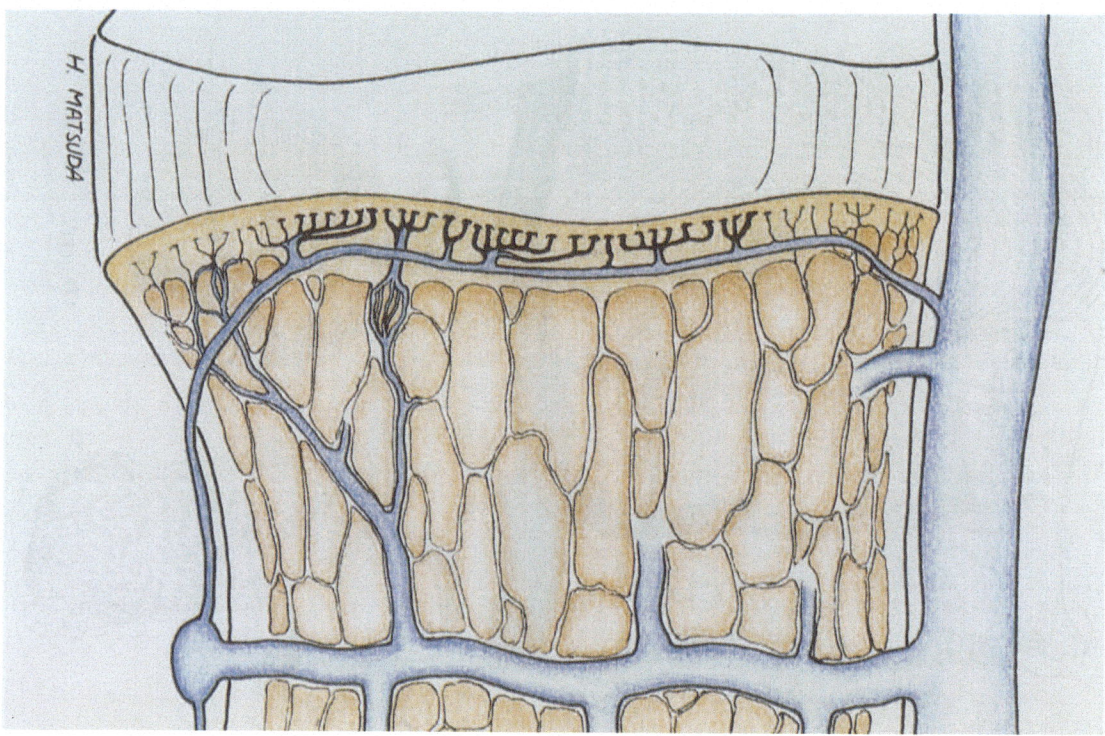

Figure 2.10. A drawing illustrating the methods of drainage of vertebral end-plate capillaries in the dog; (i) either directly into the marrow space veins or, (ii) through a sub-articular collecting vein system into a vertically orientated sub-articular vein system that will drain either backwards into the internal vertebral venous plexus or forward into the external vertebral veins

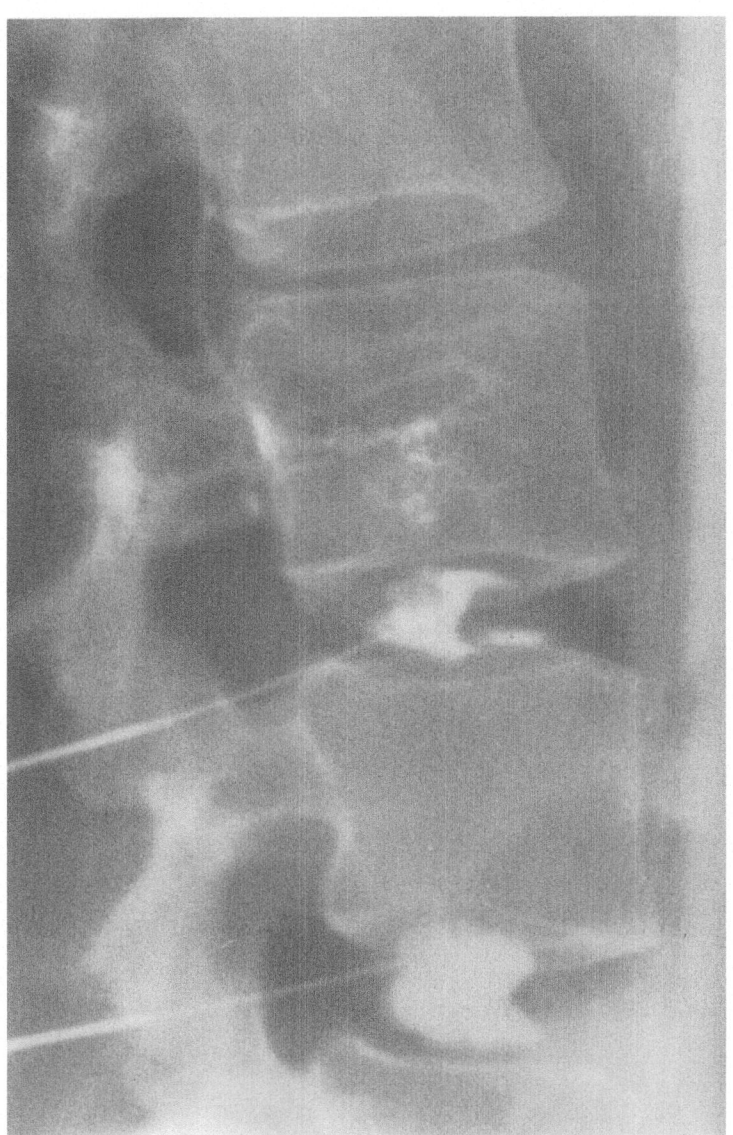

Figure 2.11. A lateral radiograph of the lumbar spine showing discograms at L 3/4 and L 4/5. The L 4/5 discogram is normal. The L 3/4 discogram shows a normal nuclear outline but note the spread of dye into the veins of the vertebral body. Batson's plexus and tributaries of the anterior internal vertebral venous plexus are filled

b) Genesis of Symptoms

Three probable causes for the symptoms are described: (i) Irritation of adjacent nerve roots and ganglia resulting from abnormal vertebral movements with or without some diffuse disc bulging, (ii) Irritation of structures adjacent to the affected disc, the spinal nerves and sympathetic nervous system, due to catabolites (noxious fluids) diffusing out of the disc, Nachemson (1969); and (iii) Leakage of discal catabolites into the general circulation via vertebral end-plate capillaries, producing features suggestive of auto-immune or hypersensitivity reactions. Some of the patients in this group suffer from profound weight loss and they are found to have abnormalities in peripheral blood smears, with rouleaux formation, altered white cell counts and elevated erythrocyte sedimentation rates (E.S.R.) (Crock, 1970).

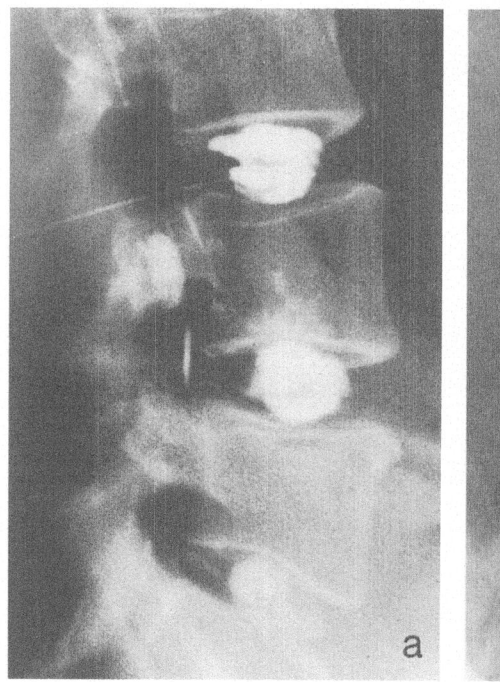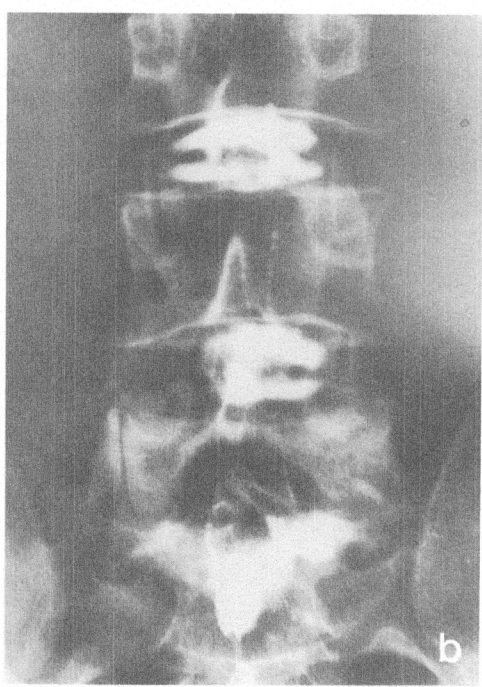

Figures 2.12 a, b. Radiographs of the lumbar spine of a man aged 37 years showing discograms at the L3/4, L4/5 and L5/S1 levels. Remnants of myodil are noted in the spinal canal from a previous myelogram performed some years earlier. The volume of dye injected at the L3/4 and L5/S1 disc spaces was approximately 1.9 ml at each disc. The volume injected at the L4/5 level was 4.5 ml. Note the flare in the body of the 4th lumbar vertebra, indicating leakage of dye through the vertebral end-plate cartilage. During injection of contrast medium at the L4/5 disc, the patient complained of severe low back pain similar to that for which he had sought treatment. The discograms appear normal in the antero-posterior view

Figures 2.13 a–c. **a** An axial view of the disc at T8/9 in a male aged 28 years showing internal disc disruption with epidural leakage of dye on the right side of the picture. **b** A lateral MRI, T2 weighted sequence in a female aged 41 years showing loss of nuclear signal at the T8/9 disc space. This patient had typical symptoms of internal disc disruption, with thoracic pain, loss of energy etc. **c** A lateral tomogram showing interbody fusion in the same patient – rib disc grafts were used

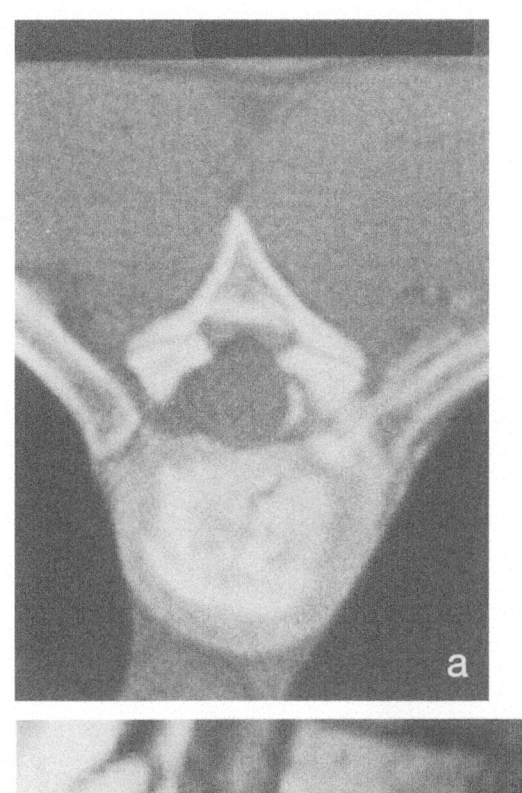

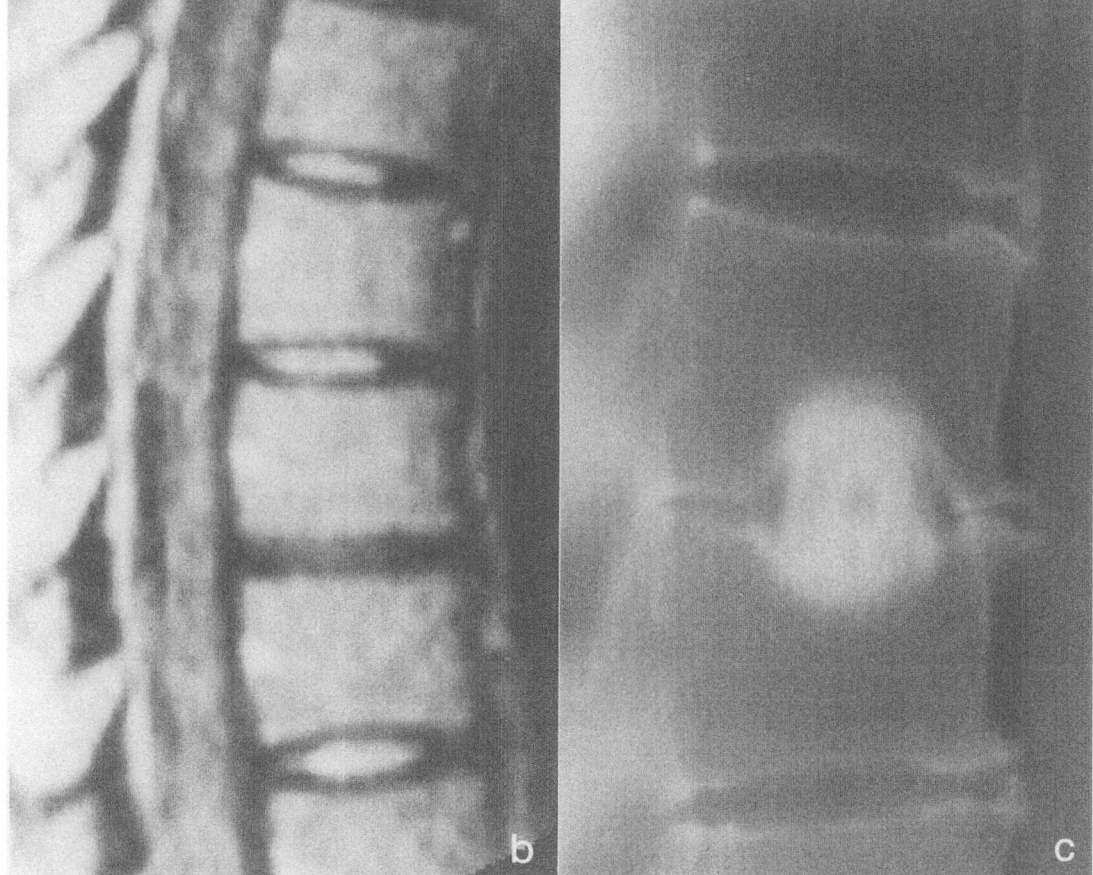

Figures 2.13a–c

2.3. Investigations

a) Plain X-Rays

Unless clear evidence of vertebral instability can be demonstrated on films taken in flexion and extension, plain X-rays are of no value in establishing this diagnosis (Morgan and King, 1957).

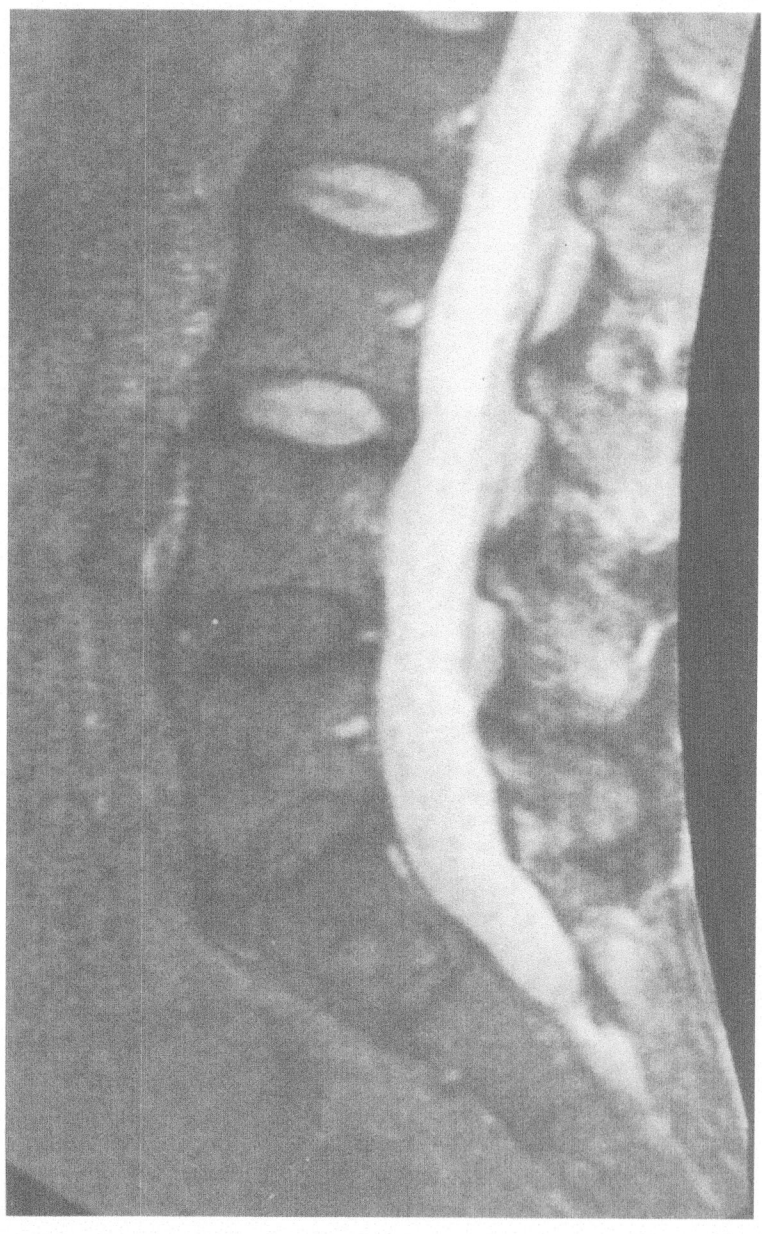

Figure 2.14. MRI, sagittal T2 weighted sequences showing internal disc disruptions at L4/5 and L5/S1 in a female aged 34 years. The disc spaces are well preserved and the nuclear signals have been lost

b) *Magnetic Resonance Imaging*

Magnetic Resonance Imaging has become the most valuable single investigation in the demonstration of changes within the disc tissues. Characteristically there is a loss of signal from the nucleus pulposus and a general greying effect involving eventually the whole disc space. The technology of magnetic resonance imaging is changing rapidly but even with recent developments *it cannot be relied upon exclusively* to demonstrate the changes which may accompany this form of disc disorder (Figs. 2.14–16 a, b).

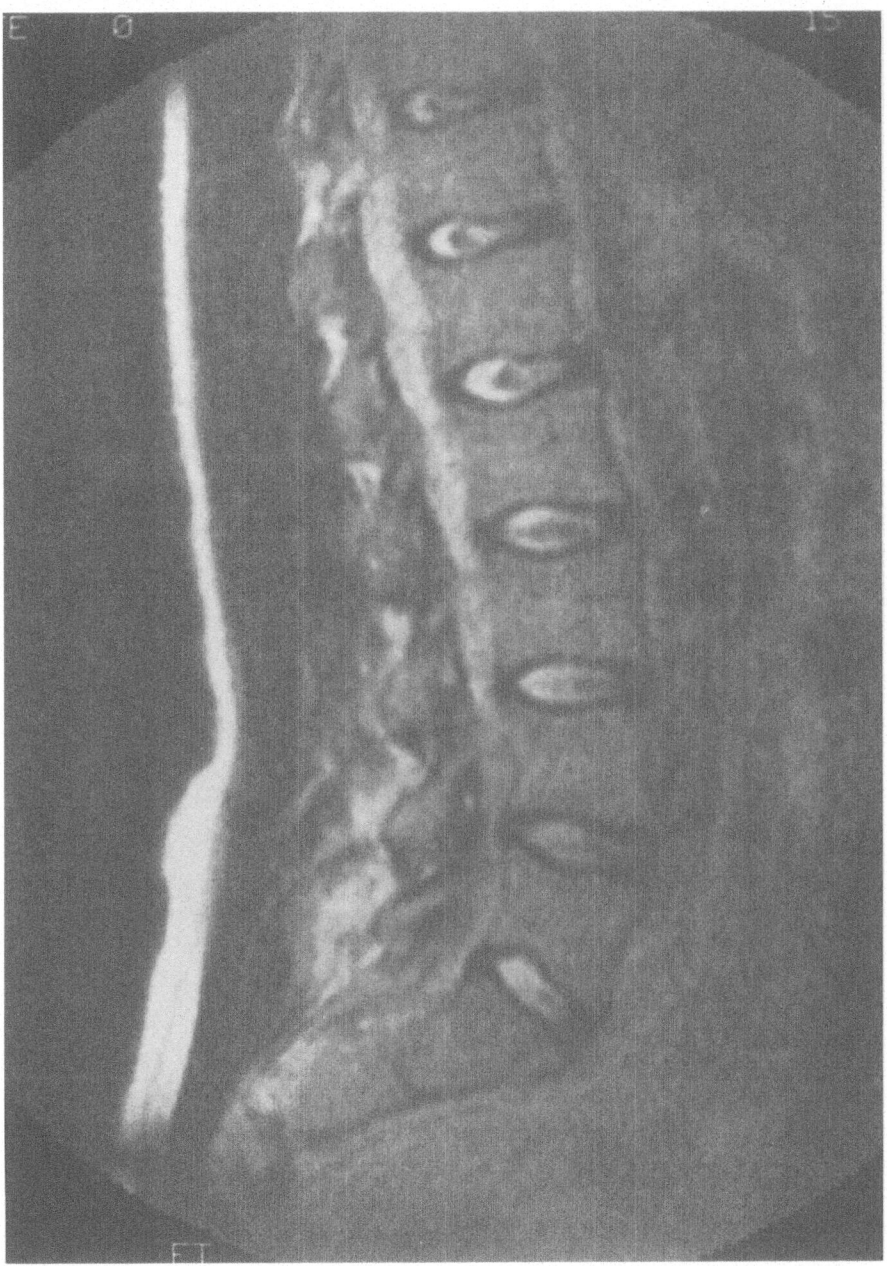

Figure 2.15. MRI, sagittal T2 weighted sequence showing internal disc disruption at L4/5 in a female aged 42 years. This diagnosis was confirmed by CT discography

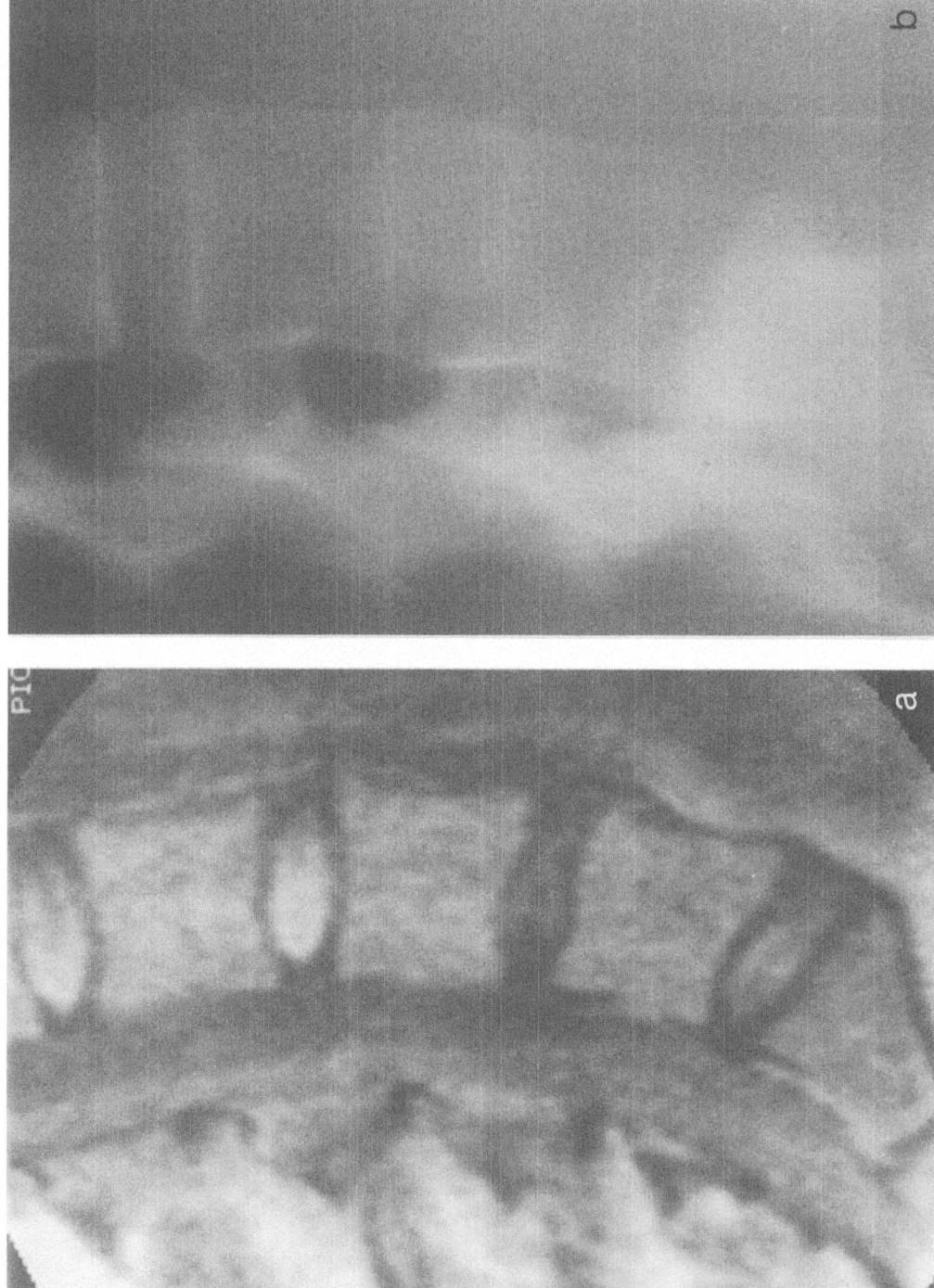

Figures 2.16a, b. **a** MRI – a detailed view of the image in Figure 2.15. **b** Lateral tomogram showing interbody fusion 9 months after operation in the same patient

c) Discography

Lumbar discography was introduced by Lindblom in 1948. *This investigation remains indispensable in the modern practice of spinal surgery,* despite the elaborate criticism which has been aimed at it, often by people who have little experience of its clinical use (Nachemson 1989). Special needles are required for its performance (Fig. 2.17). Injection of a suitable contrast medium such as Amipaque 240 should be made through a Luer-lock 1 ml syringe.

The indications for discography are: i) In suspected cases of internal disc disruption assessed on the clinical syndrome where MRI images may be equivocal; ii) In suspected cases of internal disc disruption in patients who have had "failed laminectomies"; iii) As a supplementary test following negative myelography, when in association with CT it may demonstrate some of the rarer laterally placed disc prolapses; iv) In some cases of spondylolisthesis, to determine if adjacent discs are disrupted.

Using an image intensifier X-ray machine with video storage facility, the needles may be inserted easily into the discs to be examined, the patient lying prone, sedated lightly with appropriate medication. If these facilities are not available, then X-rays in two planes should be obtained after the needles have been inserted into the discs. Injections must never be made until the needles have been placed accurately in the area of the nuclei pulposi and their positions confirmed by X-rays taken in antero-posterior and lateral views (Figs. 2.18, 2.19).

Discograms should be performed using two sets of stiletted needles. The first, a broad gauged needle, (18 gauge) is directed towards the disc surface after skin puncture, in the lumbar region, having been inserted about 4 fingers breadths lateral to the spinous process, angled towards the disc space at about 45 degrees to the horizontal axis of the spine. A fine stiletted discogram needle (22 gauge) is then passed through the "guide needle" into the disc, there being a characteristic sensation as though it were pushed into a firm mass of rubber as it enters the disc. Occasionally when the lumbo-sacral disc space is deep in the pelvis, difficulty may be experienced in inserting the discogram needle by this route. Re-placing the "guide needle" in the midline, the lumbo-sacral disc may be punctured by passing the discogram needle through the dural sac.

Injection of contrast medium into a normal disc is painless. When dye enters a disrupted disc, pain is experienced immediately. *The pain is mediated via nerve fibres*

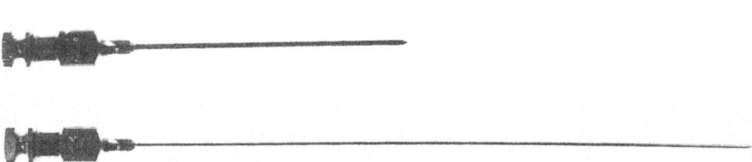

Figure 2.17. A photograph of discogram needles showing the shorter guide needle and the longer 22 gauge needle with stilette

within the disc and its pattern of radiation into the limbs is not radicular (Yoshizawa *et al.,* 1980).

The reproduced pain is usually of the same character as the patient's presenting symptom but more severe; it disappears within seconds of the injection of local anaesthetic into the disc. Pain emanating from a disrupted disc at the time of discography is not provoked by a rise in intra-discal pressure as it may come on after the injection of as little as 0.3 ml of dye, *whereas the injection of 1.5 ml of dye into an adjacent normal disc will be painless.* Notes should be made on the ease or difficulty experienced in injecting the dye, on the volume injected and on the pattern of the pain response described by the patient. In internal disc disruption, dye spreads beyond the normal confines of the nuclear zone, the radiographic patterns of the discogram varying with the anatomy of the disruption of the annular fibres of the disc or with the presence of vertebral end-plate defects (Figs. 2.20, 2.21 a, b). *Spread*

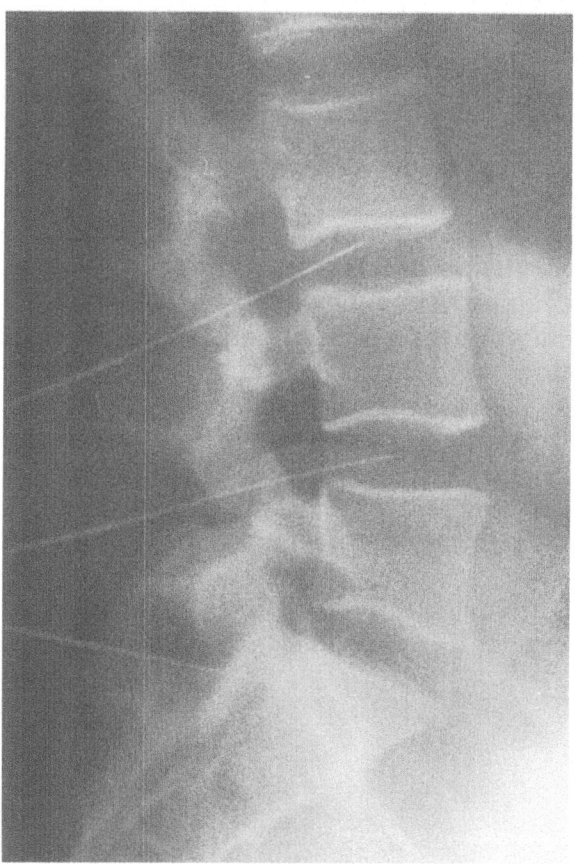
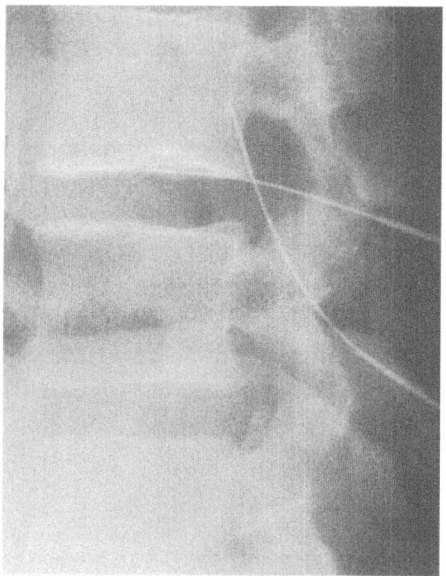

Figure 2.18   Figure 2.19

Figure 2.18. A lateral X-ray of a lumbar spine showing control X-rays with needles satisfactorily placed in the lateral view at L3/4 and L4/5 but incorrectly placed at the lumbo-sacral level

Figure 2.19. A lateral X-ray of the lumbar spine showing a control film taken after insertion of discogram needles, to illustrate the importance of obtaining X-rays to determine the position of needles before any injections are made

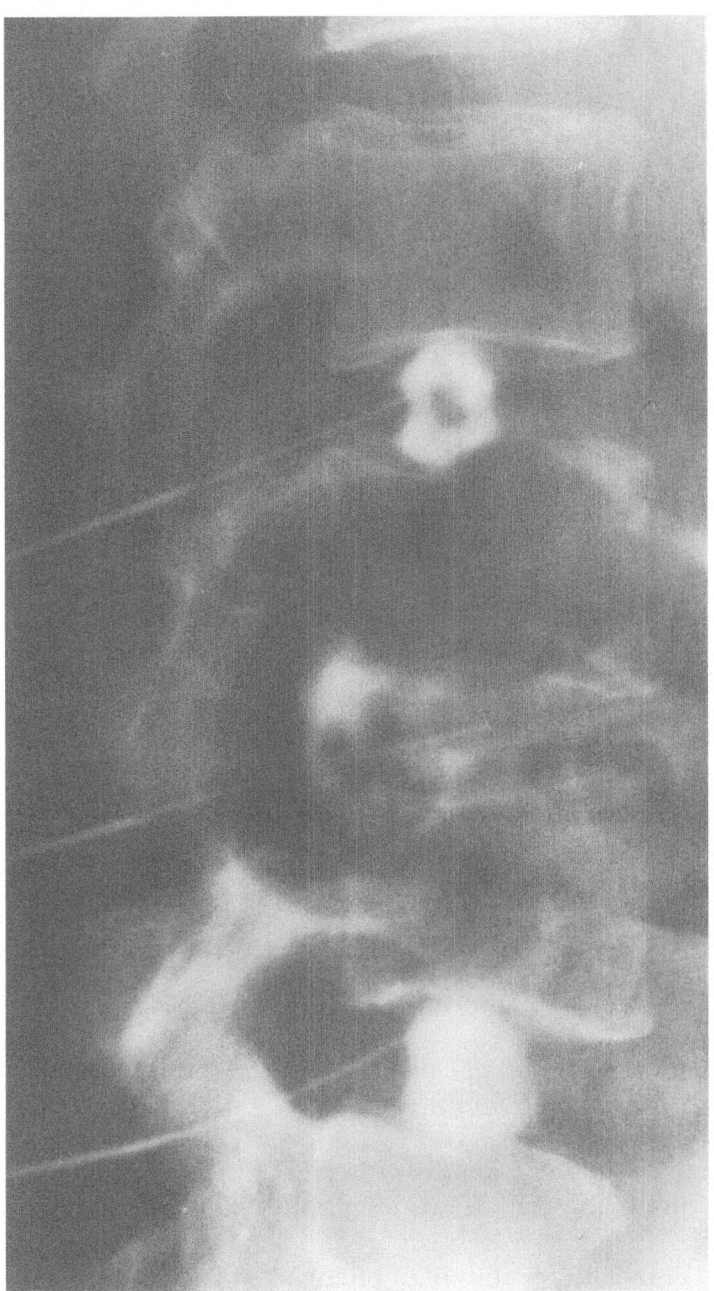

Figure 2.20. A lateral radiograph of the lumbar spine of a man aged 48 years showing normal discograms at L3/4 and L5/S1. 2 ml of dye was injected at each of these disc spaces and no pain was reproduced. At L4/5, 5 ml of dye was injected. Gross disc disruption is shown. The patient's pain was reproduced at the time of injection

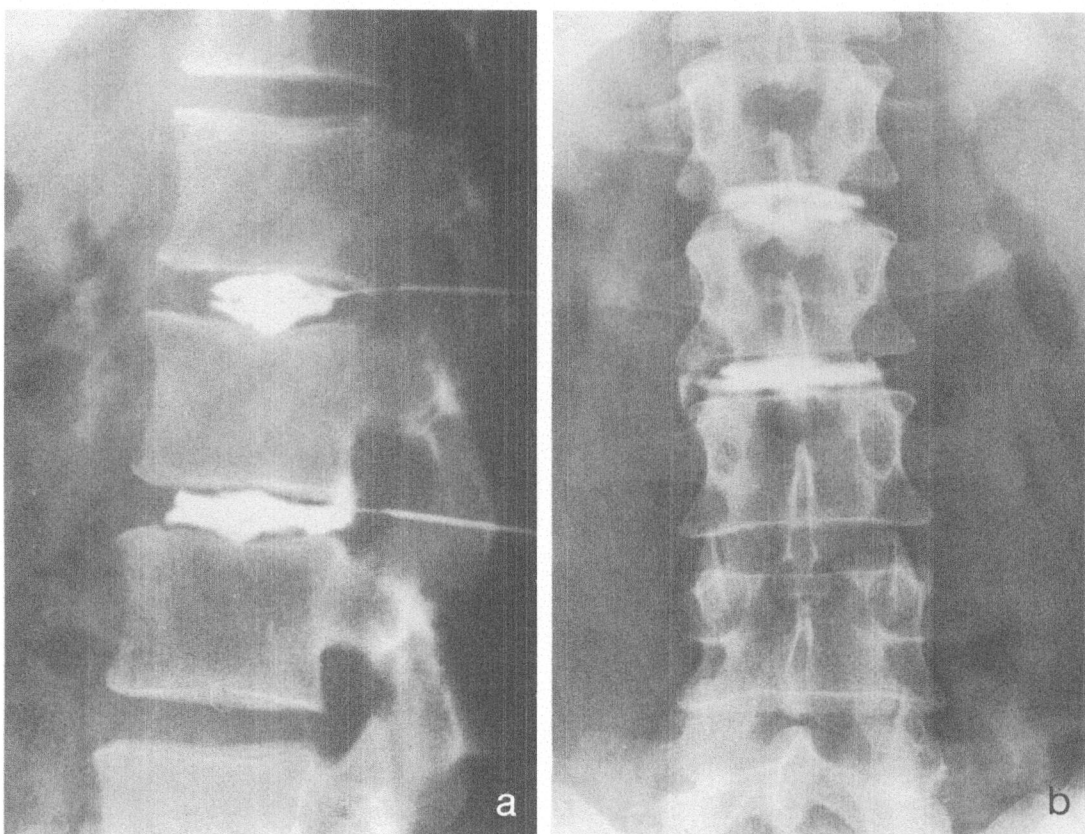

Figures 2.21 a, b. a A lateral radiograph of the lumbar spine of a man aged 42 years. Discogram needles have been inserted into the discs between L1/2 and L2/3 vertebral bodies, lateral and anterior to the thecal sac. The upper discogram is normal; that at the L2/3 level shows posterior internal disc disruption. **b** Antero-posterior view of the same case

of dye beyond the disc margins and into the spinal canal is a manifestation of abnormal permeability of the annular fibres and should not necessarily be interpreted as indicating prolapse of disc material (Figs. 2.22, a, b).

Once the injection has been completed antero-posterior and lateral X-rays should be taken and arrangements made for CT examination which will provide axial images of the affected disc.

One of the critical elements in the interpretation of the results of discography is the recording of the patients' pain response. It is usually dramatic, due to the intensity of the induced pain.

Should the patient be too heavily sedated during the procedure the observer may be unable to record any useful information in this regard. *In these circumstances the patient should be observed for 24 hours following discography.* In the presence of symptomatic internal disc disruption the clinical syndrome will invariably flare up once the effects of sedation have settled and the patient will complain of an aggravation of his or her familiar pain.

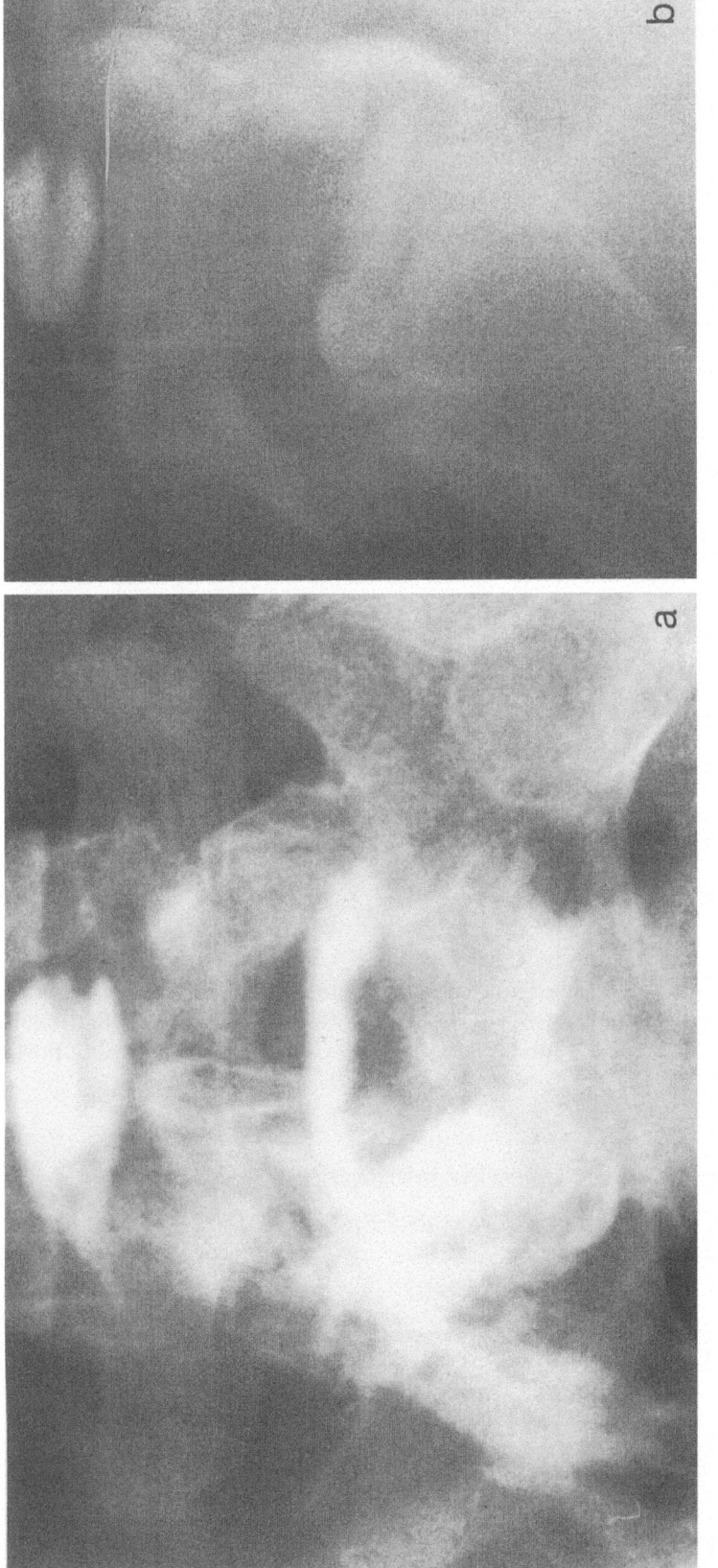

Figures 2.22 a, b. Antero-posterior and lateral radiographs of the L 4/5 and L 5/S 1 discs in a girl of 17, showing a normal L 4/5 discogram and gross disc disruption at L 5/S 1 with antero-lateral leakage of dye. This young lady had been involved in a motor vehicle accident two years earlier and presented with classical features of post-traumatic internal disc disruption, with chronic back pain, referred leg pain, loss of energy, intolerance to physical activity, and profound weight loss

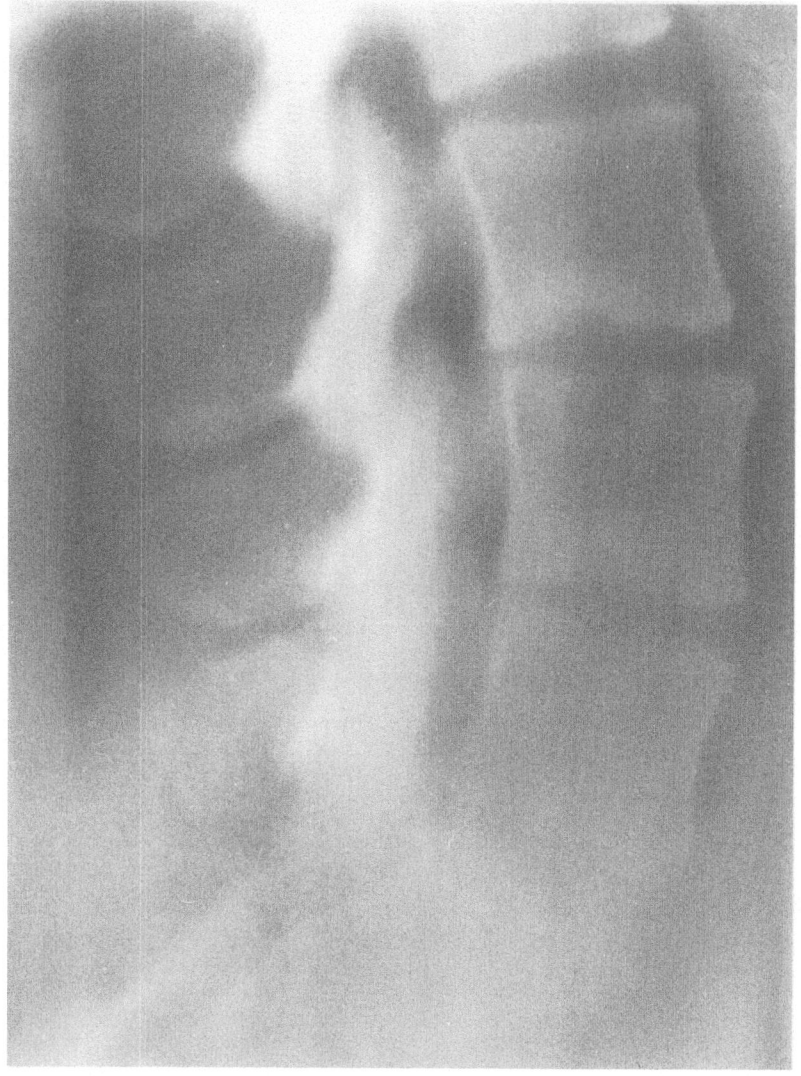

Figure 2.23. A mid-line tomogram of the lower lumbar spine from a man aged 27 years, taken three months after lumbo-sacral interbody fusion. The L 3/4 and L 4/5 discograms had been normal. Note the changes of vertebral end-plate erosion and loss of disc height typical of post-discogram discitis

A discogram report should provide the following information:

1. Details of the placing of the needles within individual discs.
2. The type and volume of dye injected.
3. The ease or difficulty of injection.
4. The patient's description of induced pain.
5. The patterns of distribution of the injected dye in antero-posterior and lateral X-rays of the disc space and in the axial plane on CT.
6. A record should be made that 0.3 ml of Zinacef[1] has been injected into each disc space at the conclusion of the procedure.

---

[1] Cefuroxine sodium for injection, Glaxo Operations UK Limited, Greenford, Middlesex UB6 OHE (Tel: 081-422-3434).

Excluding technical difficulties in its performance, discitis is the major complication which may result from discography (Fig. 2.23). The latent period between the time of discography and diagnosis of discitis varies between three to twelve weeks. For this reason, radiologists in the past have rarely reported this complication as they do not see the patients after performing the discograms. Fraser *et al.,* (1987) have made important contributions to the study of post-discogram discitis, the incidence of which has fallen virtually to zero following their recommendation for the routine use of antibiotics injected into the disc at the time of the procedure. They claim that this complication always follows the introduction of organisms from the skin surface carried into the disc on the needle point. The pattern of vertebral destruction in "post-discogram discitis" occurring in discographically normal discs, differs markedly from the more extensive and less clearly demarcated vertebral end-plate changes of vertebral osteomyelitis. In Japan it has been customary to keep patients at rest in bed for several days after discography. The rate of post-discogram discitis in that country has been very low. The classic changes of "post-discogram discitis" as seen in (Fig. 2.23) have therefore been ascribed in some cases to pressure necrosis of the vertebral end-plates and not to infection, Hijikata (1982).

d) Radiculography

Radiculography has no place in the investigation of internal disc disruption.

2.4. Surgical Treatment

a) Types

Surgical treatment is recommended after the failure of comprehensive conservative treatment. Poor results of spinal canal surgery for disc lesions other than for disc prolapse have been reported frequently (Kudelka, 1968). These poor results which are known to follow "negative laminectomies" could be largely prevented by more accurate pre-operative assessment including the use of M.R.I. and CT discography. If nothing else, the use of these investigations would restrict the extent of spinal canal explorations, as, often, more than one disc will be inspected in the hope of finding a suspected "prolapse".

i) Total Disc Excision and Interbody Fusion

Total disc excision and interbody fusion, for single or double level disc disruptions with intractable limb and spinal pain and constitutional symptoms (Debeyre and Delforges, 1959). In the lumbar region this method may be satisfactory for one or two disc levels, providing:

- the patient is not obese;
- there is no antecedent history of pulmonary embolism or deep vein thrombosis in the legs;
- lumbo-sacral articulation anomalies are not associated with great vein anomalies which may render access to the intervertebral disc space hazardous or impossible; and
- surgical technique is meticulous.

Whereas the operation of interbody fusion finds a small but undisputed role in the management of failed spinal operations (Sacks, 1965), its real place in the present state of knowledge should be for the primary surgical treatment of non-prolapsing disc lesions. Cloward (1955) has described a method of inserting grafts between adjacent vertebral bodies via the spinal canal for the treatment of lumbar disc "lesions". The operation which bears his name is not used widely because of the technical difficulties of its execution. However, there are groups of international surgeons who practice this method regularly. Exceptional surgical skill is required for its safe and effective use (Lin and Gill, 1989). For similar reasons, the operation described by Wiltberger (1957, 1958), which involves the insertion of accurately cut dowel grafts between adjacent vertebral bodies via the spinal canal, is rarely used.

When the prerequisites set out above can be met, anterior lumbar interbody fusion is a satisfactory operation which can be rapidly and safely performed by an extra-peritoneal left-sided abdominal approach, allowing ready access to more than one disc if required. Near-total disc excision can be accomplished by fashioning two parallel dowel cavities into which dowel grafts can be accurately and firmly impacted (Figs. 2.24,1–4, 25,a,b). The grafts are cut vertically downwards from the

LOWER LUMBAR DOWEL CAVITIES

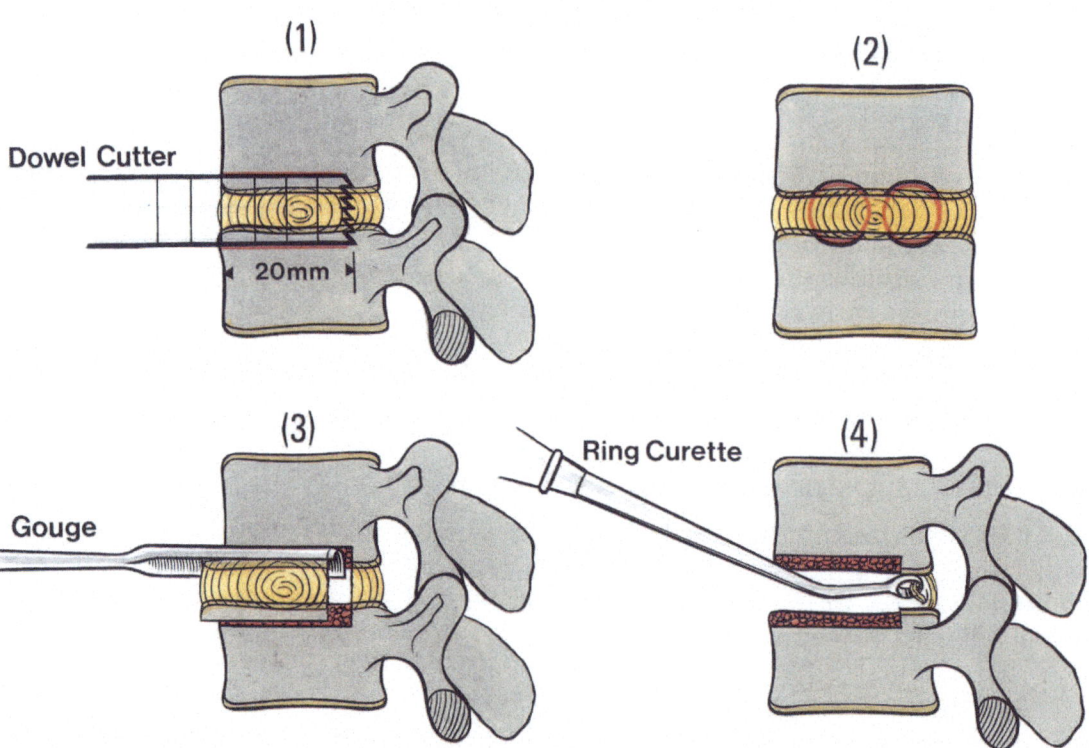

Figures 2.24, 1–4. 1 The use of a dowel cutting instrument in the lumbar spine. **2** The antero-posterior orientation of two dowel cavities in the lower lumbar area. **3** The use of the special gouge to displace the disc and adjacent fragments of the vertebral bodies. **4** The use of the ring curette for the removal of vertebral end-plate and disc tissue remnants from the interbody space

anterior third of the left iliac crest. They have tooled cancellous surfaces between the stout cortical tables of the iliac crest and their depth can be determined at will (Figs. 2.26 a, b). The final shape of individual iliac crest grafts varies with the thickness of this bone. Some will be uniformly shaped with parallel inner and outer cortical tables, while others will be wedge shaped (Figs. 2.27 a, b). Wedge shaped grafts should be impacted into dowel cavities with the flat thick iliac crest end

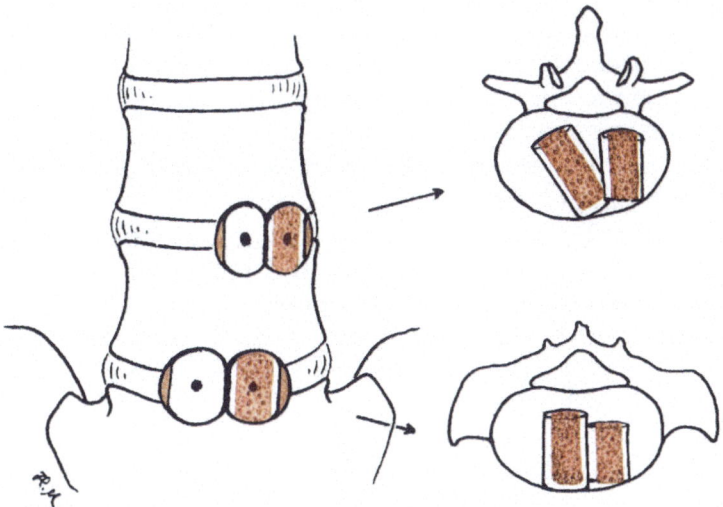

Figure 2.25. Drawings illustrating the orientation of grafts in the intervertebral spaces at L5/S1 and L4/5

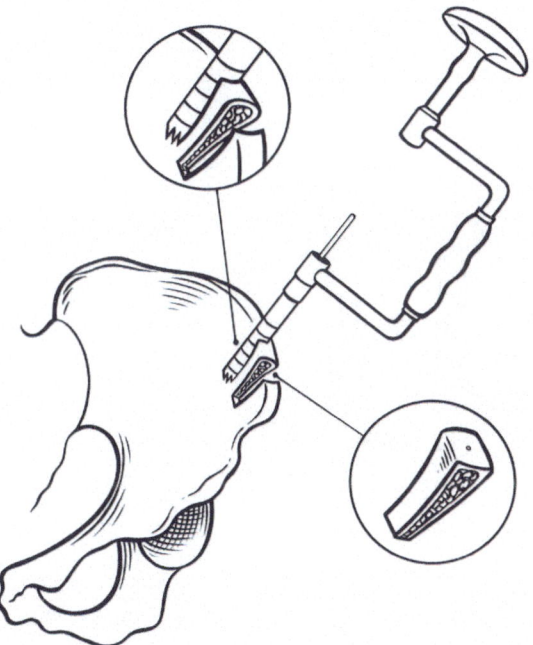

Figure 2.26. Drawing to illustrate the method of cutting grafts from the anterior third of the iliac crest. Each graft has two tooled cancellous surfaces and stout cortical faces on three sides

directed towards the depth of the cavity. Bone chips should be placed on either side of the thin wedged end to fill the dowel cavity, adding further stability to the graft. Inserted parallel to each other with their cancellous faces abutting the prepared cancellous surfaces of the adjacent vertebral bodies, these grafts are ideally situated for rapid vascularisation (Fig. 2.28). One cortical surface of each graft on either side of the disc space prevents penetration of any disc remnant which may have escaped removal by curettage before the grafts were inserted, thereby diminishing the risk of non-union.

The preparation of grafts can be time consuming and may lead to problems at the donor site or sites. North American surgeons have tended to favour the use of heterogenous bone available pre-shaped in sterile packaging, Tan *et al.* (1990). Porous ceramic and titanium implants have also been used as substitutes for autogenous interbody grafts. The titanium mesh implants are potentially dangerous if they fail in the lumbar spine (see Chapter 9).

Anterior lumbar interbody fusion being the operation of choice for the surgical treatment of lumbar internal disc disruptions, details of the technique and the assessment of results achieved will be described in detail below:

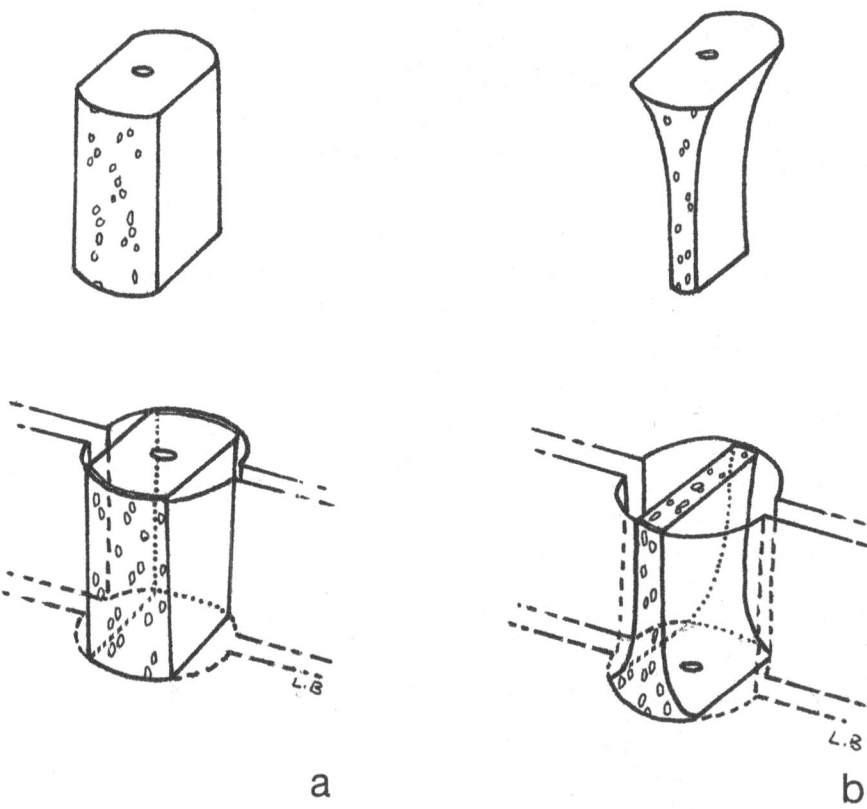

a   b

Figures 2.27a,b. **a** Top – a drawing showing a typical regularly shaped iliac crest graft. Bottom – when impacted into the prepared dowel cavity with the tooled cancellous surfaces against the cut cancellous surfaces of the vertebral bodies, it almost completely fills the space. **b** Top – a drawing showing the appearance of a wedge shaped graft. Bottom – this should be impacted into the dowel cavity as shown. Bone chips can then be packed in to the dowel cavity on either side of the thin "wedge" end of the graft

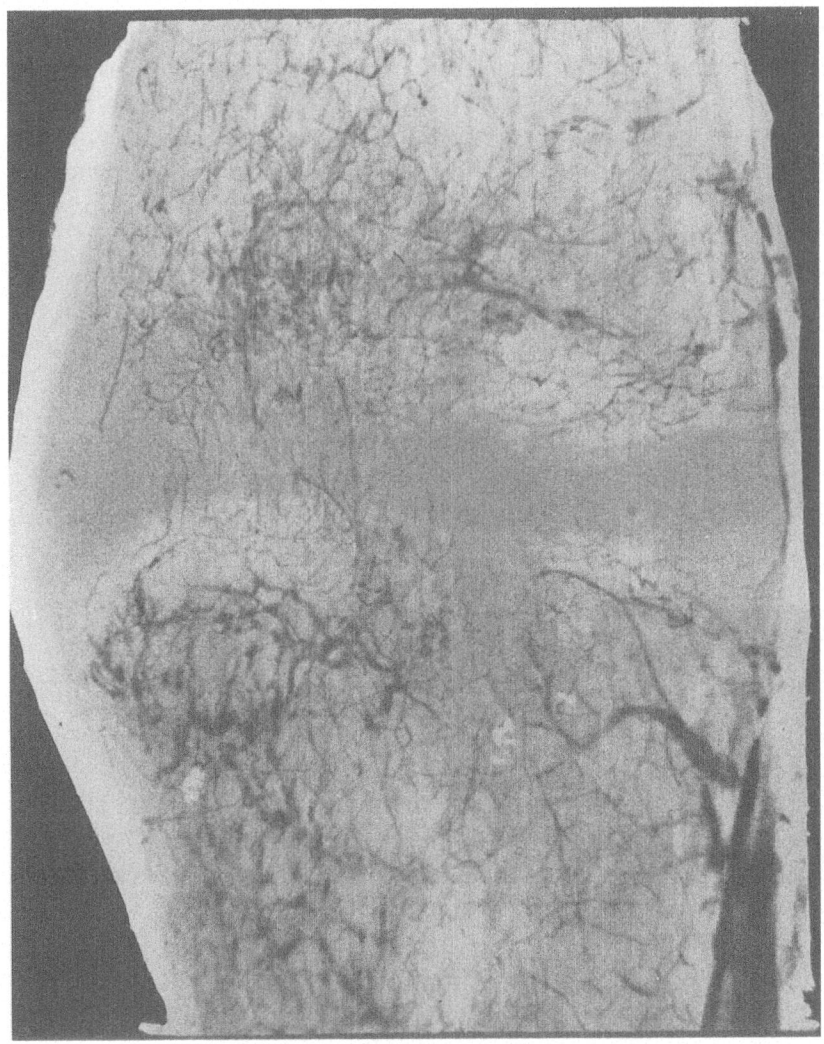

Figure 2.28. A radiograph of a thin median sagittal section of adjacent lumbar vertebrae from a dog showing the vascularization of an interbody graft 2 months after operation. The blood vessels had been injected with barium sulphate suspension

ii) Bilateral Foraminal and Nerve Root Canal Decompressions

Bilateral foraminal and nerve root canal decompressions may be indicated where a single level lumbar disc disruption has been identified in a young patient in whom the predominant symptoms are of referred leg pain without neurological abnormalities and in whom constitutional illness is not a feature. The aim in these cases is to enlarge the nerve root canals and intervertebral foramina allowing the nerve roots to accommodate to the vertebral instability resulting from the disc disruption (Morgan and King, 1957). This operation is described on pages 30–35, 127–138 (from Chapters 1 and 3).

iii) Posterior Spinal Fusion

Posterior spinal fusion, without spinal canal exploration, is still commonly practised for patients with intractable back pain and insignificant referred leg pain, in whom there is radiological evidence of multi-level disc disease. While satisfactory results often follow its use in cases with established plain X-ray changes of lumbar spondylosis, the results are far less successful when used for patients with internal disc disruption (Kostuik and Frymoyer, 1991). The procedure is most likely to succeed where a single level fusion is required. If fusion is attempted concomitantly with spinal canal exploration, methods using other than postero-lateral or inter-transverse alar grafting are likely to fail. The probability of failure is even higher if posterior fusion is attempted following earlier spinal canal surgery (Adkins, 1955).

The diagnosis of internal disc disruption is most often established by a process of exclusion after months of careful clinical observation. When first seen, patients with this condition are indistinguishable from many who present with short-lived episodes of spinal and limb pain for which, in about 80% of cases, no cause is evident

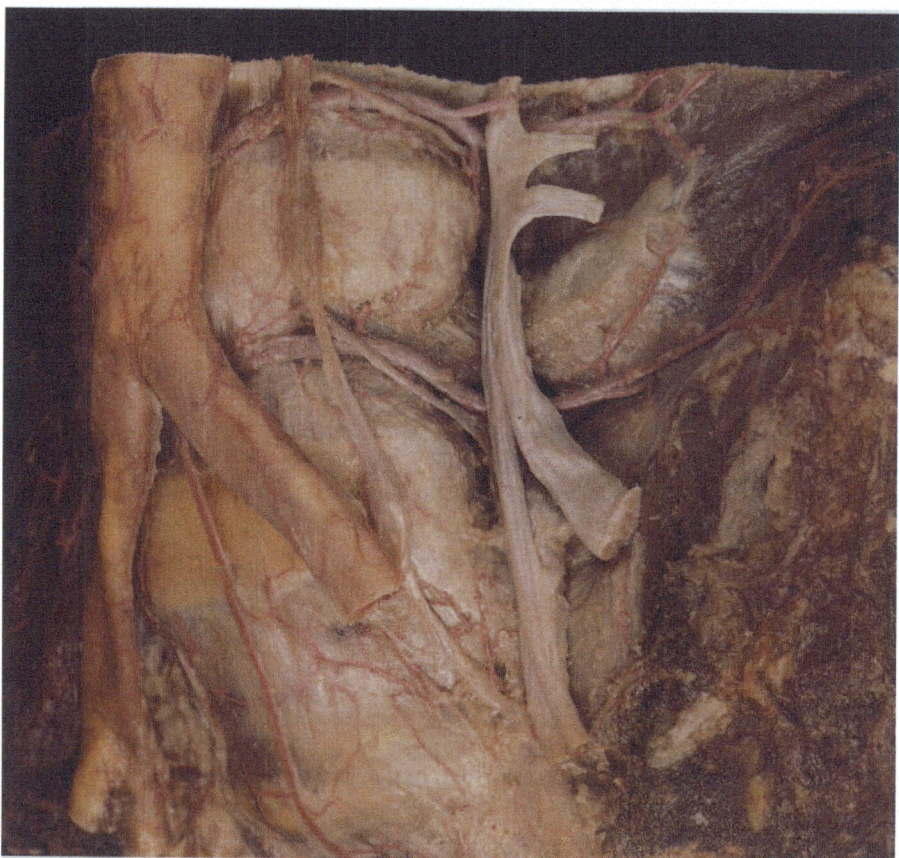

Figure 2.29. A detailed photograph of a dissection of the lumbo-sacral junction in an adult, showing the relations of the 3rd and 4th lumbar arteries to the sympathetic trunk and the pattern of branching of the median sacral artery related to the 5th lumbar vertebral body. (Dissected by Dr. S. Sihombing, of Indonesia)

(Dillane *et al.*, 1966). By contrast those patients with internal disc disruption consistently fail to respond to conservative treatment and they are often made worse by standard methods of physical therapy involving exercises and spinal manipulations. Likewise, their symptoms are aggravated by travelling in modern vehicles. It is important to distinguish these cases from disc prolapses in order to reduce significantly the "negative laminectomy" rate which accounts for many of the poor results of spinal surgery for disc lesions.

The anatomical factors pertinent to the performance of lumbar interbody fusion operations and to their ultimate success are shown in (Figs. 2.29–32 a, b).

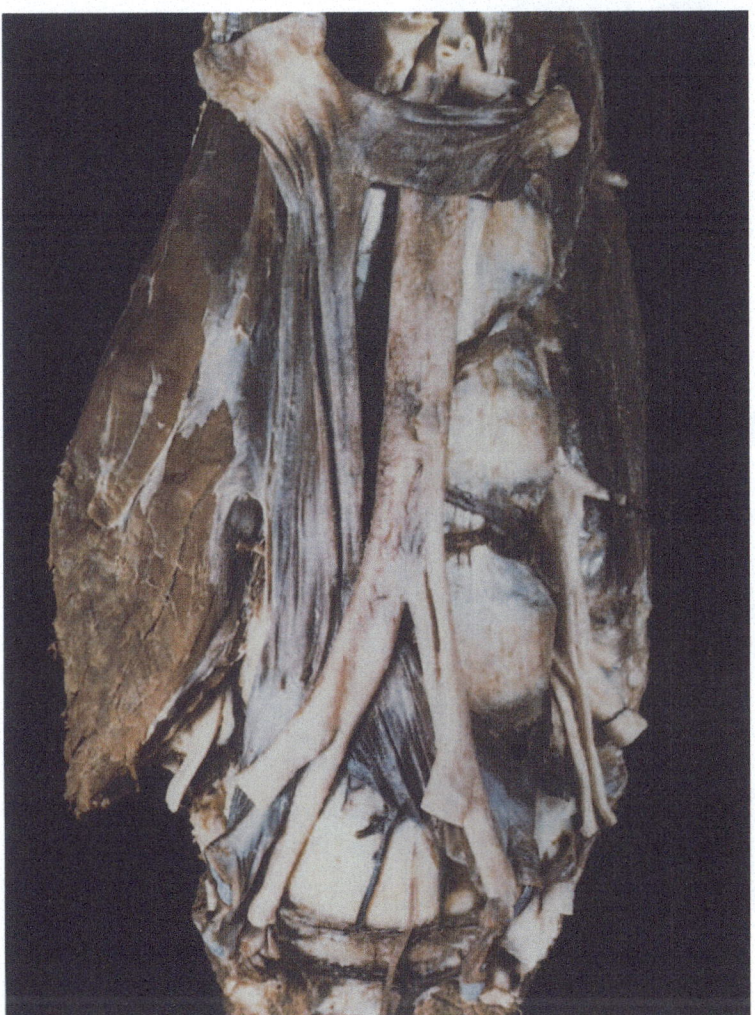

Figure 2.30. A photograph of a dissection to show the aorta and the vena cava in the abdomen. Note the bifurcation of the aorta at the lower border of the 4th lumbar vertebra. The relationship of the common iliac arteries to the common iliac veins is clearly shown. The ascending lumbar vein can be seen in the depths of the dissection, just below the disc between L4 and L5, on the right hand side of the photograph. Note that the left psoas muscle has been removed, so that the lumbar arteries and veins can be seen on the right side of the photograph.

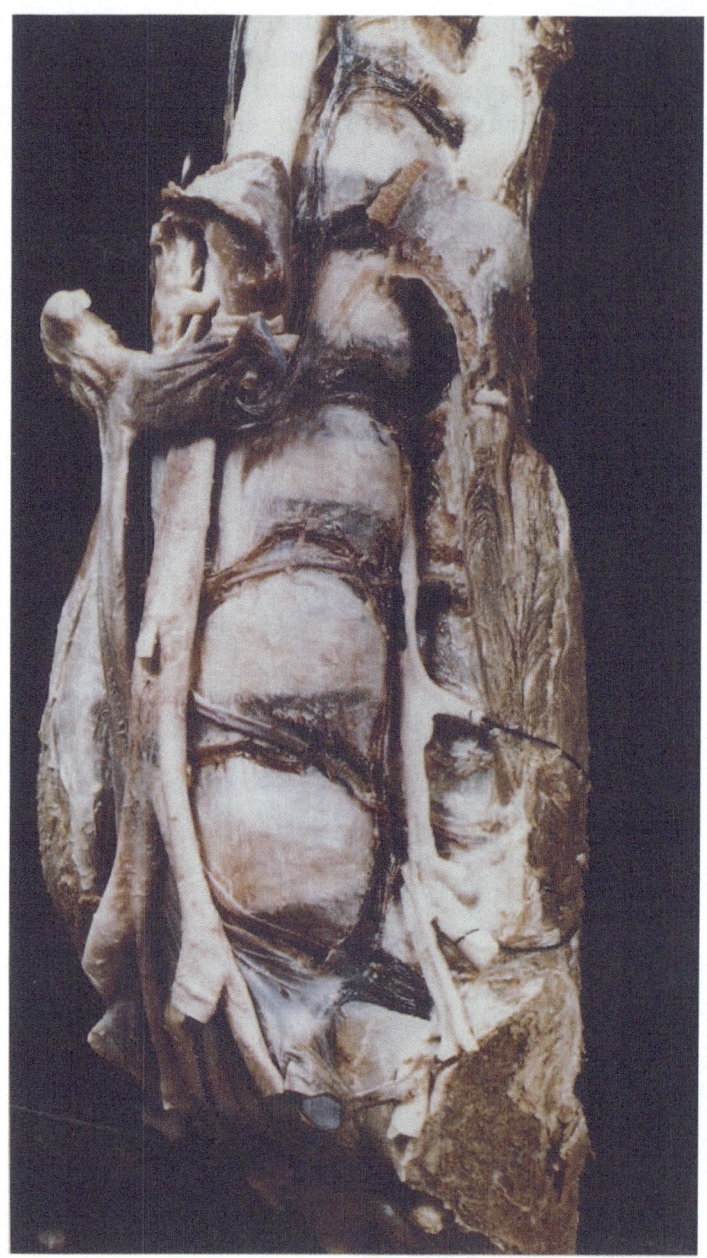

Figure 2.31. A photograph of the left side of the specimen illustrated in Figure 2.30 to show the arrangement of the left ascending lumbar vein in relation to the left common iliac vein

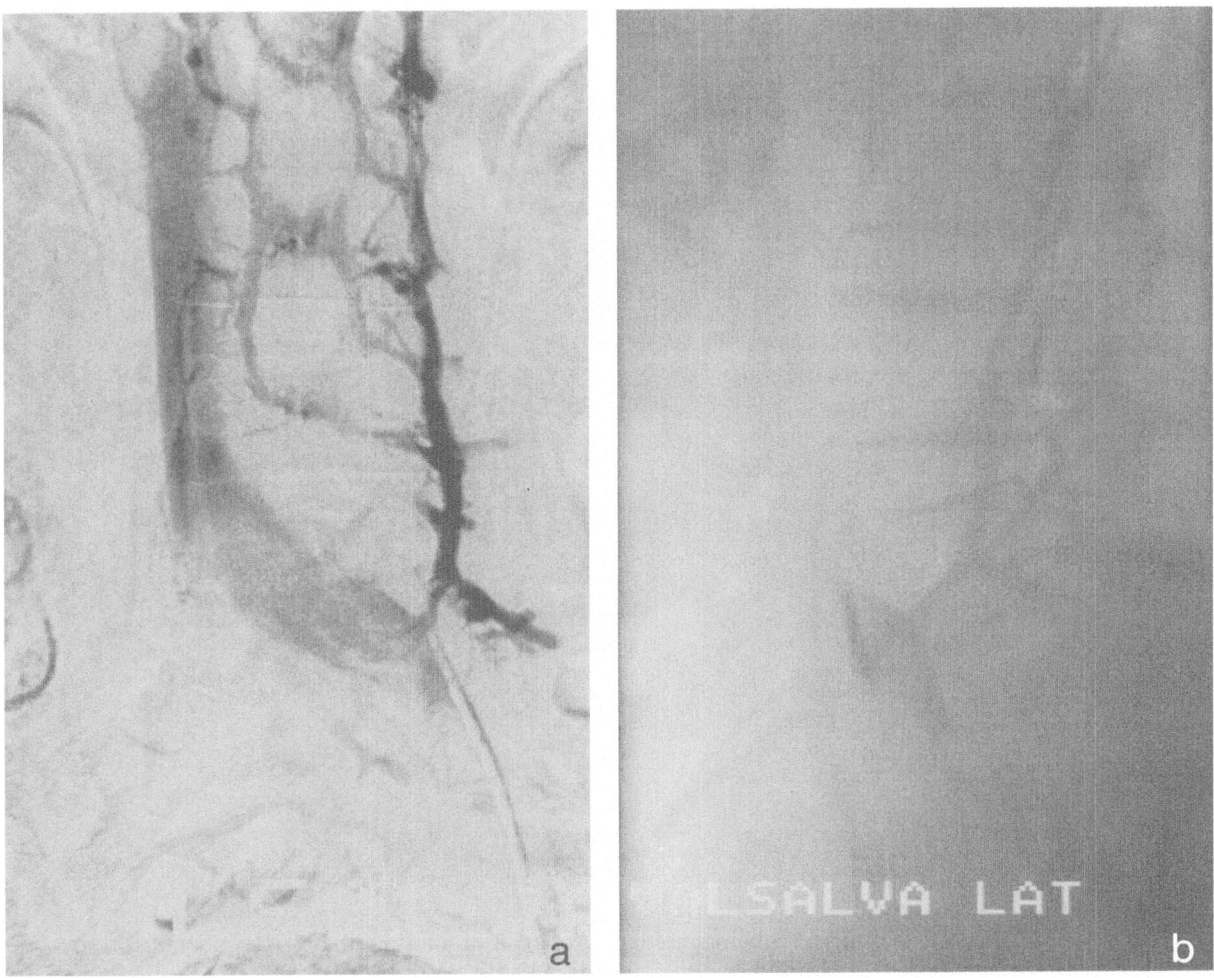

Figures 2.32 a, b. **a** An antero-posterior radiograph of the lumbar spine in a male aged 36 years, showing a venogram to demonstrate the location of the left common iliac vein and the ascending lumbar vein in the presence of a sacralization anomaly. **b** A lateral view of the same, showing the relationship of these vessels to the disc at the first mobile segment above the vertebral segmentation anomaly

b) Technique of Anterior Lumbar Interbody Fusion

i) Indications

The operation of spinal fusion was introduced first by Albee (1911) for the treatment of spinal tuberculosis. Its use was then extended by the application of anterior interbody fusion methods, popularized in Hong Kong by Hodgson and Stock (1956). In selected cases with spinal tuberculosis, anterior interbody fusion still enjoys an undisputed and favoured place in treatment (Fig. 2.33).

The role of spinal fusion in the treatment of disorders of the lumbar spine has remained vexed and confused. Apart from general agreement on the application of spinal fusion in the treatment of scoliosis, and in some cases of spondylolisthesis, there are no clear-cut published statements on indications for the use of spinal fusion techniques. With the decline in the use of fusion operations for major joints in the

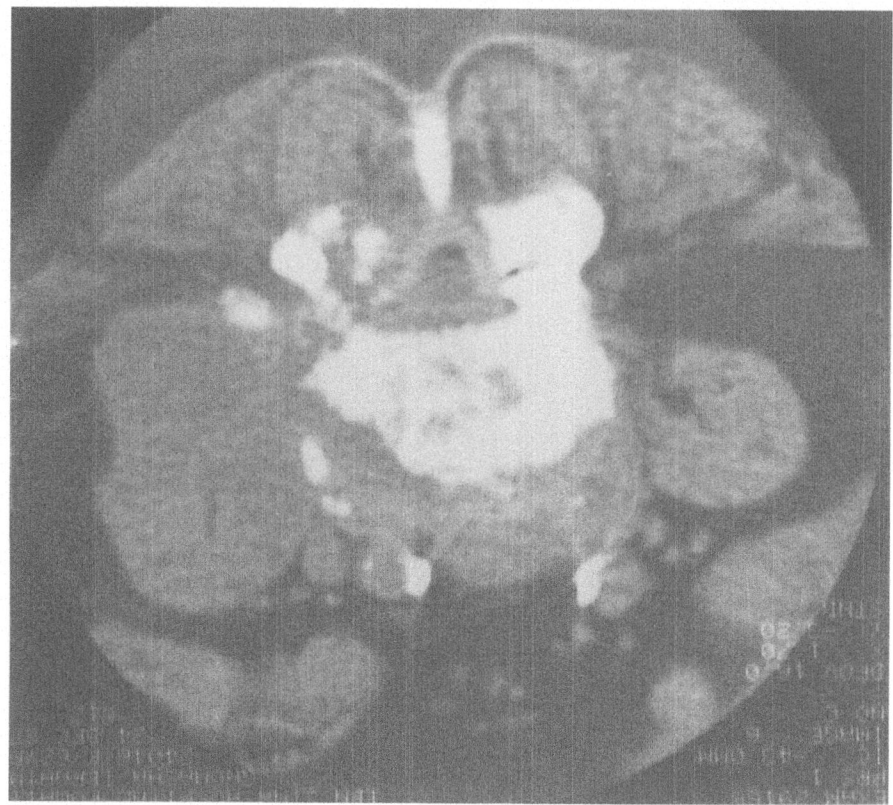

Figure 2.33. An axial CT image showing extensive destruction of a lumbar vertebra with a large left sided psoas abscess in an adult patient with tuberculosis

limbs, there has been a corresponding fall in the number of these procedures applied to spinal problems. In particular, a number of the degenerative disorders of the lumbar spine can be more effectively treated by some form of spinal canal or spinal nerve root canal decompression. Graf (1989) has introduced an operation to stabilise the lumbar spine without fusion, using pedicle screws, the adjacent heads of which are constrained by a band of woven plastic. This novel procedure requires further clinical trial before it can be confidently recommended.

In the author's opinion, the present indications for the use of anterior lumbar interbody fusion operations are as follows:

1. For the treatment of failed spinal operations;
2. For the treatment of certain disc lesions:
   a) internal disc disruption (frequently),
   b) isolated disc resorption (occasionally),
   c) nucleus pulposus calcification (rarely),
   d) disc herniation (rarely);
3. In the management of selected cases of spondylolisthesis;
4. For the treatment of certain spinal infections;
5. For the correction of selected spinal deformities;
6. For the treatment of rare miscellaneous cases, e.g. vertebral body tumours.

The operation of lumbar interbody fusion should be performed, ideally, with the aid of two competent assistants. Until the surgeon is thoroughly familiar with every aspect of the procedure, he would be wise to work with a general surgeon who has special competence in vascular surgery.

When Sir John Charnley first introduced his operation of total hip joint replacement in the early 1960's, he provoked an angry response from many surgeons by refusing to allow them to obtain the recommended instruments until they had been specially instructed in their use. The wisdom of his early caution doubtless served a good purpose in as much as total hip joint replacement operations performed by otherwise un-trained surgeons can maim. But when anterior lumbar interbody fusion is attempted by surgeons who have not been specifically trained, the results can be devastating and the patient may lose his life.

ii) General Pre-Operative Preparation

Patients should be admitted to hospital at least one day in advance of surgery. Their medical assessment before operation is of great importance and will be discussed in detail in Chapter 10. The patient's X-rays including MRI and CT Discography, where appropriate, should be clearly displayed on viewing boxes in the theatre. Facilities should be available for taking control X-rays on the theatre table when fusions above the lumbo-sacral junction are to be performed. The quality of spinal images obtained in operating rooms even with modern image intensifiers is often poor. Good quality films of the patient's spine must therefore be available in the theatre for comparison with those taken at the time of surgery. Problems in identifying vertebral levels with radiographic control in operating theatres may be challenging in the presence of lumbar segmentation anomalies, in identifying thoracic disc levels and in the neck when the patient's shoulders obstruct the view of lower cervical vertebrae, or the neck is unduly long. In this last case, for example, when using an image intensifier, it may not be possible to see C2 when a needle has been inserted at C6/7. Errors in counting disc space levels are then very likely to be made.

iii) Positioning

For approaches to any of the lower three lumbar intervertebral discs, patients are placed supine on the operating table. For rarer upper lumbar fusions, they are placed in the lateral position with the left loin uppermost. The surgeon should pay particular attention to the placing of restraining devices and arm supports, ensuring that the patient's trunk is held in a stable position and that undue pressure is not exerted on the peripheral nerves or veins in the legs. Calf stimulation during the operation is strongly recommended.

iv) Abdominal Incision

In the lower lumbar region, oblique, left-sided incisions are made, commencing at the mid-line between the umbilicus and symphysis pubis and extending upwards and laterally, parallel to the level of the iliac crest. The accompanying illustrations show the steps in the muscle splitting approach devised by Fraser (1982) which allows wide extra-peritoneal approach to the lumbar spine, without division of the rectus abdominis muscle (Figs. 2.34–37).

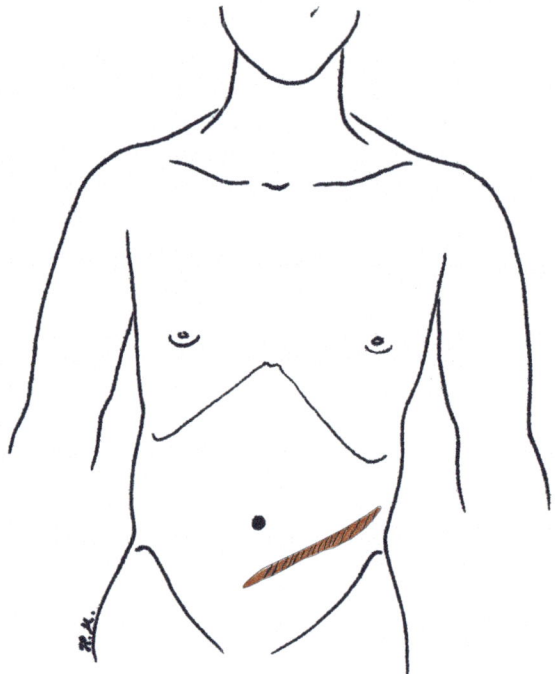

Figure 2.34. A drawing to show the line of the skin incision for a left-sided extra-peritoneal approach to the lower lumbar vertebral column (Dr. H. Matsuda)

The fibres of the external oblique muscle are incised in the line of the skin incision and the margins separated to expose the internal oblique muscle, the fibres of which are then separated by blunt dissection medially from the lateral edge of the rectus sheath, laterally for several centimetres. Retractors are then inserted beneath the upper and lower margins of this muscle to expose the underlying transversus abdominis muscle. Elevating the internal oblique muscle with retractors, the surgeon is then able to grasp the transversus aponeurosis and incise it carefully, separating it from the underlying peritoneum.

A vertical incision is then made along the lateral border of the rectus sheath dividing the fibres of the internal oblique and transversus abdominis muscles together. When this abdominal wall incision has been completed, the peritoneum is further separated from the abdominal wall and psoas muscles by digital dissection. A small Raytec pack is inserted into the para-colic gutter and pushed upwards for some distance until the psoas major muscle is clearly defined. The ureter can be seen lying adherent to the peritoneum. It is carried forward when a large modified Deever-type retractor is inserted, resting on the anterior surface of the lumbo-sacral disc or on the antero-lateral edge of the L4/5 or L3/4 discs at the anterior edge of the left psoas major muscle, depending on the level to be fused (Figs. 2.38, 2.39). Fraser (1991) has recently described an extra-peritoneal approach involving a vertical incision in the left rectus sheath, avoiding altogether splitting of the fibres of the external oblique, internal oblique and transversus abdominis muscles. This is similar to an incision recommended by Selby and Henderson (1991), in which a transverse incision is made in the left rectus sheath with vertical extensions medially and inferiorly and laterally and superiorly (Figs. 2.40 a, b).

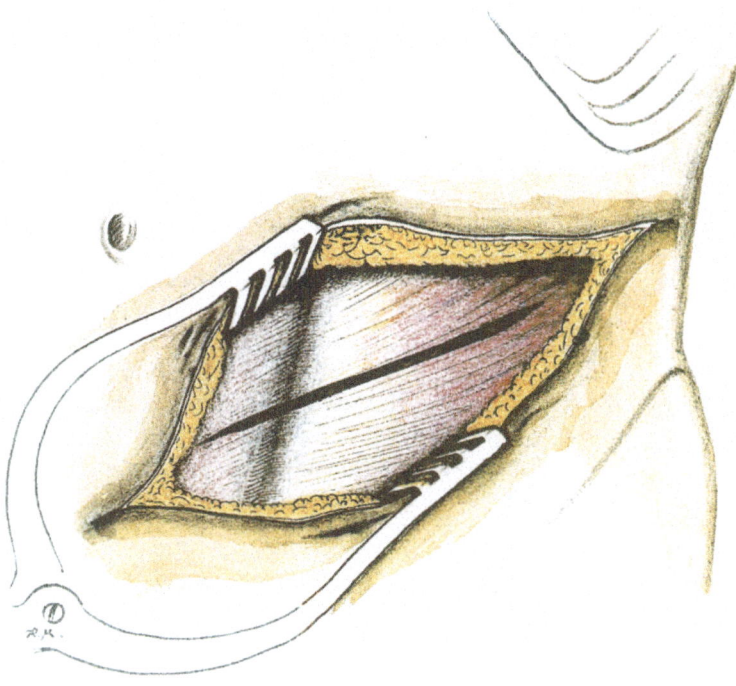

Figure 2.35. A drawing to show the line of division of fibres of the external oblique muscle (Dr. H. Matsuda)

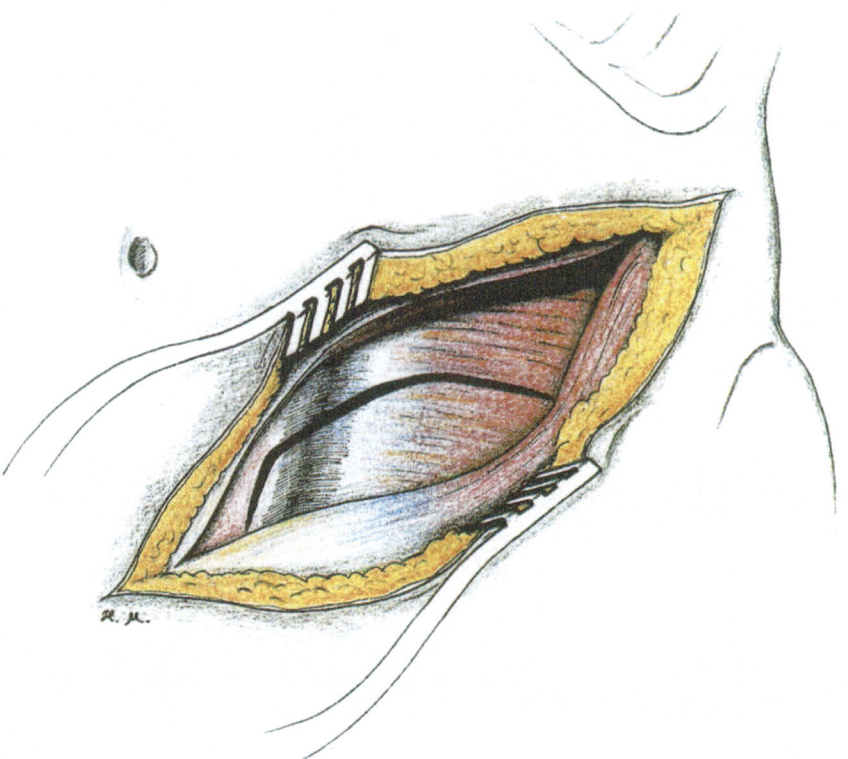

Figure 2.36. A drawing depicting the division of the rectus sheath vertically downwards at its lateral edge (Dr. H. Matsuda)

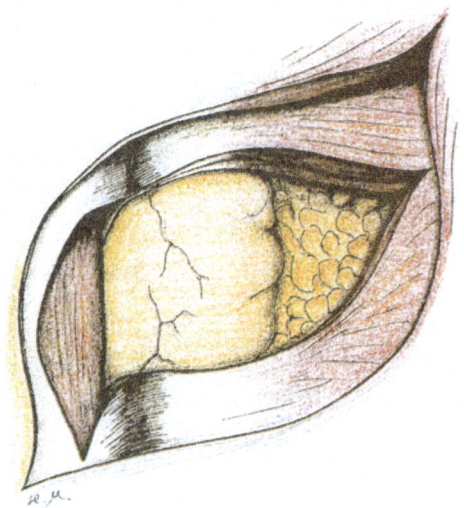

Figure 2.37. A drawing illustrating the splitting of the fibres of the internal oblique and transversalis muscles to expose the extra-peritoneal space on the left side of the abdomen. Division of the anterior layer of the rectus sheath vertically downwards then permits wide exposure of the extra-peritoneal space without division of the rectus abdominis muscle

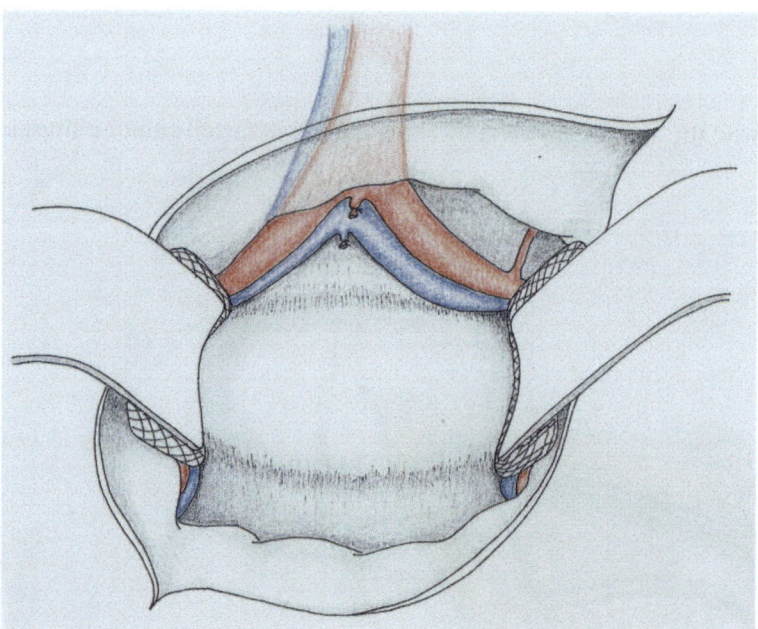

Figure 2.38. A diagram illustrating the use of the retractors at the lumbo-sacral space, with loose Raytec swabs beneath them protecting the walls of the great vessels (Miss L. Butler after Dr. H. Matsuda)

Figure 2.39. A drawing to illustrate the principal anatomical features at the L4/5 level, showing the modified Deever's retractors in place. Note the retraction of the psoas muscle at the bottom of the drawing, with the outline of the sympathetic trunk (in yellow) anterior to the retractor (Miss L. Butler after Dr. H. Matsuda)

Figures 2.40 a, b. a A drawing depicting a transverse incision in the left rectus sheath in preparation for an extra-peritoneal approach to the lumbar spine. **b** A detailed view to show the ascending and descending limbs of the z-shaped incision in the fibres of the anterior rectus sheath

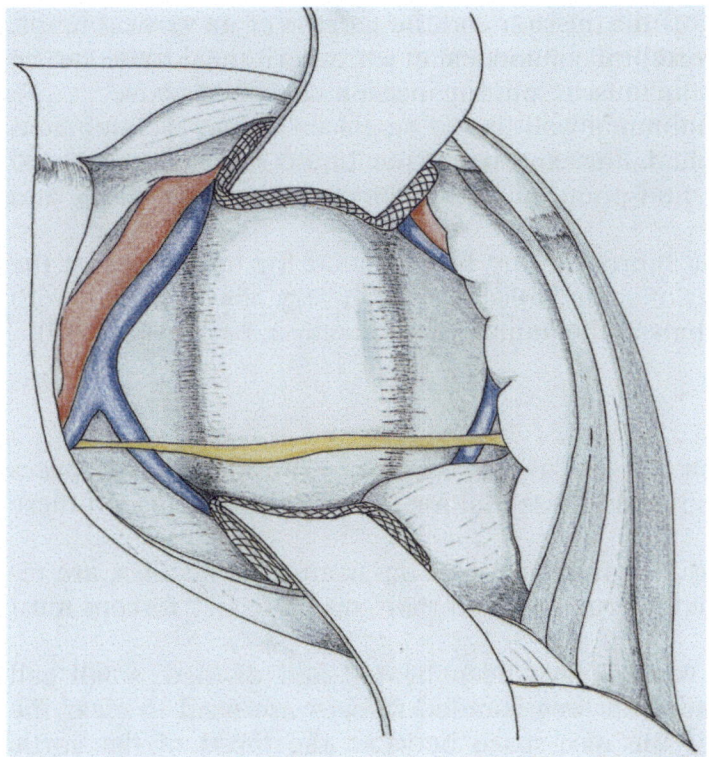

Figure 2.39

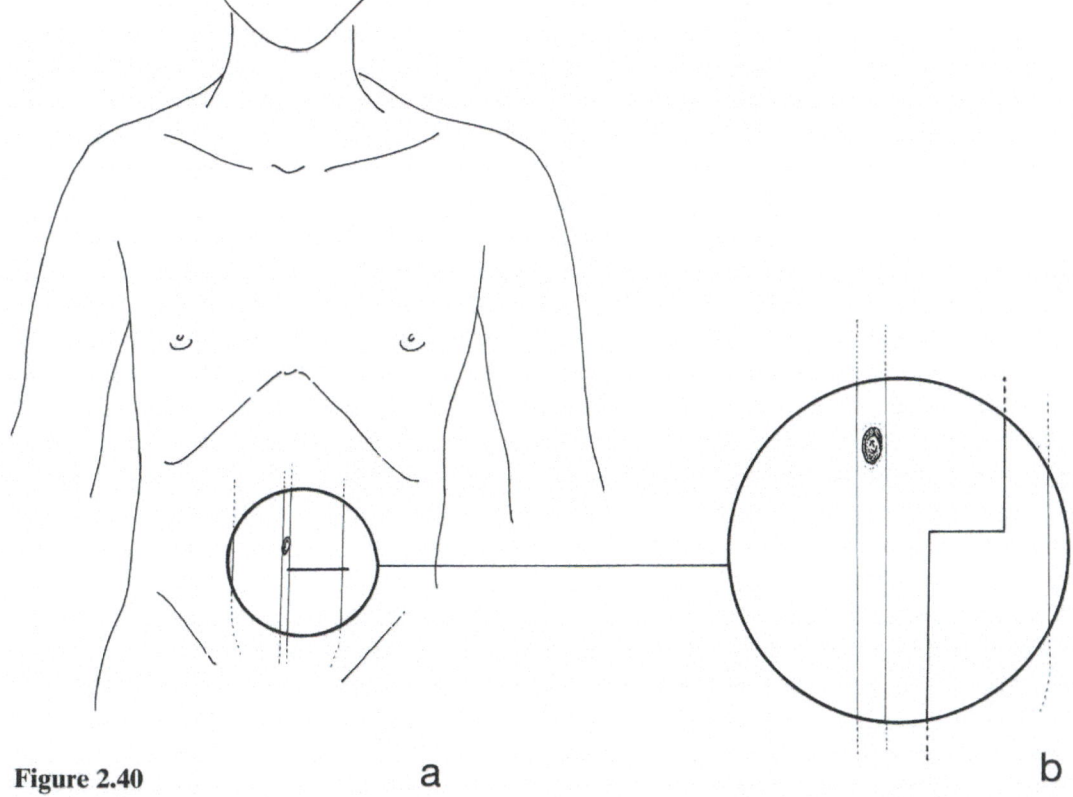

Figure 2.40   a   b

Depending on the placing of this incision and the lengths of its vertical limbs, wider exposure of the lumbar vertebral column via an extra-peritoneal route can be more easily achieved than with the muscle splitting incision described above.

The skin incision on the abdominal wall should be placed nearer the umbilicus if the L 3/4 disc is to be approached. For exposure of the lumbo-sacral disc it should be placed slightly below the mid-point of a line between the umbilicus and symphysis pubis.

A mid-line transperitoneal approach may be indicated for operations at the lumbo-sacral level in some cases of spondylolisthesis or in very obese patients with high Ferguson angle measurements at the lumbo-sacral junction, Ferguson (1949).

v) Haemostasis

The techniques of vessel ligation are vital to the success of exposing the disc spaces at various levels in the lumbar spine and essential for the safe performance of these operations.

Vascular sutures, including 5/0 suture material on atraumatic needles, are required. In addition, long-handled instruments and right-angled artery forceps must be available for use.

When the median sacral vessels have been ligated and divided, small gall bladder dissecting swabs mounted on long-handled forceps are used to clear the loose tissues from the front of the disc space between the limbs of the aortic bifurcation and the right and left common iliac veins, thus clearly exposing the anterior longitudinal ligament (Fig. 2.38). In retro-peritoneal approaches to the L5/ S1 disc space, the filaments of the presacral sympathetic plexus are rarely seen; the danger of damaging these nerves in the male has been exaggerated by opponents of this method of spinal fusion (Flynn and Hoque, 1979). The thin anterior longitudinal ligament is then divided transversely across the middle of the disc space and the ends are swept upwards and downwards to expose the junction of the vertebral end-plate and the disc on either side of the disc space. The cuff of tissue formed by its rolled edges helps to protect the walls of the great veins at the sides of the disc space.

Retro-peritoneal fibrosis is seen without exception when anterior interbody fusion operations are performed following previous explorations of the spinal canal. Of variable density in cases of isolated disc resorption or internal disc disruption, this fibrotic tissue may make it very difficult to separate the common iliac veins in the midline, even rendering access to the disc impossible. In such cases damage to the thin wall of the left common iliac vein is likely to occur unless the surgeon is aware of this potential problem. The application of artery forceps or vascular clips, such as Weck clips, to this large thin-walled vein must be avoided. Repair of this vessel requires adequate exposure of the bleeding site to be made. Digital pressure above and below any tear in the vein will control the blood flow to allow identification of the defect in its wall until it can be repaired with a fine atraumatic vascular suture.

The left common iliac vein is sometimes very large, measuring 3 or 4 cm from lateral to medial edge, rendering access to the lumbo-sacral disc between the medial edges of the right and left common iliac vessels impossible. In such circumstances, the medial border of the left psoas muscle should be retracted carefully. Un-named arteries and veins often pass into the muscle directly from the lateral walls of the adjacent left common iliac artery and vein. These small vessels can cause trouble-

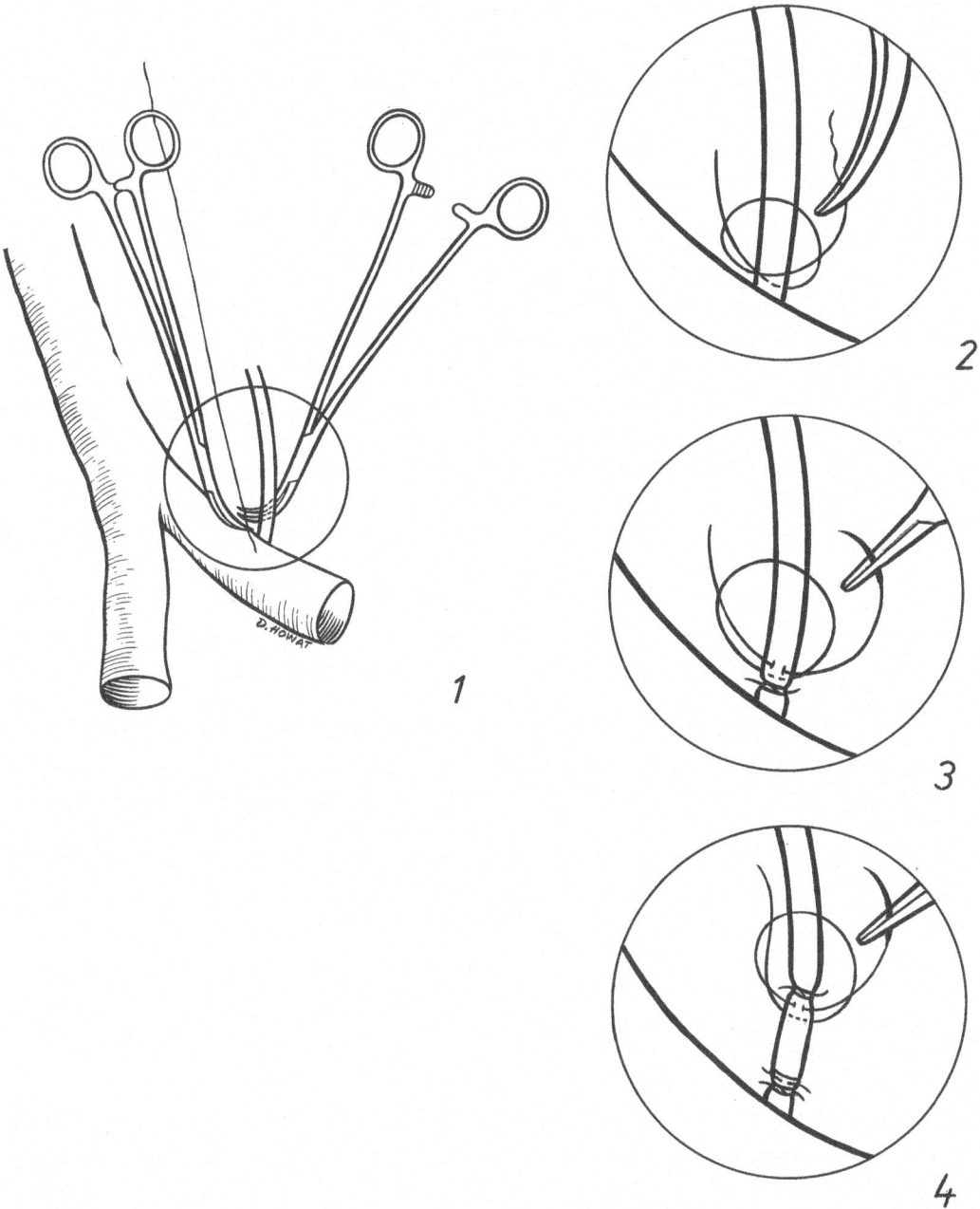

Figure 2.41, 1–4. 1 A drawing to illustrate the passage of a ligature beneath the ascending lumbar vein on the left side. **2** Tying the ligature on the ascending lumbar vein adjacent to its entry point into the left common iliac vein. **3** Showing the passage of a transfixion circumferential locking suture beyond the first tie placed on the ascending lumbar vein near its junction with the left common iliac vein. **4** Showing the insertion of a transfixion circumferential locking suture further along the course of the ascending lumbar vein. The vessel may then be divided without risk of the ties slipping after the vessel has been cut

some haemorrhage. They should be carefully isolated and coagulated with diathermy well clear of their origins from the great vessels, before being divided.

The lateral wall of the left common iliac vein should then be exposed by careful
blunt dissection aided with the use of a sucker to remove surrounding loose fat. The
left sympathetic nerve trunk should be identified and small regional lymphatic
channels coagulated if necessary before the edge of the left common iliac vein can be
clearly seen. *The ascending lumbar vein will be seen at this stage* and the decision
taken to ligate and divide it, depending on its length. If it becomes tightly stretched,
preventing retraction of the common iliac vein across the front of the L5/S1 disc
space, it must be divided. Details of this manoeuvre are outlined below.

To expose the disc between the L4 and L5 vertebral bodies, it may also be necessary to ligate and divide the left ascending lumbar vein. The sympathetic trunk is
first identified where it lies along the anterior margin of the psoas major muscle, on
the side of the vertebral body (Figs. 2.29, 2.39). The fibres of the fibrous arcade,
which attach the psoas muscle to the superior and inferior vertebral margins at the
disc space, are divided and the psoas muscle is retracted laterally.

The ascending lumbar vein is often quite large, with a diameter at its entry
point into the lateral wall of the left common iliac vein of between 3 and 5 mm
(Figs. 2.30, 2.31). The techniques for the safe handling, dissection and ligation of
this vessel are among the most critical manoeuvres to be performed in the whole of
this operation. Whether or not ligation is required depends on the length of the
vessel and its site of entry into the left common iliac vein. In patients with
sacralization anomalies, vertebral venography should be performed before embarking on anterior lumbar fusions (Figs. 2.32 a, b). This vein is usually surrounded
by fatty tissues from which it must be dissected free. This can be done by using a
blunt probe and a smooth-ended fine sucker.

The vessel is ligated with sutures of 3/0 black silk, just beyond its entry point
into the left common iliac vein and again, further along its course, deep to the psoas
muscle. It is essential to lock these black silk sutures on to the wall of the ascending
lumbar vein with 5/0 sutures, transfixing its wall and encircling the vessel adjacent to
each suture. The vessel is then divided between these locking sutures with a fine
scalpel blade, mounted on a long handle (Figs. 2.41, 1–4). With these precise manoeuvres safely completed, the great vessels may then be retracted towards the mid-
line from the antero-lateral surface of the L4/5 disc space (Fig. 2.39).

Exposure of the L3/4 disc space can be achieved often without division of any
significant vessels, although, on occasions, the lumbar vessels lying on the side of the
body of L4 may need to be separately ligated near the anterior margin of the psoas
major muscle before the great vessels can be safely retracted from the antero-lateral
surface of this disc.

Exposure of upper lumbar discs is best done with the patient in the lateral
position on the operating table and with the incision running through the bed of the
twelfth rib to allow extra-peritoneal exposure of the upper lumbar vertebral column.

vi) Preparation of the Interspace for Graft Insertion

The preparation of dowel cavities in the intervertebral space is carried out with the
use of special cutters supplied in six sizes for use at any vertebral level. Each cutting
cylinder has circumferential markings clearly visible on its external surface. These
rings are separated from each other by 5 mm (Figs. 2.42, 2.43).

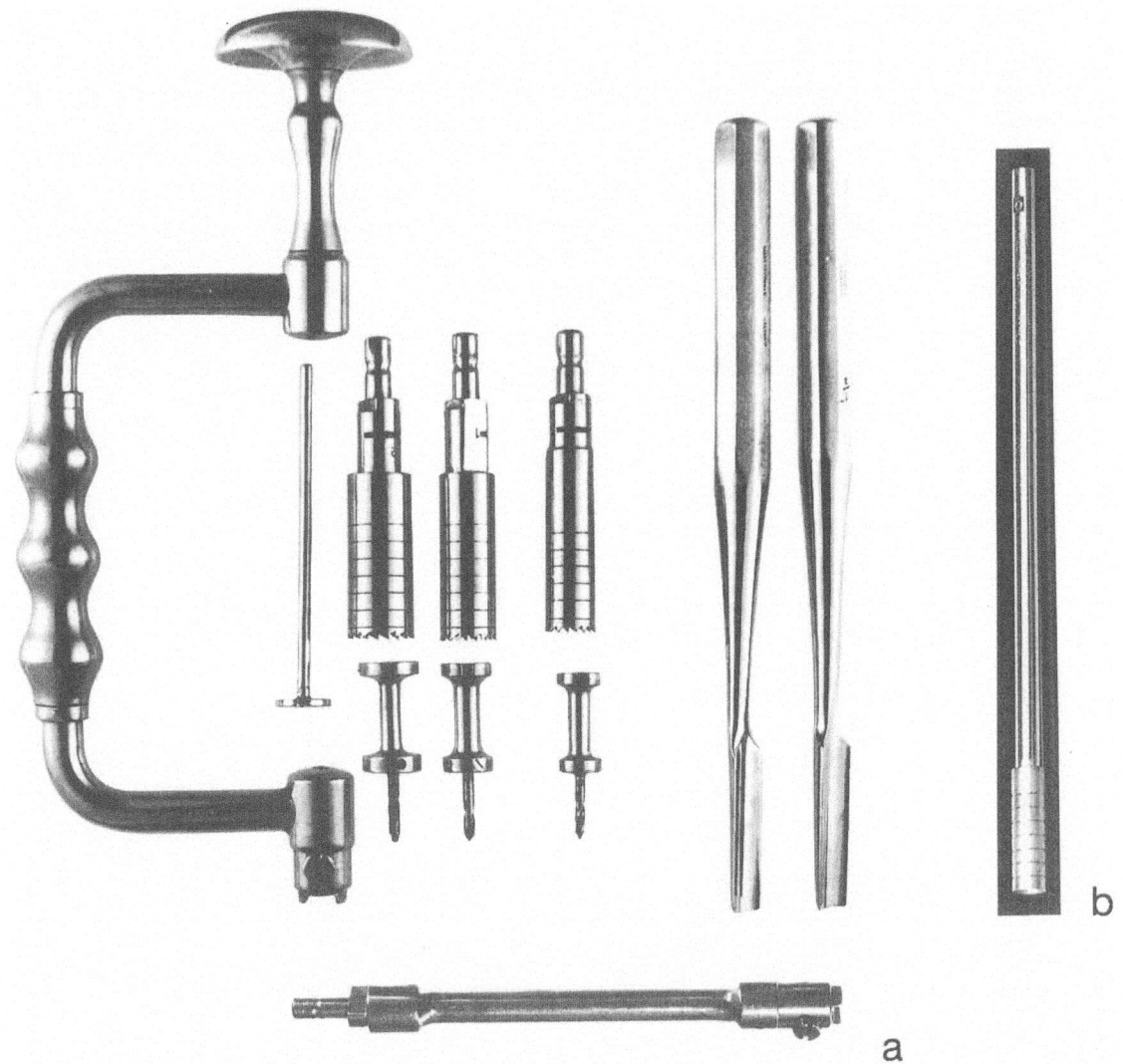

Figures 2.42 a, b. a A photograph showing a modified Hudson brace and three toothed dowel cutting instruments, with starter centre pieces and one graft ejector. Each "toothed dowel cutter" is designed to be used initially with a "starter centre-piece" inserted. The pointed centre piece perforates the intact disc thereby anchoring the cutter so that when it is oscillated in its fixed position, the margins of the proposed vertebral dowel cavity can be scored. Symmetrical ellipses should thereby be cut into each vertebral body. The centre-piece is then ejected from the cutter, which is re-inserted and further oscillated until the dowel cavity has been cut to its desired depth. On the right side, note the special gouges which are used with the cutters. At the bottom of the picture, an extension piece is shown for use during lumbar interbody fusion operations. **b** A photograph of a *"tubular smooth-ended dowel cutter"*. These are available in the same range and sizes (0–6) as *the toothed dowel cutters*. If there is any doubt about the orientation of the vertebral end-plates, the intervertebral disc should first be excised and the end-plate cartilages curetted from the vertebrae. A tubular cutter of appropriate size can then be placed accurately on the adjacent vertebral margins and tapped into place, producing the desired symmetrical elliptical margins of the proposed dowel cavity. It is then easier to re-insert the same sized toothed dowel cutter with which to complete the preparation of the dowel cavity. If the smooth-ended tubular cutter is punched into the final desired depth it may be difficult and potentially dangerous to withdraw it from between the vertebrae. This important addition to the instrumentation was introduced by Dr. D. Selby of Dallas Texas.
These instruments are manufactured exclusively by the Thomson and Shelton Instrumentation Company, 6119 Danbury Lane, Dallas, TX 75214, U.S.A.

In due course, *grafts are cut using the cutting cylinder that is one size larger than that used to cut the intervertebral dowel cavities.* When the cutting instruments are in use in the disc spaces, the surgeon must at all times have the undivided attention of his two assistants, to ensure that the great vessels are protected from injury. Specially modified Deever's retractors, which have smooth excavated ends, are held in place with loose Raytec swabs positioned to prevent the edges of the great vessels or adjacent soft tissues from herniating beneath them.

The surgeon must be thoroughly familiar with the measurements of the intervertebral space in each patient when preparing the dowel cavities. Measure-

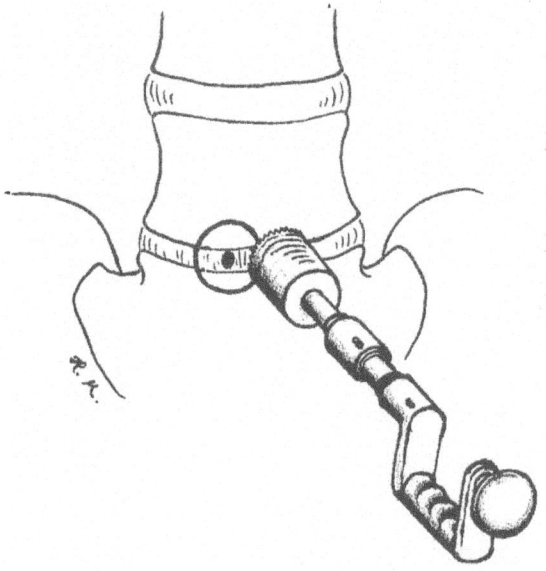

Figure 2.43. A drawing to illustrate the use of the Hudson brace, with the extension piece and the cutter, to prepare a dowel cavity at the lumbo-sacral junction

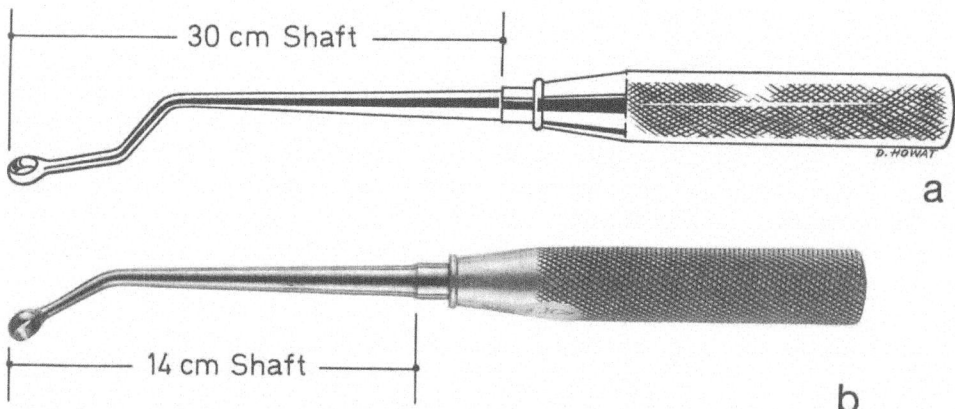

Figures 2.44 a, b. **a** A drawing of a long handled ring curette with a double-angled shaft, suitable for curettage of the vertebral end-plate and disc remnants in lumbar interbody fusions. **b** A photograph of a Cloward-type ring curette with single angle on the shaft, suitable for use in smaller patients

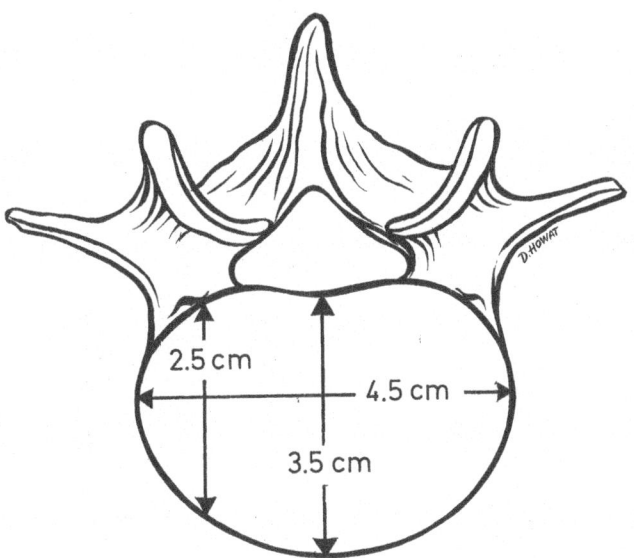

Figure 2.45. A drawing to illustrate the measurements of the L5 vertebral body in an adult of average size

ments of the vertical height of the disc space and the antero-posterior depth should be available from pre-operative roentgenograms. In addition, it is to be noted that the antero-posterior measurements vary, being greatest in the mid-line and smallest laterally because the shape of the disc bearing surface of the vertebral body is oval, not rectangular (Fig. 2.45).

When the parallel plugs of the adjacent vertebral body fragments and the intervening intervertebral disc have been displaced from the interspace using a gouge specially tooled to match the size of the cutter (Figs. 2.24, 1–4), the disc remnants are then removed from the interspace with rongeurs. In addition, vertebral end-plate remnants should be removed with ring curettes (Figs. 2.44 a, b). Aided by the use of a vertebral spreader, it is possible to remove the bulk of the disc tissue and vertebral end-plate cartilages from the interspaces (Figs. 2.46 a–c). However, during these manoeuvres the surgeon must avoid penetrating the spinal canal or damaging the great vessels, which may have slipped out from beneath the retractors (Fig. 2.47).

The graft beds prepared by this method are well-vascularized. Indeed, one of the great advantages of this operation is that the blood supply of the vertebral bodies is not disturbed; thus, vascularization of appropriately placed grafts is assured (Crock and Yoshizawa, 1977).

Graft Preparation

The use of autogenous bone grafts is strongly recommended. The left iliac crest is exposed by retracting the infero-lateral edge of the abdominal skin incision and a separate incision is then made through the tendinous fibres covering its upper border. The muscles are then separated from the crest and from the inner and outer tables of the ilium. Retractors are inserted to expose the area of the bone from which grafts are to be cut. Dowel cutting instruments one size larger than those used to prepare the dowel cavities in the intervertebral space are then used to cut grafts from

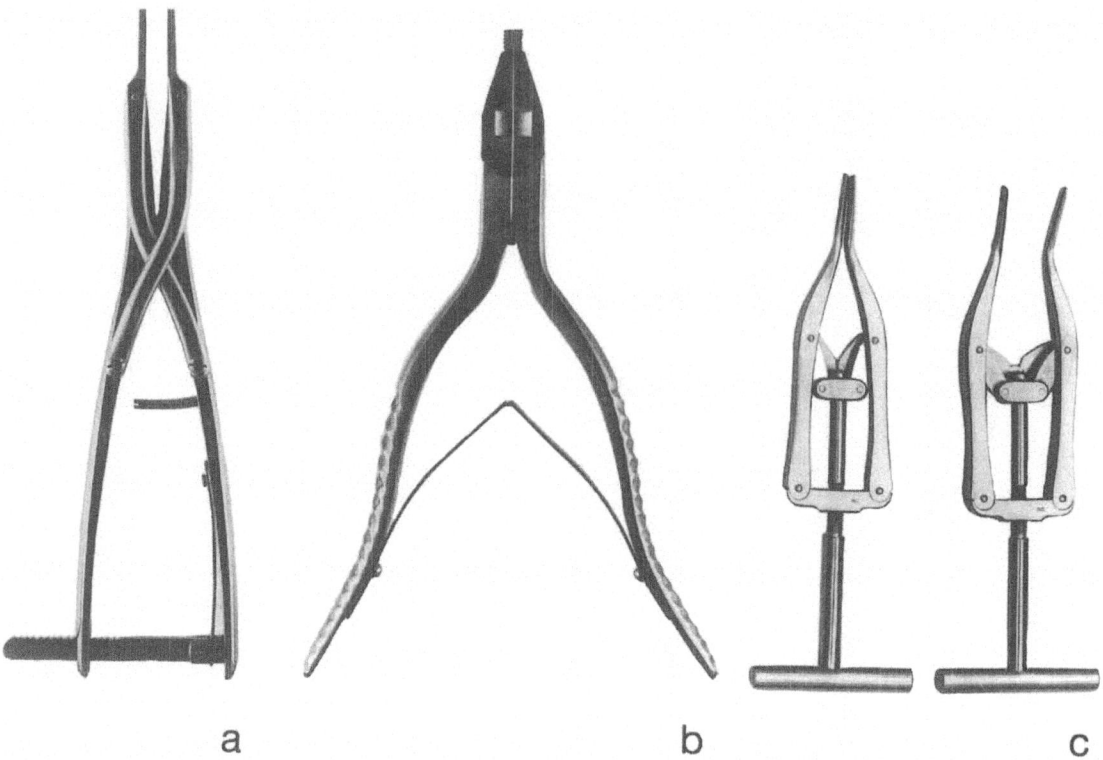

a   b   c

Figures 2.46 a–c. Photographs of different types of vertebral spreaders. The central instrument is of Cloward design and is not self-retaining. It is suitable for use in interbody fusions, though it was not designed for that purpose. The instruments in **a** and **c** are of Japanese design

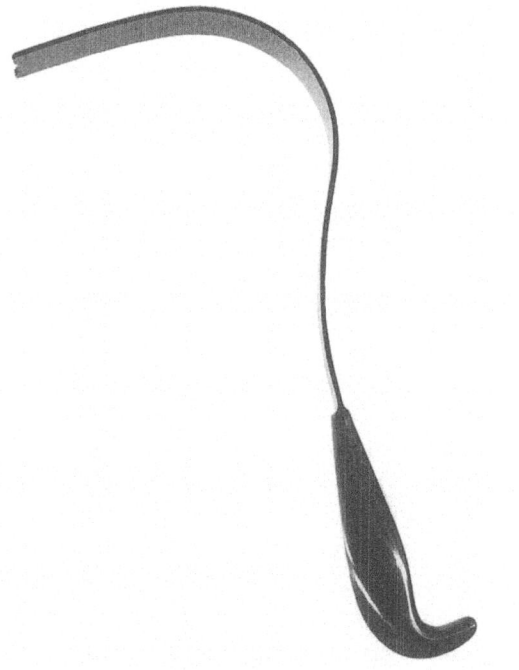

Figure 2.47. A photograph of a modified Deever's type retractor with a smooth excavated end, suitable for retraction of the great vessels across the front of the disc space in the lumbar region

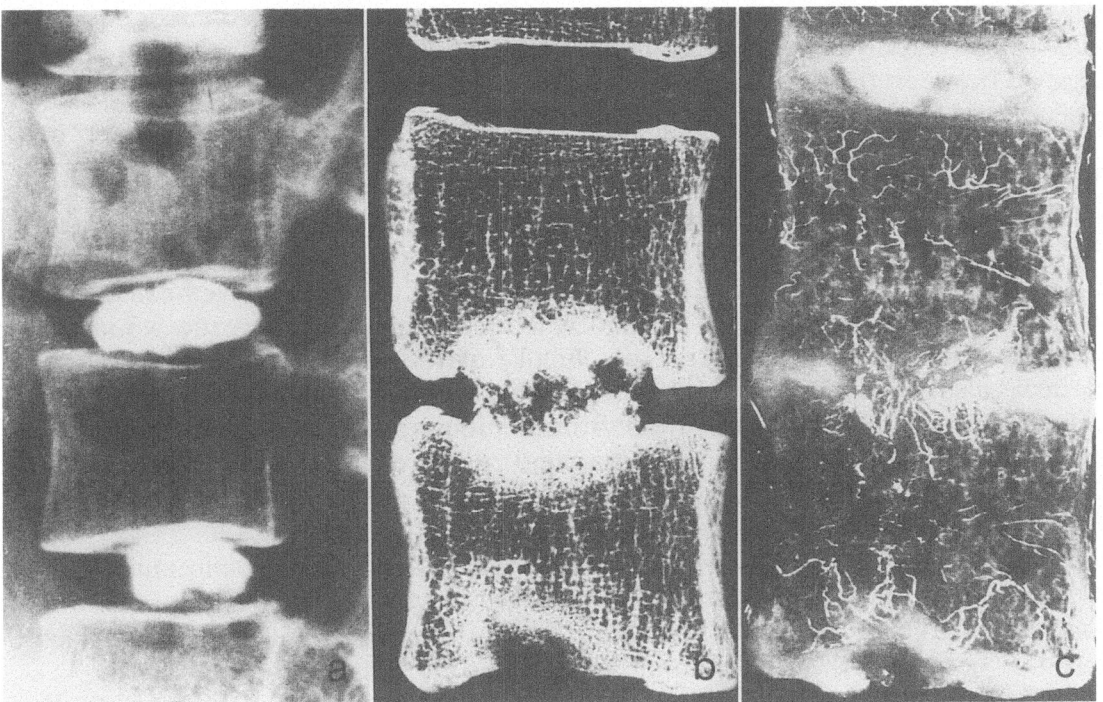

Figures 2.48 a–c. a A normal discogram at L 1/2 and internal disc disruption at L 2/3 in a female patient aged 37 years – she committed suicide 3 months after operation. **b** At the L 2/3 level, union of the graft is incomplete, and the cancellous bone of the graft has been infiltrated by disc tissue remnants. **c** Photograph of a thin sagittal section of the lumbar spine taken at necropsy. The L 1/2 disc is shown at the top of the specimen. At L 2/3, vessels in the interbody graft can be seen. On the right, tufted vessels abut against invading disc tissue. Centrally, the graft is vascularized

the iliac crest, passing vertically downwards to the required depth. Grafts of 2.5–2.8 cm in depth are of satisfactory size in most patients. On occasion, cancellous chips may be cut from the bony fragments of vertebral bodies obtained from the dowel cavities. (These fragments may be used to supplement the iliac crest grafts in larger patients). The iliac crest grafts have three cortical faces and two "tooled" cancellous faces (Figs. 2.25–27 a, b). They are designed to be impacted adjacent to each other with the cortical faces orientated laterally in the disc space and the cancellous surfaces facing the vertebral bodies. Purely cancellous grafts inserted into the intervertebral disc space have been shown by Crock (1976) to be liable to invasion by disc remnants, thus predisposing to non-union (Figs. 2.48 a–c). This complication has been largely obviated by the use of grafts cut from the anterior iliac crest in the manner just described.

vii) Graft Impaction

In the last phase of this operation, the intervertebral disc space is again carefully exposed by the assistants. A vertebral spreader is inserted into one of the dowel cavities and opened to allow a final inspection of the interspace. *The depth of the dowel cavity is checked with a depth gauge and ruler and the first graft then impacted.* This is a potentially dangerous manoeuvre as the edge of a great vessel may become trapped between the graft and the wall of the dowel cavity. Successful retraction at this critical stage of the operation calls for strict attention to detail (Figs. 2.50a–c).

Following impaction of the first graft, the vertebral spreader is removed from the second dowel cavity and the second graft is then impacted. Some haemorrhage will then occur from the vertebral bodies, oozing from the junctions of the grafts on either side. This is never severe and usually ceases in two or three minutes.

Attention is finally focussed on the donor site. If two grafts have been cut from the iliac crest the bony defect is filled with bone cement before the wounds are closed in layers with suction drainage. Small cavities are curetted out between the cortical faces of the iliac crest at the anterior and posterior limits of the pelvic defect left after removal of the dowel grafts. Bone cement pushed into these cavities helps to maintain the stability of the newly moulded "pelvic crest" and diminish pain in the post-operative period. In Japan "ceramic spacers" specially designed to fill the defect and maintain the outline of the iliac crest are frequently used[2].

The method of operation described here has been used by the author since 1961. *Of approximately 1500 operations performed in 30 years mortality at operation has been nil.* Three patients have died; two in the post-operative period of acute coronary occlusion; the third committed suicide four months after operation.

No major urological complications have been encountered with this method of spinal fusion. Retention of urine occurs in some patients, but its management only rarely involves the use of a catheter for one or two days.

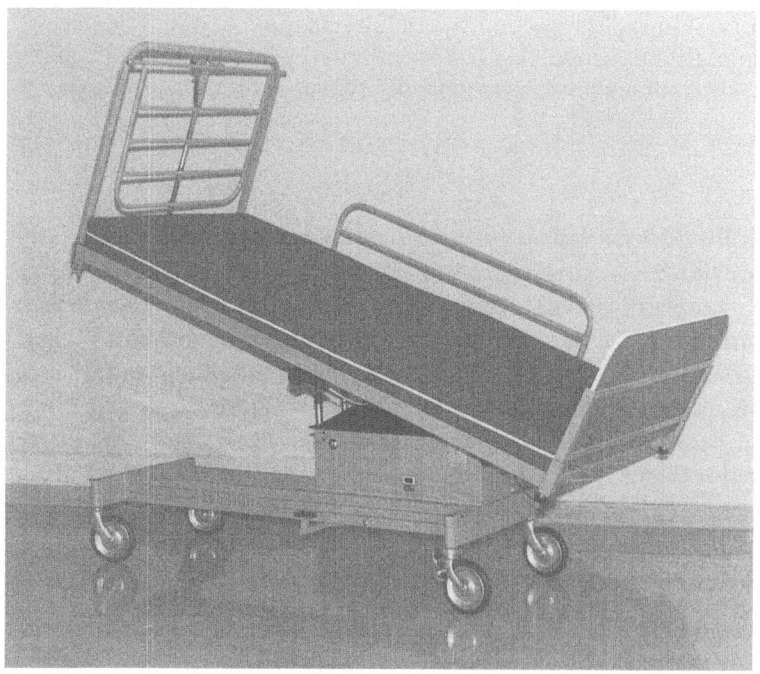

Figure 2.49. A photograph of an electrically operated bed which can tilt to the vertical position, allowing patients to stand in comfort early after spinal operations

---

[2] Kyocera Corporation, Kyoto, Japan.

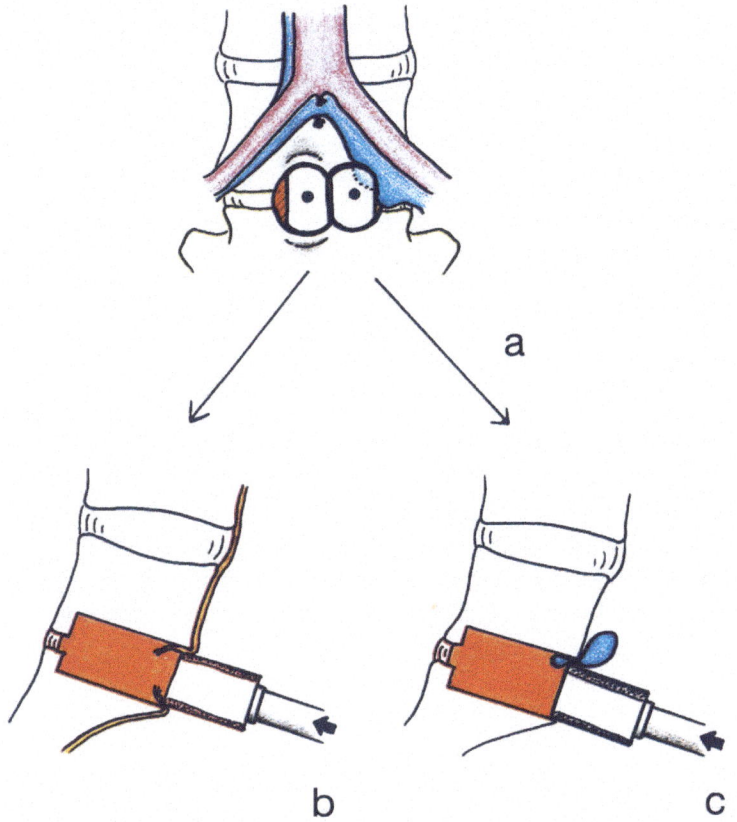

Figures 2.50 a–c. a A drawing illustrating entrapment of part of the medial wall of the left common iliac vein after graft impaction. **b** A lateral view of the lumbo-sacral space depicting the rolling inwards of the free margins of the anterior longitudinal ligament during graft impaction. This should be avoided by proper retraction of all soft tissues adjacent to the dowel cavity before grafts are impacted. **c** A lateral view of the lumbo-sacral space demonstrating the hazard of trapping the medial edge of the left common iliac vein during graft impaction. This problem should be avoided at all times by careful retraction of the vessels at the time of graft impaction

In exposing the lumbo-sacral intervertebral disc space in the male, the use of diathermy in the presacral area should be avoided. The author is aware of complaints of sterility in only two patients, both of whom had complained of impotence before operation.

viii) Post-Operative Care

Patients are nursed supine with one or two pillows, and rolled from side to side several times a day with a pillow placed between their legs. We recommend the use of beds[3] which can be tilted vertically to allow patients to stand and to get out of bed with little assistance from the nursing staff. Intravenous therapy is continued until bowel sounds are heard or flatus has been passed (Fig. 2.49).

---

[3] Edgerton Vertically Tilting Beds, Edgerton Hospital Equipment Ltd., Farwig Lane, Bromley, Kent BR1 3TU, United Kingdom.

Prophylactic anticoagulant therapy is used routinely. Subcutaneous Calciparine[4] 5000 iu twice daily or the recently introduced Clexane[5] in a single daily dose, may be administered until the patients have become fully mobile.

Lumbar Supports

Except for patients having single level interbody fusions at L5/S1, all are fitted, before surgery, with plastic supports moulded to their iliac crests. These are applied within a few days of operation and worn for three or four months afterwards.

ix) Complications

1. Deep vein thrombosis

Using the surgical techniques described above and the prophylactic measures of calf stimulation during surgery, with elastic stockings post-operatively and prophylactic anticoagulant therapy I have seen *no cases of deep vein thrombosis in the past five years*. At operation an important step in its prevention is to avoid entrapping the edge of a great vein during graft impaction (Figs. 2.50 a–c).

2. Non-union of grafts

a) The use of purely cancellous grafts may lead to non-union following infiltration of the grafted bone by reactive disc tissues which also prevent vascular penetration of the graft (Figs. 48 b, c).

b) Special surgical techniques will be required to prevent non-union in the following circumstances:

i) When the vertebral end-plates are widely separated. The disc tissues should be excised with a scalpel and the vertebral end-plate cartilages curetted. The disc space is thereby narrowed. A dowel cutter of appropriate size should then be selected. The starter centre piece should be removed and the cutter, affixed to the extension piece alone should be placed across the disc space and tapped into place with a hammer. The Hudson brace is then fitted and the cutter oscillated, at first counter-clockwise, then clockwise, until an accurate circular dowel cavity is cut between the vertebral bodies. Alternatively the long dowel tube cutters may be used (Fig. 2.42 b).

ii) When the vertebral end-plates are of irregular shape, the cutters may fail to remove a segment of vertebral end-plate cartilage. This area should be identified, by using a dental mirror. After curettage of the "uncut" vertebral end-plate remnants, cancellous chips should be placed in the cavity, preliminary to graft impaction (Figs. 2.51, a, b).

c) During impaction, care should be taken to avoid rotation of the graft. If this occurs, the dimensions of the second dowel cavity will be larger than required and the second graft will fit loosely (Figs. 2.52a, b).

---

[4] Heparin, Difrex Australian Laboratories Pty. Ltd., Glebe Street, Glebe, N.S.W.
[5] Rhone-Poulenc Sante Propharm, 180 Rue Jean Jaures, B.P. 37, 94702 Maisons Alfort Cedex, France.

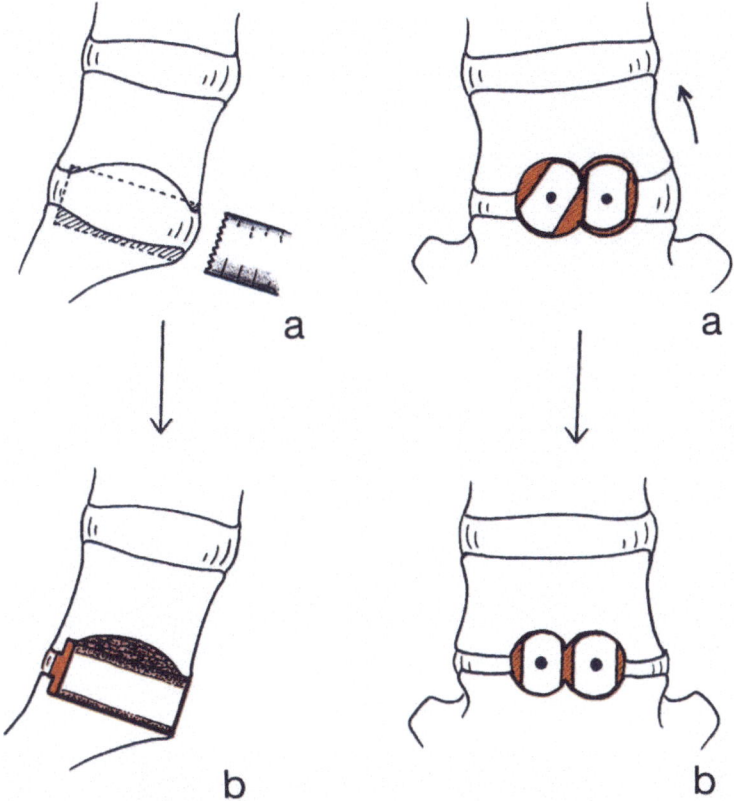

Figures 2.51 a,b   **Figures 2.52 a,b**

Figures 2.51 a,b. a A drawing of a lateral view of the lumbo-sacral space to illustrate the problem created when the vertebral end-plate of L5 is "ballooned". Cutters may then fail to remove the "ballooned segment" when they are inserted in the course of preparing the dowel cavity. **b** A drawing to show that the area needs to be separately prepared with a curette and grafted with cancellous chips before dowel grafts are impacted

Figures 2.52 a,b. a A drawing to illustrate the problem of inserting a graft eccentrically, as on the left-hand side. This will distort the outline of the other cavity so that the second graft will not fit firmly into it. **b** A drawing to demonstrate the correct placing of grafts parallel to each other, so that each fits snugly in the intervertebral space

3. Infection at the graft site

This is a rare complication after interbody fusion operations. If it occurs it may be very serious. Management of this problem is discussed on p. 314.

4. Iliac crest fracture (Fig. 2.53)

5. Post-operative entrapment of the lateral femoral cutaneous nerve of the thigh

Meralgia paraesthetica due to fibrosis around the iliac crest donor site occurs occasionally. Symptoms may be relieved by local steroid injections, though sometimes surgical release of the entrapped nerve may be necessary.

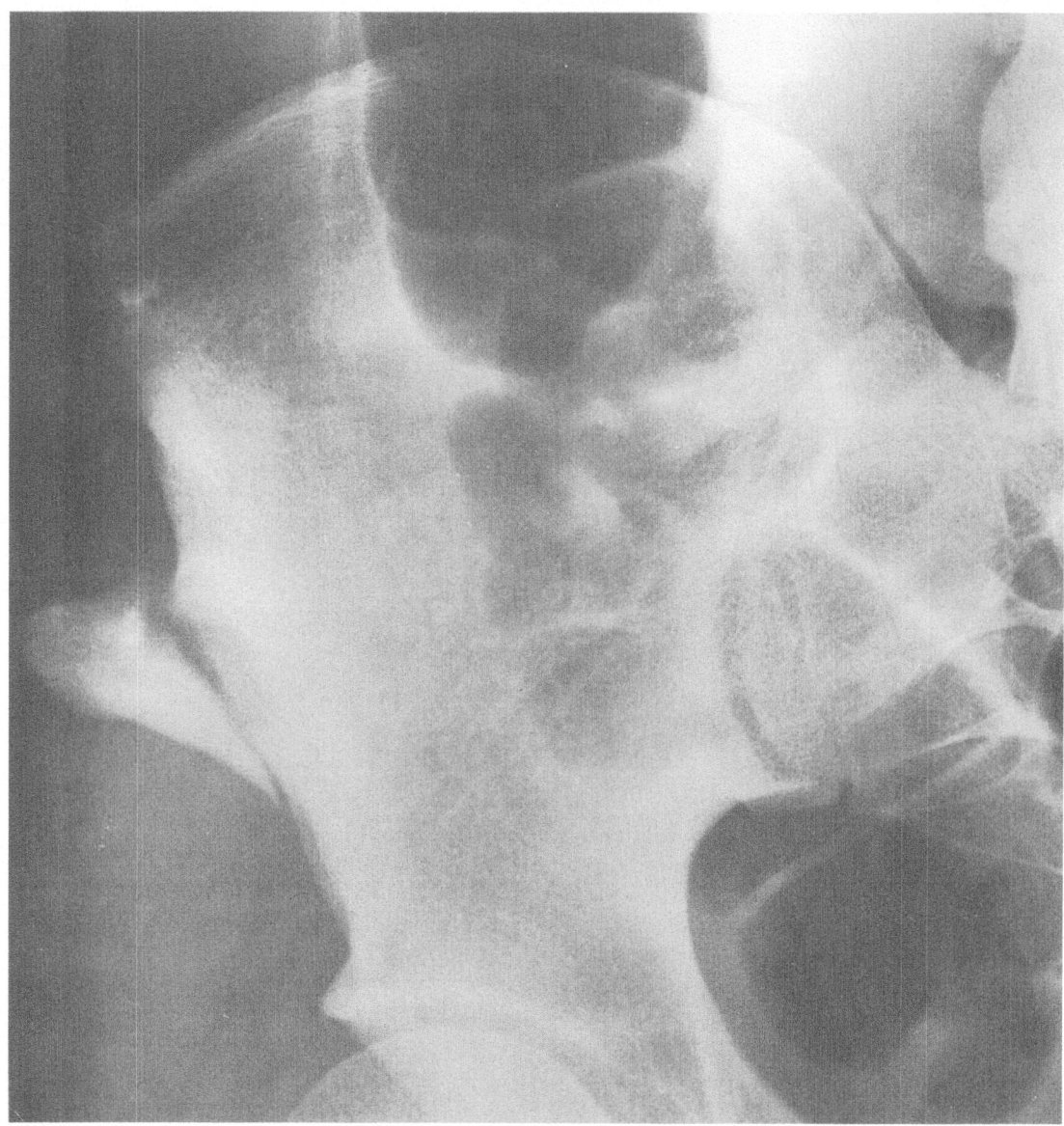

Figure 2.53. A radiograph of the ilium to show a fracture in the region of the anterior-superior iliac spine which occurred following removal of grafts for interbody fusion. This healed without incident

c) Results of Anterior Interbody Fusion

With the use of this technique which allows repeated, reproducible accuracy, lumbar interbody fusions can be achieved in a high percentage of cases in a wide range of disorders of the lumbar spine.

The results of 150 anterior lumbar interbody fusion operations performed by two surgeons in Australia (H. V. Crock and G. M. Bedbrook) were published by Fujimaki et al. (1982).

The data on these patients was gathered, analyzed and classified into three groups: Group I (84 cases); those patients in whom their first and only spinal operation had been an interbody fusion; Group II (38 cases); those patients in whom interbody fusion had followed some other spinal operation; and Group III (28 cases); those patients in whom supplementary operations had been performed following lumbar interbody fusion operation.

The results, including information on occupation, time lost from work and on ultimate re-employment are listed for each group in Table 2.1.

The radiological assessment in these cases is set out in Table 2.2.

Examples of the radiological appearances in lumbar interbody fusions are shown in Figs. 2.54–58 a, b).

Table 2.1. Summary of findings

Group	Occupation		Time off (months)	Resumed same occupation	Commenced other occupation	Did not return to work
1	Non-sedentary	49	11.8	39	7	3
	Home duties	18	3.3	16	1	1
	Sedentary	17	7.4	17	0	0
		84				
2	Non-sedentary	23	24.0	14	6	3
	Home duties	7	5.6	6	0	1
	Sedentary	8	6.5	7	0	1
		38				
3	Non-sedentary	19	16.5	10	3	6
	Home duties	5	11.5	3	1	1
	Sedentary	4	12.5	2	0	2
		28				

Table 2.2 Radiological assessment

	Group	G.M.B.	H.V.C.
1.	84 Cases	26 cases	58 cases
	Union	24	56
	Non-union	2	2
2.	38 Cases	16 cases	22 cases
	Union	16	21
	Non-union	0	1
3.	28 Cases	8 cases	20 cases
	Union	8	19
	Non-union	0	1
Total union		48 (96%)	96 (96%)

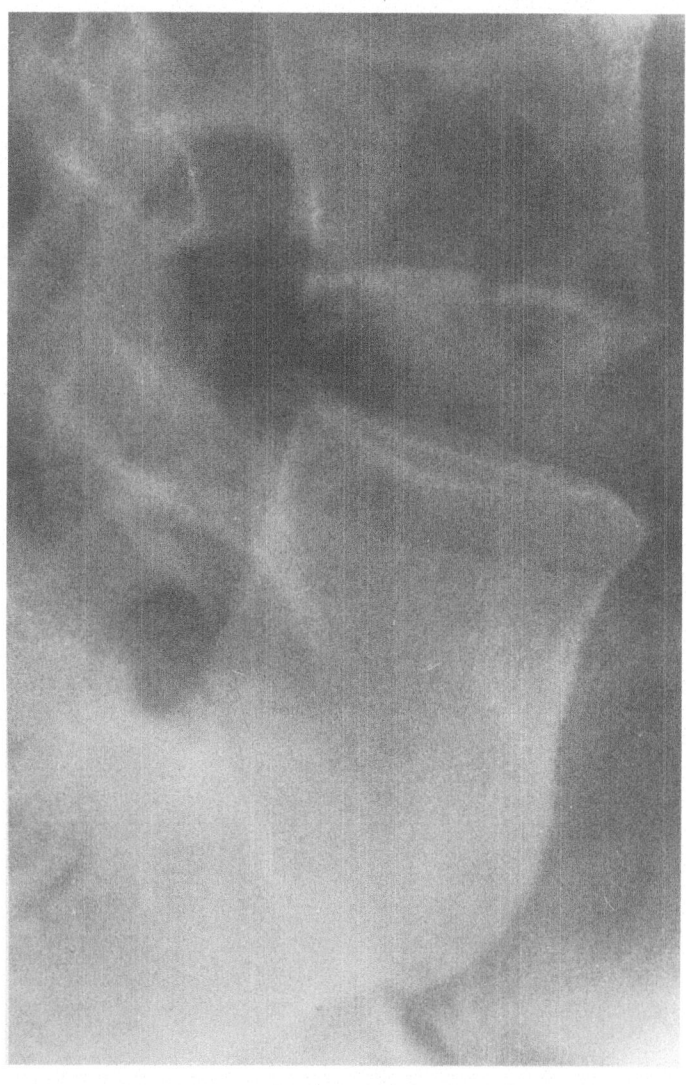

Figure 2.54

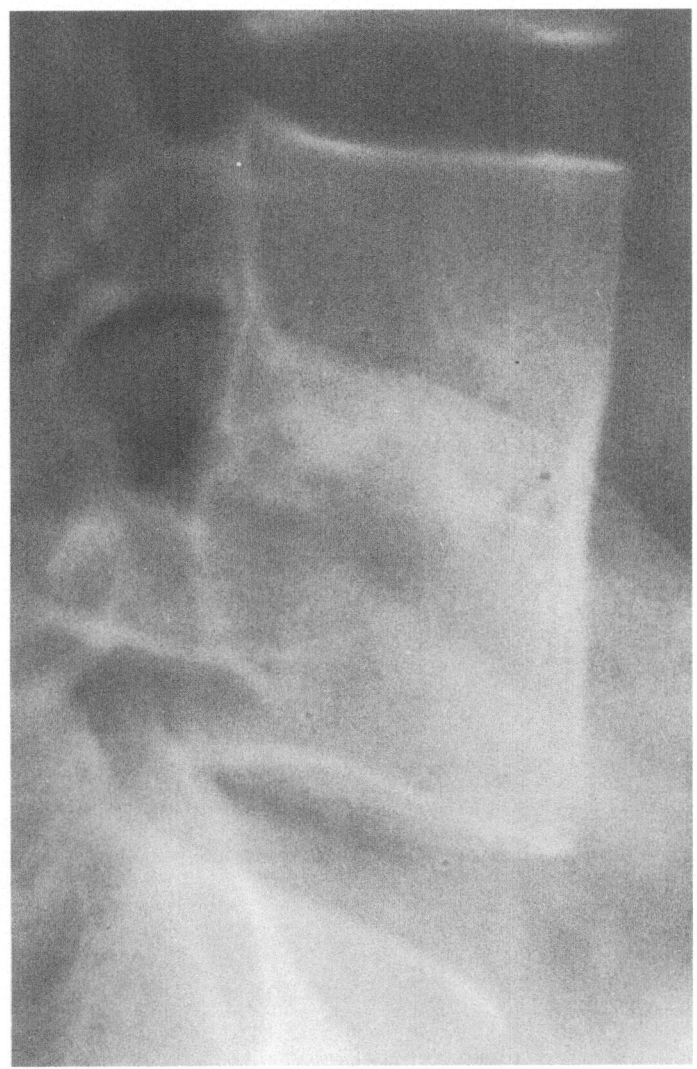

Figure 2.55. A lateral view radiograph showing an L4/5 interbody fusion in a 46 year old woman ten years after operation

Figure 2.54. A lateral radiograph to show an L5/S1 anterior interbody fusion in a male aged 30 years, taken ten years after operation

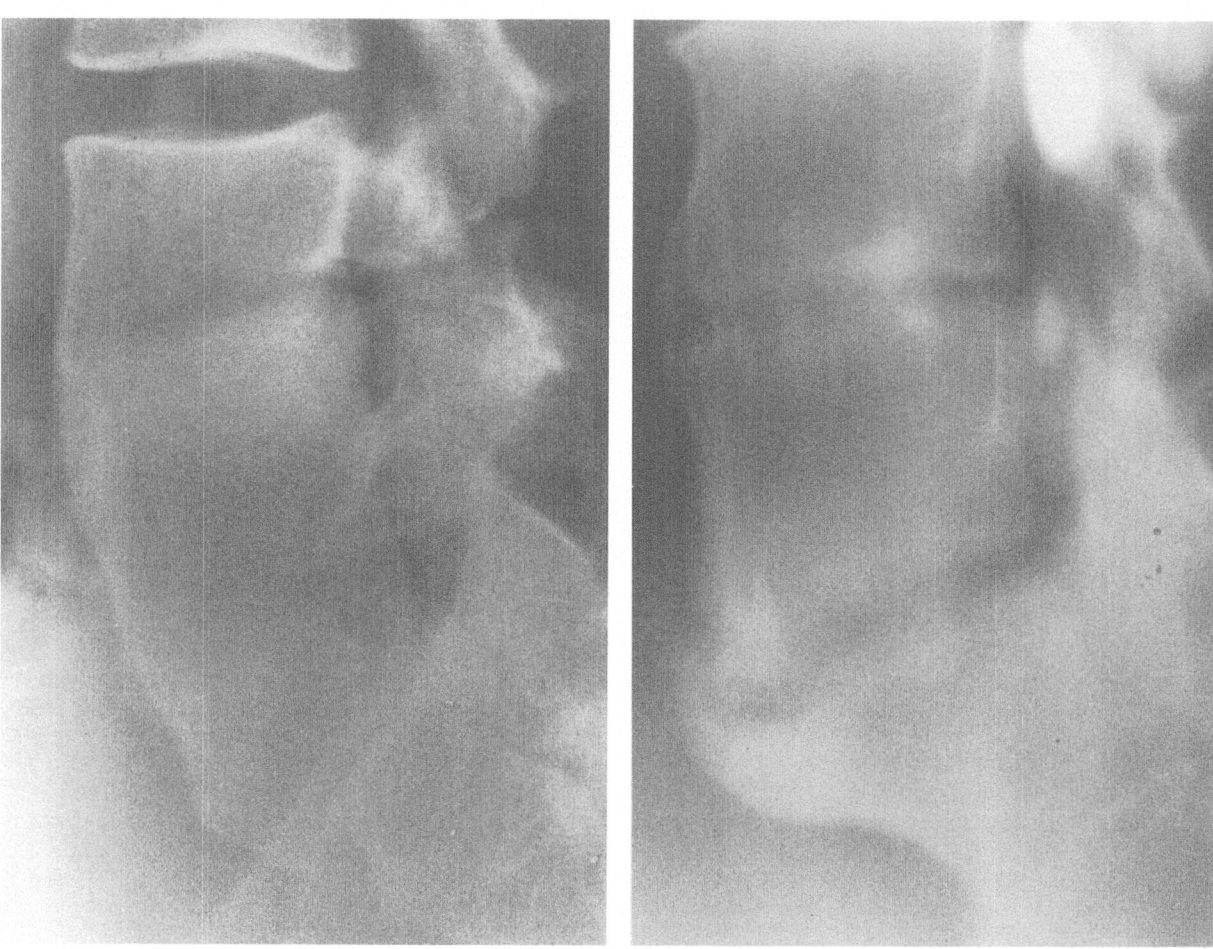

Figure 2.56   **Figure 2.57**

Figure 2.56. A lateral radiograph showing L4/5 and L5/S1 interbody fusions in a 48 year old man five years after operation

Figure 2.57. A lateral radiograph of the lower lumbar spine showing a sound L4/5 interbody fusion and an un-united L5/S1 interbody fusion, with sclerosis anteriorly in the intervertebral disc space

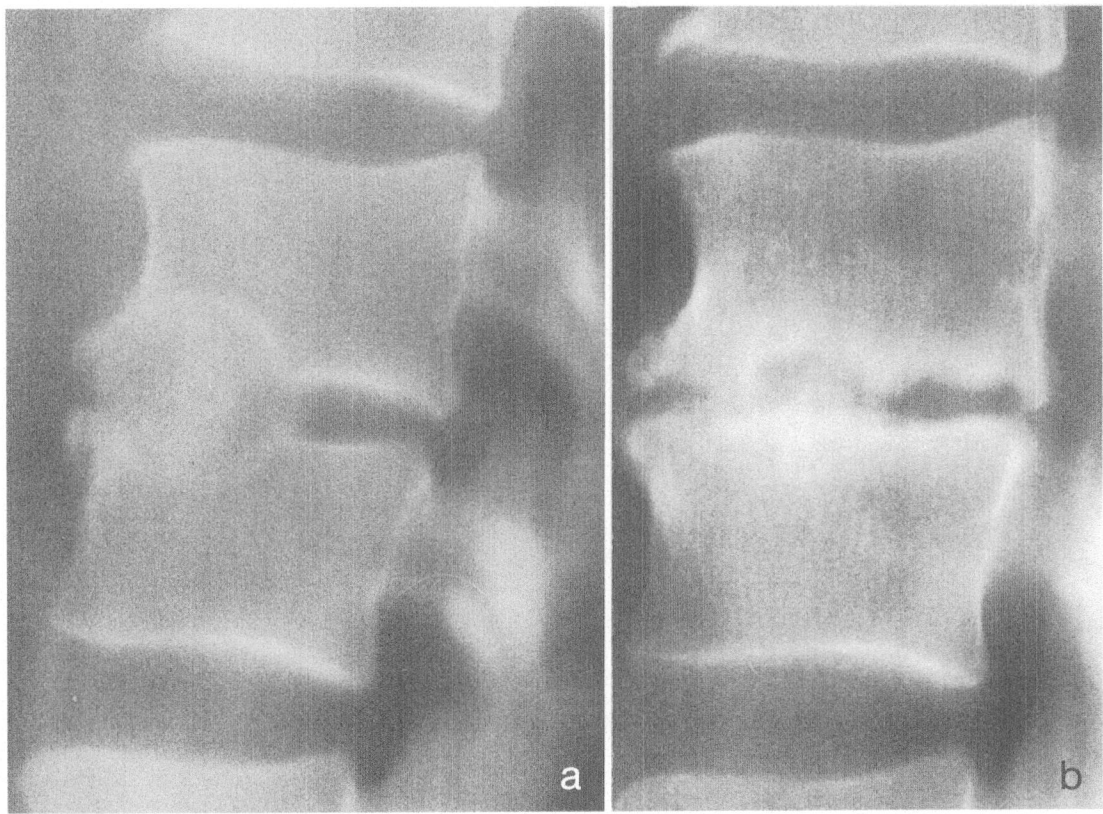

Figures 2.58 a, b.   Lateral tomographs of the upper lumbar spine of a man aged 46 years. **a** Three months after operation. A circular cancellous graft has been inserted transversely at the L 3/4 level. **b** One year later. There is collapse of the graft and established non-union

3

Disc Prolapses

3.1. Introduction

Despite the fact that Mixter and Barr published their description of rupture of the intervertebral disc with involvement of the spinal canal in 1934, confusion still exists about the diagnosis of this lesion and there is often uncertainty about which cases should be treated surgically. The fact that disc prolapses which require surgery are not common is still not widely accepted. In the past ten years extraordinary advances have been made in the development of instruments, lighting, photographic and video recording systems relative to endoscopic surgical equipment and operating microscopes. While large joint surgery has already been revolutionised as a result of the wider use of this technology in orthopaedic surgery, its application in spinal surgery has not yet been clearly established. Until that goal has been reached, the principles that govern surgical approaches to the spinal canal deserve to be restated in the interests of sound surgical education and for the benefit of young surgeons in parts of the world where advanced medical technology may not be available to benefit them and their patients. Even from the vast literature on this subject the synthesis of practical guidelines to diagnosis and surgical management can be made only with difficulty.

Careful neurological examination is the cornerstone of clinical diagnosis, although it may not be possible to distinguish between disc prolapses at the L5/S1 or L4/5 levels on neurological grounds.

When a surgeon operates on a patient for a suspected disc prolapse, assuming that the correct spinal level has been exposed, finding that the exposed disc seems unduly soft on palpation or merely bulging, obsession with the diagnosis of disc prolapse in these circumstances often leads to removal of disc tissue. The patient's symptoms will usually be worse after the operation. Against this background, what then constitutes a useful guide to the management of lumbar disc prolapses?

In the lumbar region, disc prolapses are most commonly seen at either the L4/5 or L5/S1 vertebral interspaces or at both of these levels. Higher in the lumbar region they may present with unusual symptoms and signs mimicking intra-spinal tumours. In this region they are rare and usually occur in elderly people (Aronsen and Dunsmore, 1963).

The initiating factors are probably multiple, but trauma may precipitate the prolapse. The physical force of the precipitating trauma is often mild, though its influence varies inversely with the extent of pre-existing pathological changes in the affected disc. In normal discs, tensile forces of considerable magnitude (60–80 kg/cm^2) exist in the posterior part of the annulus, this fact giving strong support to the mechanical theory of the production of ruptures of the posterior annulus (Nachemson and Morris, 1964). In young subjects, heavy lifting while bending may lead to the formation of a small prolapse, whereas in older patients massive disc sequestration may follow simple bodily movements such as bending or twisting of the spine. Disc prolapse may be a complication of posturing of the trunk under anaesthesia for other surgical procedures, such as gall bladder, renal or gynaecological operations.

3.2. Pathology

The pathological features of disc prolapse have been described by many writers (Coventry et al., 1945; Reynolds and Katz, 1969; Taylor and Akeson, 1971). The characteristics of prolapses vary with the physical qualities of the affected disc tissue. Knowledge of the varying relationships which prolapsed disc tissue may bear to the neural contents of the spinal canal is essential to the understanding of the varied clinical pictures which many present (Fig. 3.1). In young persons, discrete, small,

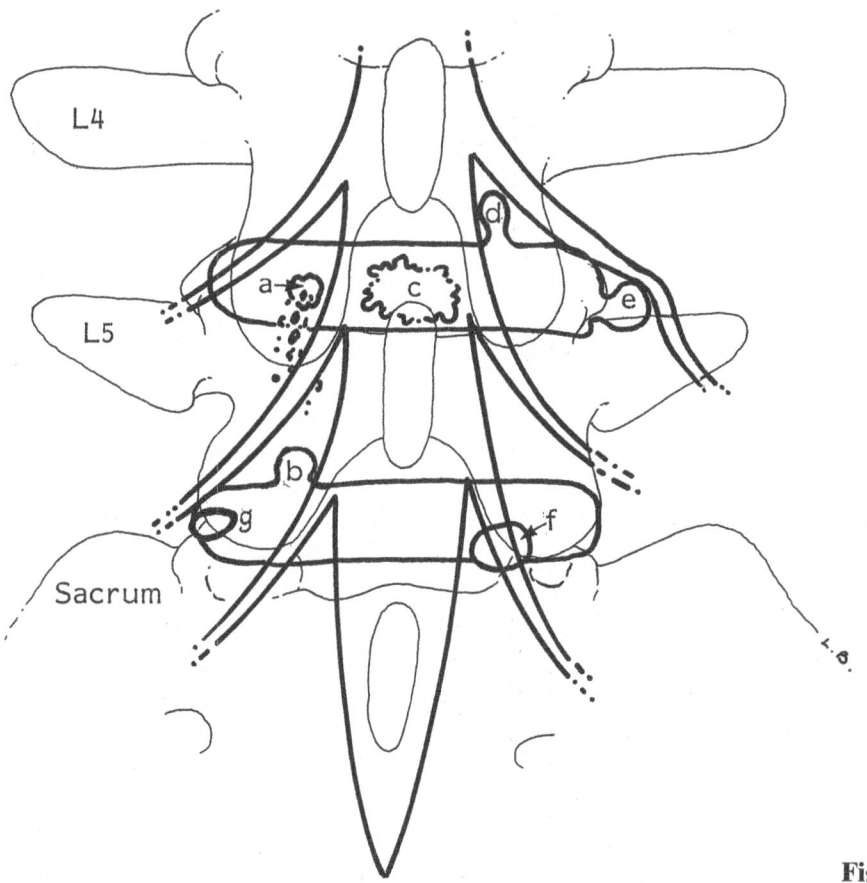

Figure 3.1

rounded, firm or fluctuant protrusions are found with stretched but intact annular fibres and, when incised at operation, only a small quantity of disc tissue may escape and be removed, leaving in the disc a defect which admits neither curettes nor disc rongeurs easily. The consistency of such discs is often described as rubbery. Some degenerative annular fibres are usually found with the extruded nuclear tissue in these cases.

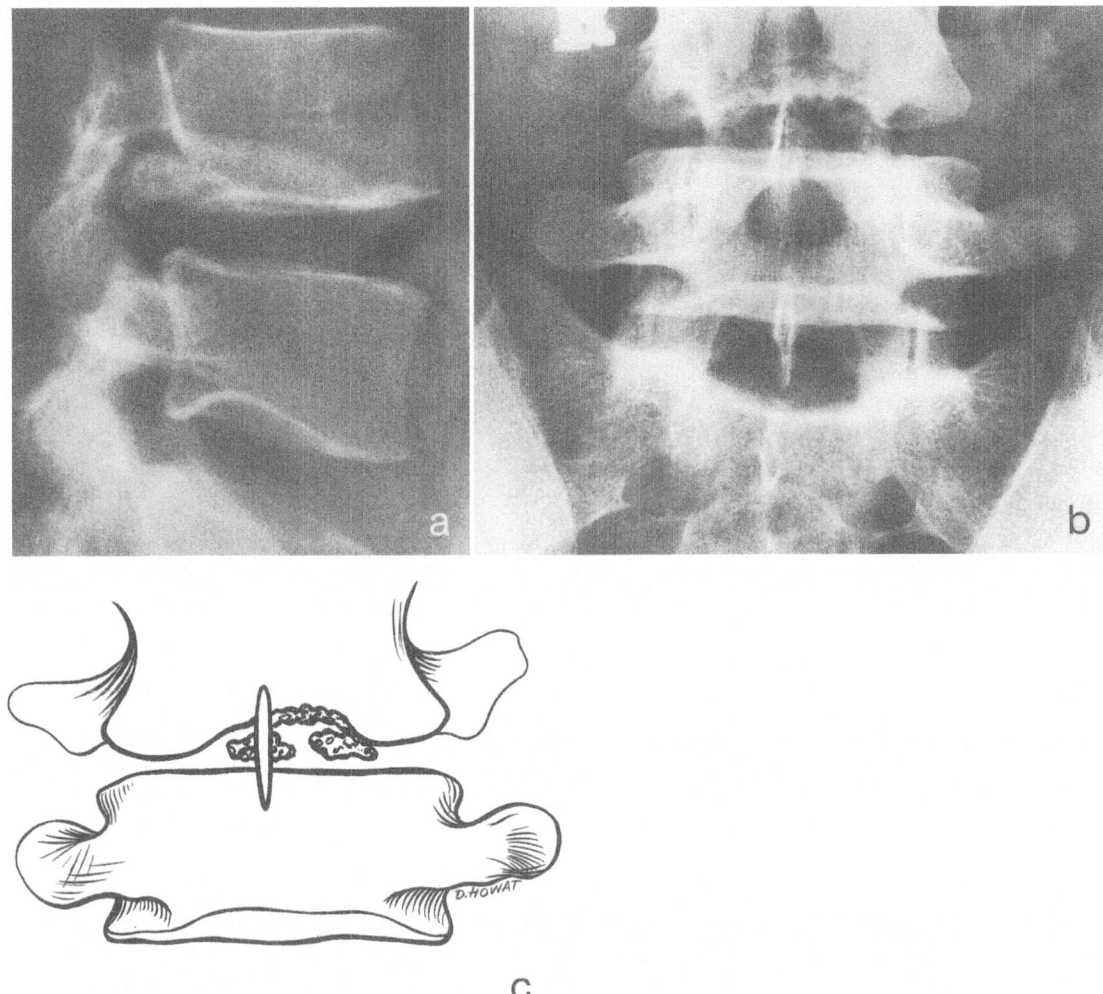

Figures 3.2 a–c. Intra-spongeous disc herniation with fracture of the vertebral body margin and sequestration of disc fragments into the spinal canal. **a** Lateral radiograph. A large bony fragment separated from the posterior-inferior margin of the 4th lumbar vertebral body. It projects into the spinal canal. **b** Antero-posterior view. The L4/5 disc space is narrowed and tilted. There is a defect in the central zone of the vertebral end-plate area of the 4th vertebral body. Below this, two bony fragments can be identified. These findings were confirmed at operation. **c** Drawing of the position of these fragments. (Courtesy of Mr. K. Mills)

Figure 3.1. A drawing depicting various types of disc prolapses which may be encountered in the lumbar region. *a* A sequestrated disc with fragments migrating distally from its origin at the L4/5 interspace. *b* "A shoulder" prolapse related to the S1 nerve root at its take off point from the dural sac. *c* A central disc prolapse. *d* An axillary prolapse. *e* An extra-foraminal prolapse. *f* The common sub-rhizal prolapse. *g* An intra-foraminal prolapse

Extrusion of variable quantities of disc tissue (1.1–13.5 g) into the spinal canal may be seen when gross degenerative changes have occurred in the disc as a whole. The description of "sequestrated disc fragments" is then applied. The components of such fragments may include nuclear, annular and end-plate material.

Between these two extremes, a variety of pathological changes may be noted. Incomplete sequestration may be associated with marked peri-neural fibrosis, a finding related to physico-chemical changes in the disc (Nachemson, 1969). Calcified nuclear tissue may herniate, or calcification may occur in prolapsed tissue leading occasionally to erosion of the dural sac (Blikra, 1969).

A sequestrated fragment may migrate to another level from the disc of its origin, leaving a clearly defined oval defect in the posterior annulus (Fig. 3.1). Sequestrated disc tissue may present posterior to the dural sac (Hooper, 1973).

Rarely, disc tissue may prolapse into the vertebral bodies and re-enter the spinal canal, pushing ahead of it a small fragment of vertebral end-plate bone and cartilage (Figs. 3.2 a–c).

In a sub-rhizal prolapse, the disc fragment lies anterior to the affected nerve root, and this usually causes severe pain with objective motor and sensory signs distally, in the part of the limb supplied by the compressed nerve root.

Prolapses situated between the dural sac and the nerve root sheath, axillary prolapses, or these lying on the outer side of the nerve root sheath, para-rhizal prolapses, may produce symptoms of severe sciatica without abnormal objective physical signs.

Centrally placed prolapses or a large migrating sequestrated fragment in the spinal canal may give rise to physical signs including bowel or bladder dysfunction and neurological signs or symptoms which vary from day to day in one leg or the

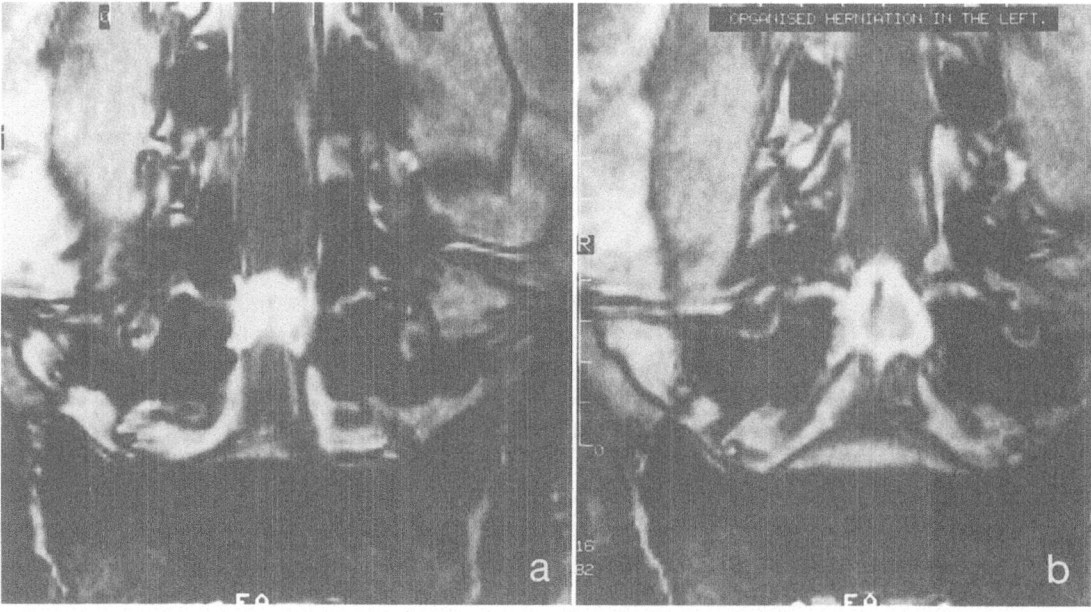

Figures 3.3 a, b. MR images with gadolinium enhancement showing marked oedema and venous engorgement at L4/5 with an organised left sided sub-rhizal disc prolapse

other. In the lumbar region, cauda equina claudication with the onset of buttock or leg pains after walking short distances may also be found (Verbiest, 1955).

In considering this pathology, the clinician should always give some thought to the shape and size of the patient's spinal canal (Figs. 3.3 a, b).

3.3. Clinical Features

The classic features of lumbar scoliosis, depression of one or more reflexes in the affected limb, muscle weakness or wasting, gross limitation of straight leg raising and the finding of areas of impaired sensation over affected dermatomes are all well known.

Perhaps less well appreciated is the reported observation that the pattern of pain radiation into the leg does not differ appreciably in L4/5 and L5/S1 disc lesions. In fact, clinical signs caused by lumbar disc prolapses may be misleading. Brown and Pont (1963) observed in a review of 570 patients that the ankle jerk may be absent in cases of prolapse at L4/5 or at L3/4. They found that sensory changes in the foot were more accurate aids in diagnosis than were changes in the leg as a whole.

In eliciting the physical sign of limitation of straight leg raising as an index of sciatic nerve irritation, attempts to lift the leg quickly from the extended position, with the patient supine, frequently evoke such a painful response that the straight leg can be raised only a few degrees from the examination couch. On the other hand, if the knee and hip are cautiously flexed and the knee then extended slowly with the examiner's thumb in the popliteal fossa exerting some pressure on the terminal branches of the sciatic nerve, and these manoeuvres are combined with dorsi-flexion of the foot, even minor degrees of sciatic nerve irritation can be appreciated. This is commonly known as Lasègue's sign. A patient with convincing sciatica is unable to sit upright with both knees fully extended. In the presence of sciatic irritation he will automatically flex the hip and knee on the affected side when attempting to adopt this posture. This has been described as the "bath-tub sign" by Pennybacker (1959).

Changes in the clinical features referred to above are all important in assessing the progress or failure of recovery of sciatica due to disc prolapse. Of particular importance is the severity of pain, especially when it reaches a level which consistently disturbs sleep at night.

3.4. Investigations

a) Plain X-Rays

These X-rays always provide essential information on the bony anatomy of the vertebral column particularly in regard to the arrangement of laminae and the site of the lumbo-sacral junction. They are also important for the exclusion of other lesions such as spondylosis which may cause confusion in diagnosis. Usually they do not provide any useful guide to the site of prolapse.

b) MRI

This is already established as the investigation of choice in the diagnosis of lumbar and thoracic disc prolapses. In the cervical spine it is often useful, but CT radiculography is more accurate in helping to localize smaller and laterally situated disc prolapses.

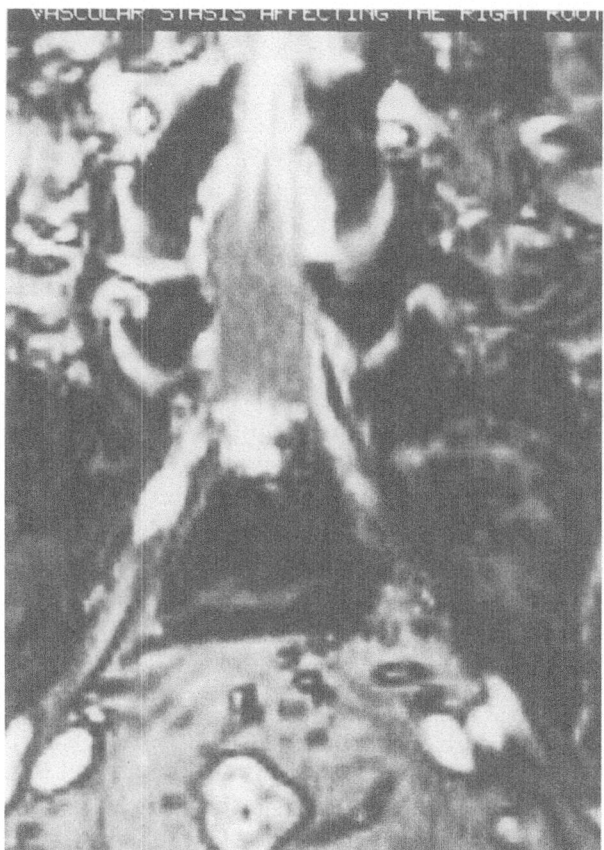

Figure 3.4. Coronal reconstruction of a lumbar MRI showing vascular stasis affecting the right sided lower lumbar nerve root due to a disc prolapse related to the take off point of this nerve root with surrounding oedema spreading centrally

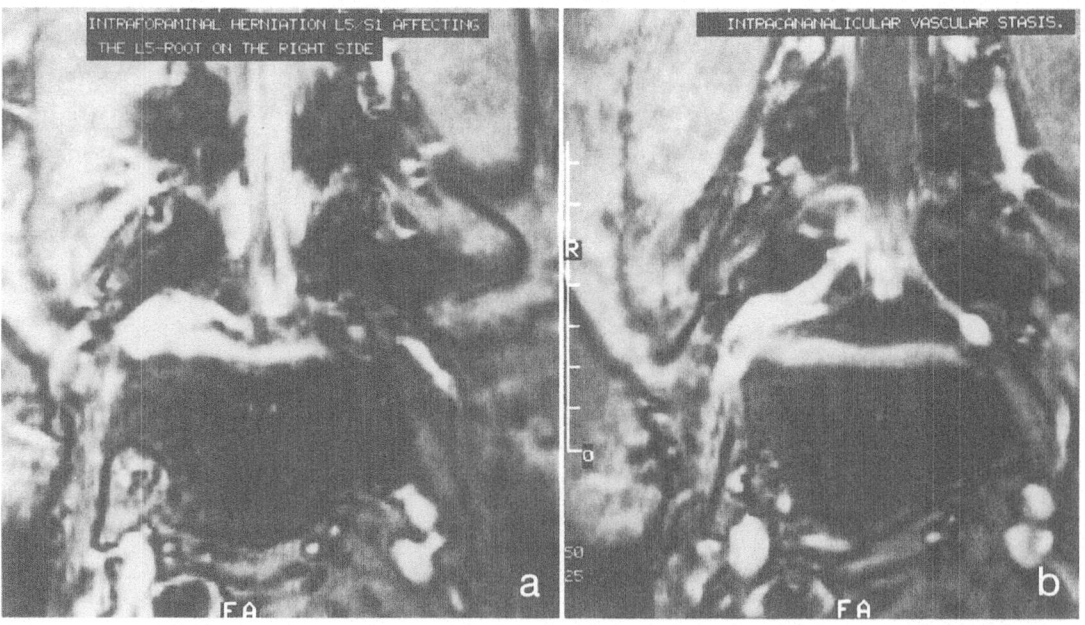

Figures 3.5 a, b. Coronal reconstructions of MR images showing: **a** an intra-foraminal herniation at L5/S1 affecting the right sided L5 nerve root with **b** marked intra-canalicular vascular stasis

Used with gadolinium enhancement it gives accurate definitions of foraminal, extra-foraminal, intra-canalicular and sequestrated disc prolapses and shows the amazing extent of root oedema or vascular engorgement that occurs adjacent to many of these lesions (Figs. 3.3–3.11).

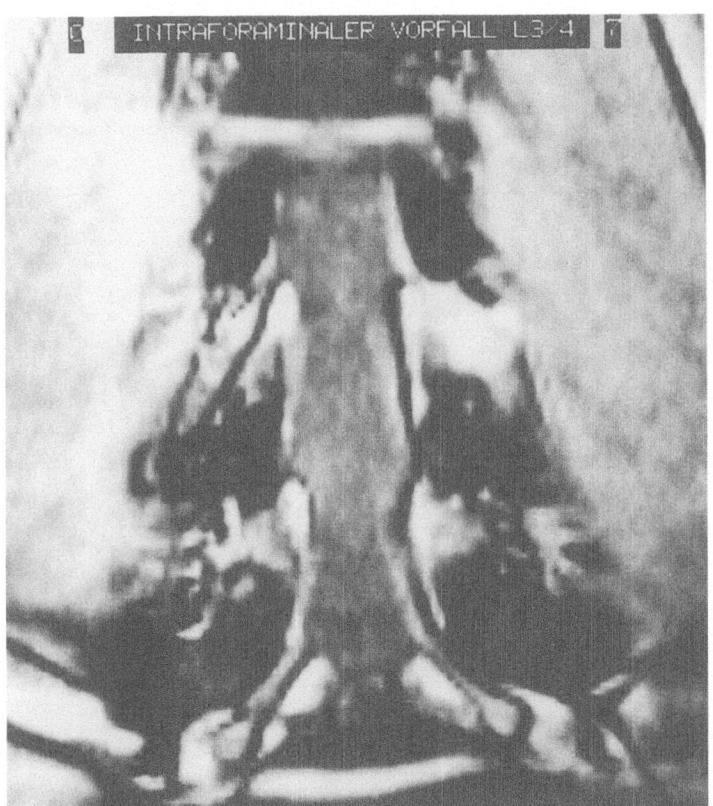

Figure 3.6. MRI – coronal reconstruction showing an intra-foraminal prolapse at L3/4

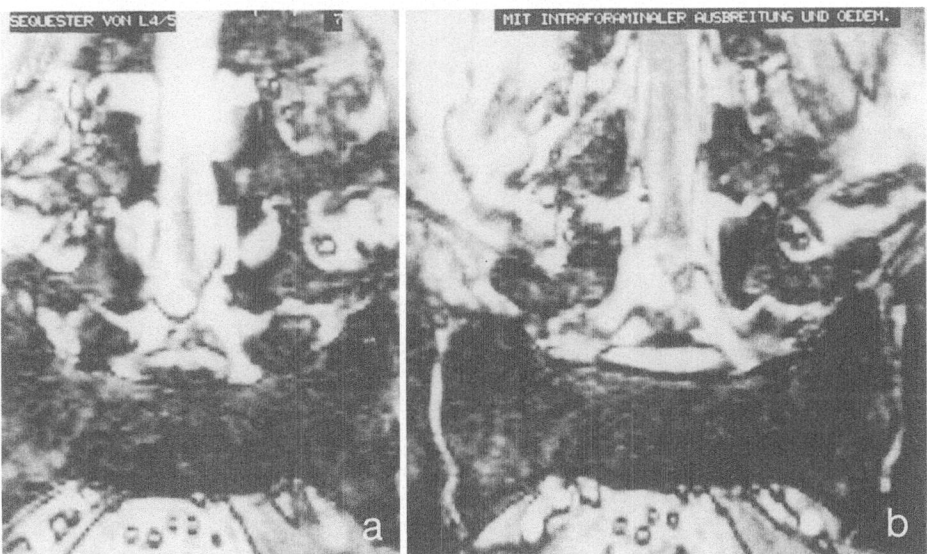

Figures 3.7a,b. Coronal reconstructions of MR images showing: **a** sequestration of the L4/5 disc with **b** an intra-foraminal sequestration and surrounding oedema

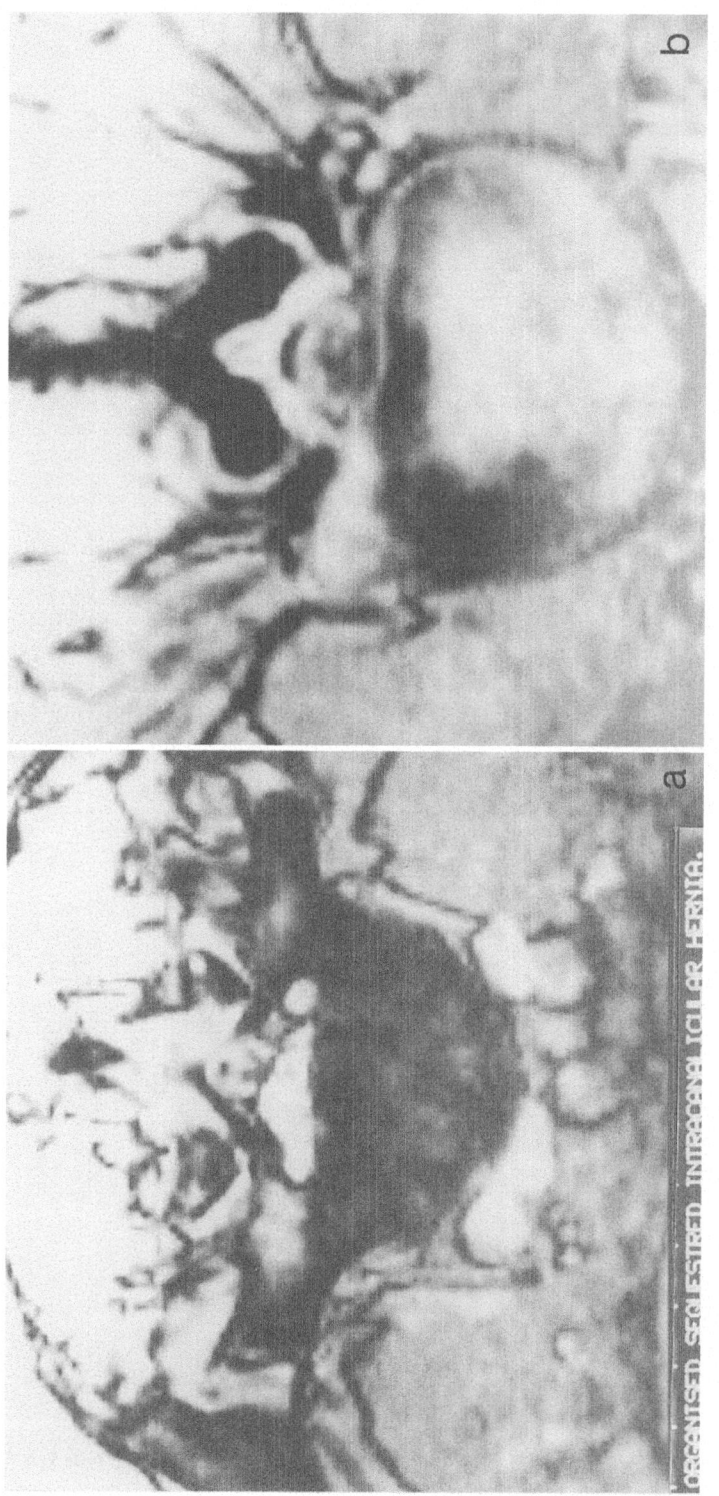

Figures 3.8a,b. a An axial MR image with gadolinium enhancement in the case of an organised sequestrated intra-canalicular hernia. Note the surrounding oedema and in particular the oedema in the pedicle of L5 due to venous obstruction in the intervertebral foramen. **b** A large intra-foraminal hernia with surrounding oedema

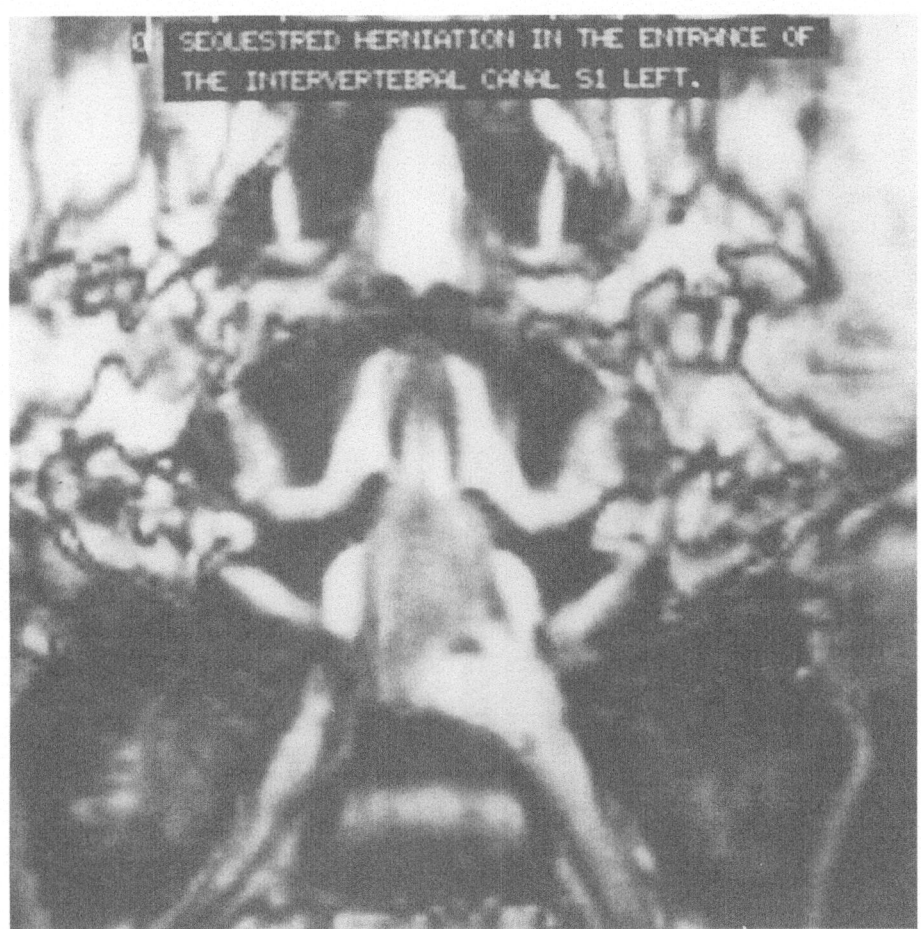

Figure 3.9. A coronal reconstruction showing a sequestrated herniation extending along the nerve root canal of S1 on the left side

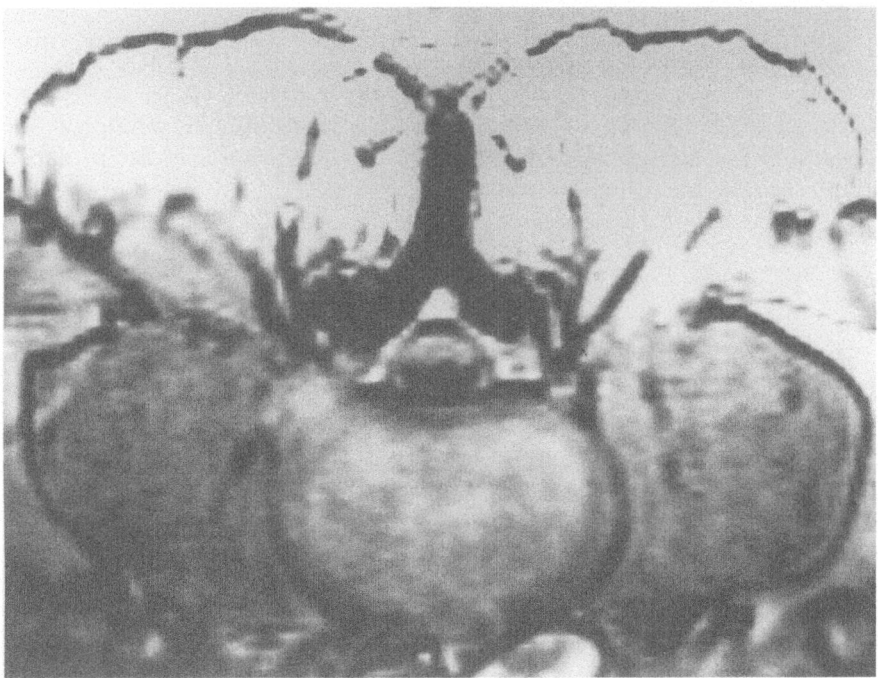

Figure 3.10. An axial MR image showing an extra-foraminal prolapse in the lumbar region

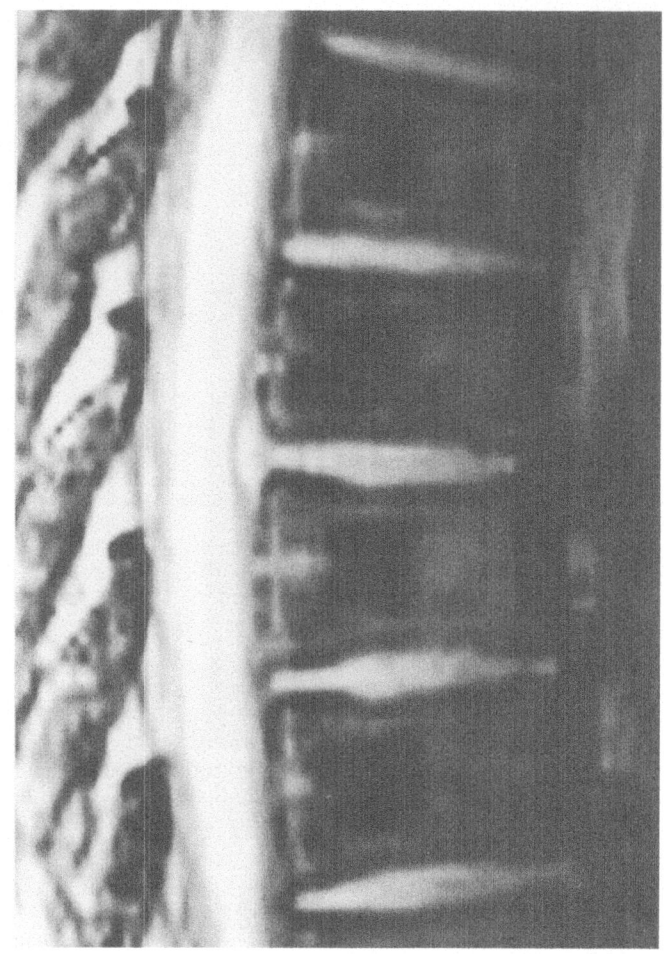

Figure 3.11. A mid-sagittal T2 weighted MR image showing a large thoracic disc prolapse projecting on to the dural sac and indenting the spinal cord

c) Myelography

The introduction of water soluble myelographic media such as Metrizamide or Omnipaque in recent years has greatly enhanced the accuracy of diagnosis of disc prolapses, particularly in combination with CT examination.

When MRI and CT examinations are not available, myelography should be used as a routine pre-operative investigation in cases of suspected disc prolapse. It is invaluable in the investigation of any atypical case and is especially useful in cases of suspected disc prolapse where there is advanced spondylosis shown on the plain x-rays, or in the presence of bony anomalies such as lumbar sacralisation. In these cases it will aid in the diagnosis of associated spinal canal stenosis (Fig. 3.12 a,b), or it may help to identify the level of origin of a disc sequestrum and its distribution in the spinal canal (Figs. 3.13–3.15).

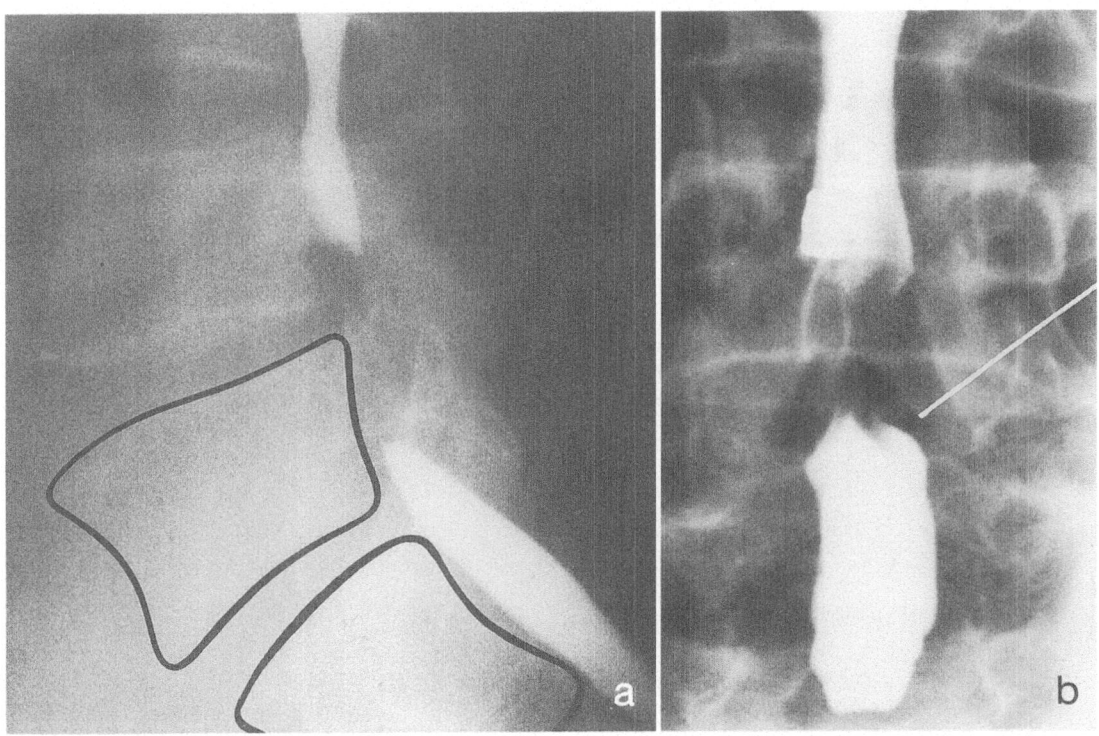

Figures 3.12 a,b. Disc prolapse into a congenital narrow lumbar canal. A 62 year-old man (weight 110 kg) lifted a bag of cement, flexing and rotating his spine. He developed back pain and severe bilateral leg pain; these symptoms were relieved following excision of a small disc fragment and bilateral nerve root canal decompression laminectomy. **a** Lateral and **b** antero-posterior radiographs of the lumbar myelogram, showing gross obstruction of the iofendylate column. Note the symmetrical indentation at the upper end of the lower iofendylate column in (**b**) (marker), suggesting the association of true spinal stenosis. (Courtesy of Mr. B. Davie)

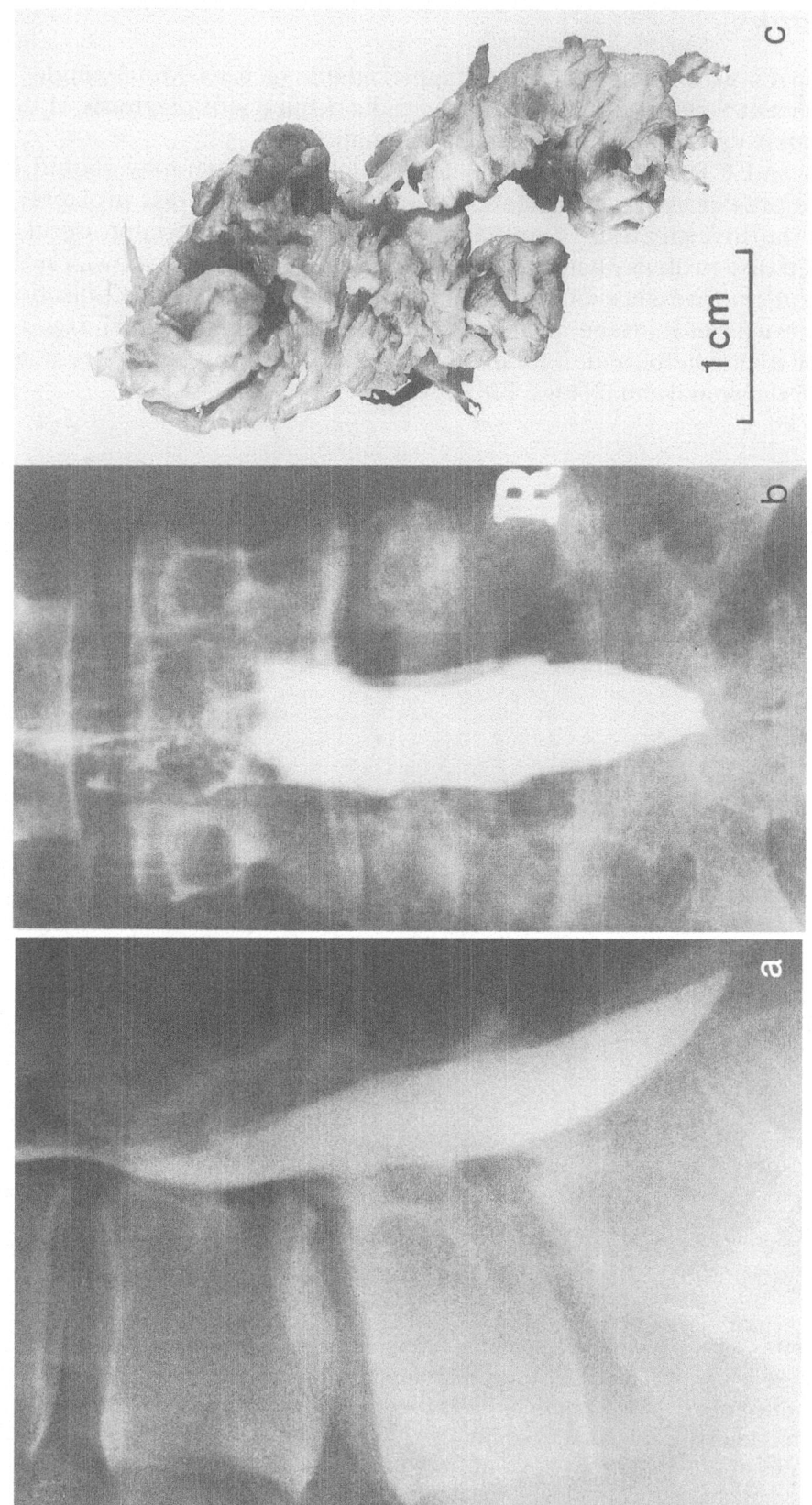

Figures 3.13a–c. Sequestrated L4/5 disc with migrating fragments. **a** and **b**: Lateral and antero-posterior radiographs of the lumbar myelogram of a woman, aged 39 years, who had severe right-sided sciatica. The deformation of the dural sac is consistent with the presence of migrating sequestrated disc fragments. It is best seen in the antero-posterior view. **c** The photograph shows the appearance of the sequestrated disc material which was removed at operation, orientated to correspond with its position in vivo

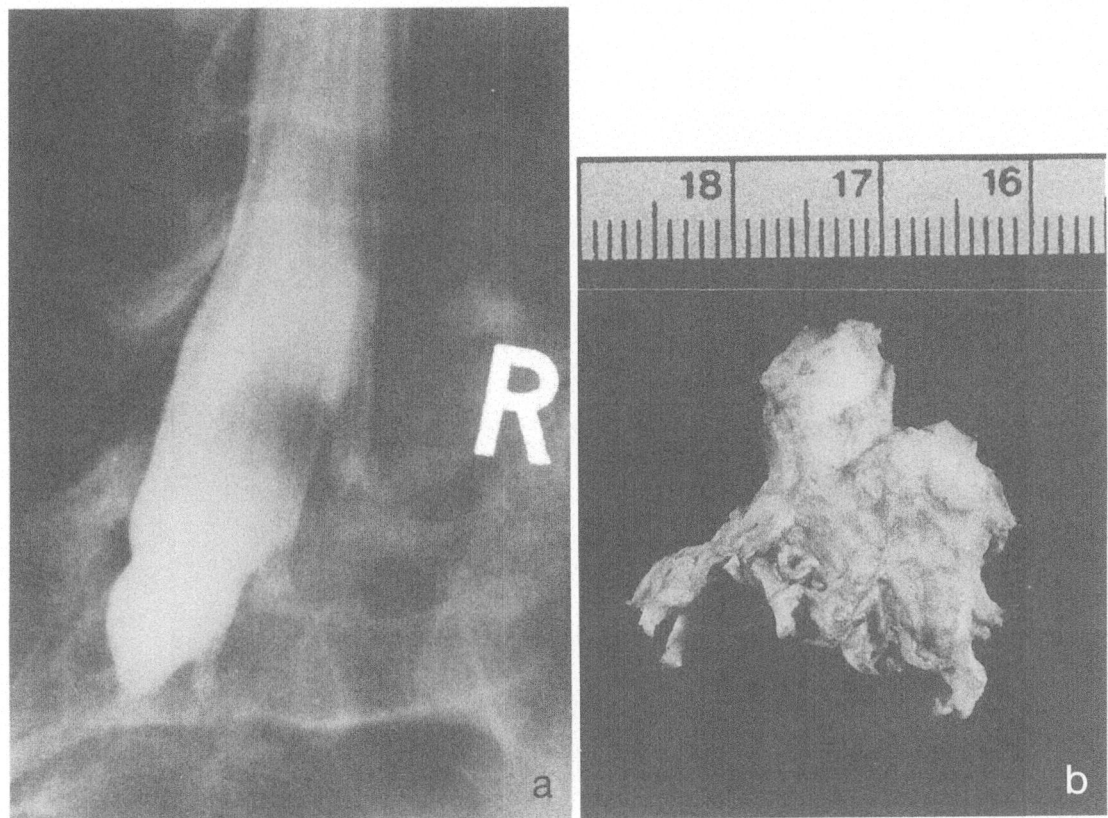

Figures 3.14a,b. a A right-sided, slightly oblique view of a radiculogram in a 27 year old male showing a large central and right sided filling defect at L5/S1. This represented a massive disc sequestration stemming from the L5/S1 disc and extending distally in to the sacral spinal canal between the S1 and the S2 nerve roots. **b** A photograph of the specimen removed at operation. This consisted of mixed elements of disc tissue including vertebral end-plate cartilage

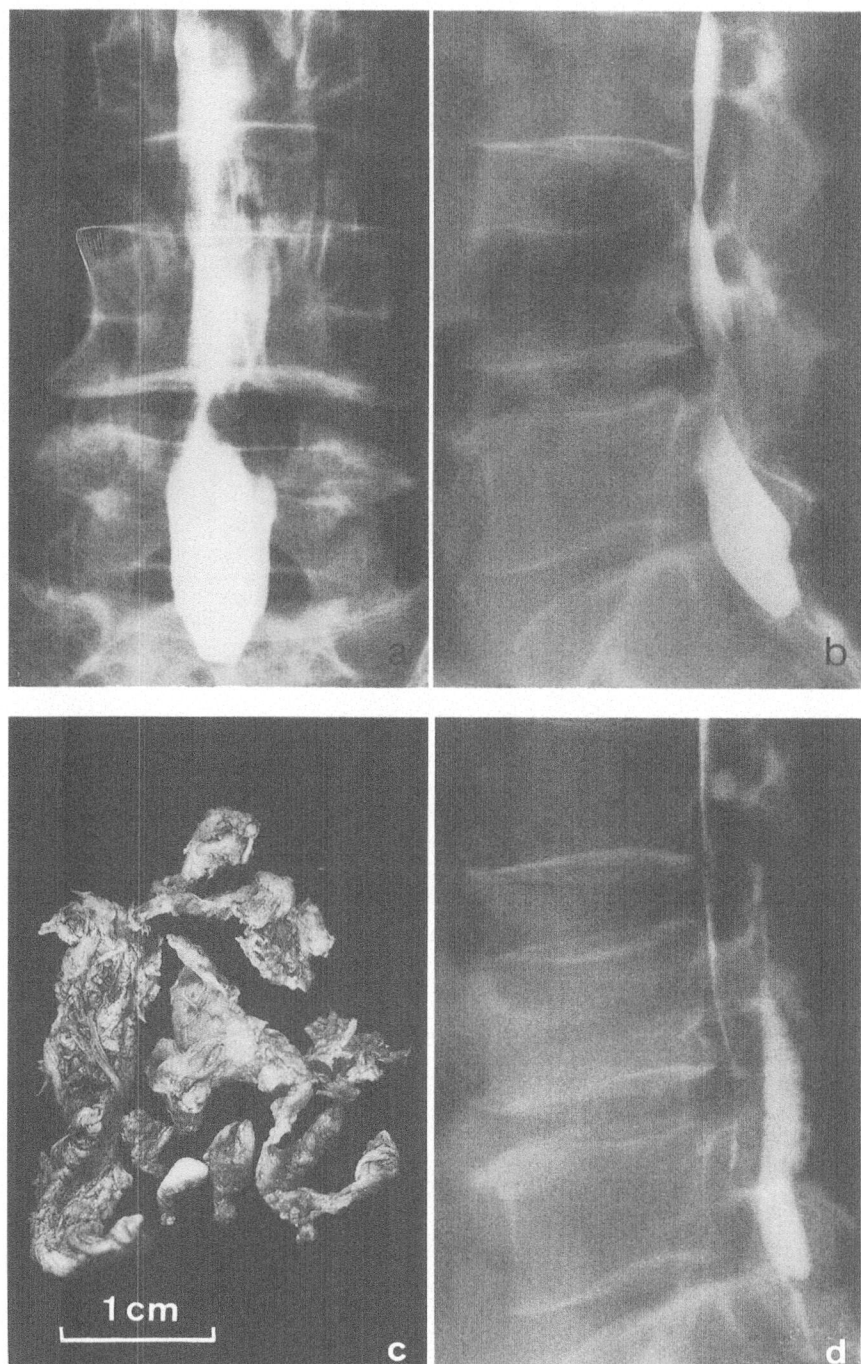

Figures 3.15a–d. Massive disc sequestration following twisting of the lumbar spine treated by disc excision and posterior interbody fusion. A 53 year-old male jeweller suffered from intermittent back pain for 13 years. While using a powered floor-standing machine, he twisted his spine and suddenly developed severe left-sided sciatica. **a** and **b** Antero-posterior and lateral radiographs of the lumbar myelogram, showing a large filling defect at the L4/5 disc space. **c** The sequestrated disc fragments removed at operation. **d** Lateral radiograph taken after operation showing the restored normal outline of the dural sac. Bone grafts are seen between the vertebral bodies of L4 and L5; they were inserted through the spinal canal following disc excision

d) C.S.F. Examination

Some authors recommend routine examination of the C.S.F. in the investigation of disc lesions, to test its dynamics and contents (Mercer and Duthie, 1964), while others with extensive experience in the management of spinal conditions rarely do so (Armstrong, 1965; Northfield and Osmond-Clarke, 1967).

The normal protein content of C.S.F. lies between 15 and 40 mg/ml (Bickerstaff, 1973). In lumbar disc prolapses rises up to 100 mg/ml may be seen, with figures as high as 1,000 mg/ml in the presence of marked spinal block. However, many would hold the view that changes in the protein content are rarely of practical use in diagnosis. Johnson (1972) discusses the mechanisms of absorption of C.S.F. and states: "It appears that a subsidiary pathway is via the large spinal veins around the emerging nerve roots". Abnormalities of serum albumin may be found in collagen diseases, those changes being reflected in the C.S.F. with the appearance of abnormal albumins, "para-albumins", in it. With advances in the understanding of C.S.F. physiology, it is logical that surgeons should make greater use of more recent biochemical techniques of analysis of this fluid, especially in some of the non-prolapsing varieties of disc lesions discussed in this chapter. Whenever myelography is undertaken, a sample of C.S.F. should be obtained for cytological and chemical testing.

e) Discography

This investigation is rarely indicated as an aid to the diagnosis of disc prolapses. In atypical cases of severe sciatica with minimal abnormal physical signs and normal myelographic findings, a discogram may help to clarify the diagnosis (Wilson and McCarty, 1969). In combination with CT examination foraminal and extra-foraminal disc prolapses at unusual sites can be identified.

f) Intra-Osseous Spinal Venography

Intra-osseous spinal venography has not been used widely in the English-speaking world. German observers claim that when it is used with tomography it is just as reliable as myelography in the diagnosis of lumbar disc protrusion and prolapse. The special value of this procedure is noted in acute cases of massive midline prolapses involving the cauda equina (Vogelsang, 1970). MRI with gadolinium enhancement has rendered this investigation almost obsolete (see Chapter 2).

g) Electrodiagnostic Tests

Technical and interpretative difficulties in the use of electromyography have been described by Simpson (1972).

3.5. Indications for Surgical Treatment

Absolute indications for operations are:

a) Major neurological deficits, such as: Acute cauda equina compression due to massive disc sequestration or the prolapse of a small fragment of disc tissue into an abnormally small lumbar spinal canal; paraparesis due to thoracic disc prolapse, brachial paresis or quadriparesis due to cervical disc prolapse.
b) Persistent or recurrent pain, with or without abnormal physical signs, in the extremities. This is the most common indication for surgery after an adequate trial of conservative treatment in cases of lumbar or cervical disc lesions.
c) Progressive neurological deficits, such as paraparesis, foot drop or quadriparesis.
d) Persistent spinal deformity, such as lumbar scoliosis or marked lumbar flexion deformity which may be found in certain cases of lumbar disc prolapse or spinal tumour.

3.6. Treatment for Lumbar Disc Prolapses

a) Discussion

i) Surgery

In the lumbar region, a limited unilateral inter-laminar approach may suffice for the removal of discrete small rubbery disc prolapses, but it can only be recommended in young people. Where disc sequestration has occurred or in cases where rather desiccated disc tissue is found, more extensive intra-disc space curettage should be carried out and at the same time a careful bilateral nerve root canal decompression performed. Such a procedure performed at the time of laminectomy for disc fragment excision reduces the late problems of recurrent nerve root irritation that may arise from nerve root canal stenosis on one or both sides, resulting from secondary disc space narrowing. In these circumstances, there is little justification for extending the operation to include posterior spinal fusion (Spurling, 1949). Indeed, the failure rate is high, graft resorption being very common when inter-laminar fusion has been attempted after exploration of the spinal canal. In addition, late spinal canal stenosis may lead to recurrent symptoms which are difficult to manage. Postero-lateral inter-transverse fusion is more reliable in these circumstances if spinal fusion seems warranted because of gross vertebral instability (Watkins, 1959).

From the point of view of the relief of sciatic pain, recent long term reviews indicate that "laminectomy" alone will produce good results (Jackson, 1971; Naylor, 1974), variations in the actual technique of laminectomy exerting little effect on the outcome.

Where most of the disc remnants are removed in some cases of massive disc sequestration, gross vertebral instability can occur. Posterior interbody spinal fusion performed through the spinal canal, either by the technique described by Cloward (1952) or that recommended by Wiltberger and Abbott (1958), offers a solution to a difficult problem (Fig. 3.15 d).

Numerous reviews analyzing the results of various forms of treatment for disc prolapse and spondylosis in the lumbar region are available. Basically it is impossible to compare series published by different authors for two reasons: firstly, because indications for operation vary so widely; secondly, because the operative techniques and pathological findings described are also variable.

Authors everywhere agree on a number of matters:

- compensation patients always respond more slowly to treatment than do private patients;
- the results of simple disc fragment excision for frank disc prolapse are good in more than 80% of cases;
- prolonged paralysis before operation may not recover completely following it; and
- paralysis seen for the first time after operation usually recovers rapidly and completely.

Cervical disc prolapses can be treated almost exclusively by anterior disc excision thereby avoiding the more painful procedure of posterior exploration of the cervical canal.

Thoracic disc prolapses are rare. They are usually found between T9 and T12 vertebrae though upper thoracic lesions do occur. MRI has increased the rate and accuracy of their diagnosis (Fig. 3.11).

ii) Chymopapain

Intra-discal injection of chymopapain (Discase), a proteolytic enzyme, was introduced into clinical practice in 1963 for the treatment of disc prolapse (Smith and Brown, 1967). Clinical diagnosis is confirmed by discography, following which the enzyme preparation is injected through the discogram needle.

Biochemists have been sceptical of its use because of the difficulty of standardization of the enzyme preparations and the potential for damage of tissues other than nucleus pulposus, should it escape from the intervertebral disc space (Lowther, 1972). Chymopapain, nonetheless, found its way into quite wide use especially in some parts of the U.S.A. and Canada. The difficulties in assessing its efficacy in treatment have been highlighted by MacNab (1973), because there is no general agreement on clinical syndromes presented by a disc herniation. He quotes the following results assembled from a nationwide review undertaken by Lyman Smith in 1972: in 2,557 patients there was marked improvement in 1,769 (70%), slight improvement in 340 (13%) and no improvement in 448 cases (17%).

Although chemonucleolysis is no longer widely used in North America even by its former most ardent proponents, persistent interest in this method of treatment has led to the establishment of a Society for Intradiscal Therapy.

A number of controversies continue to provoke debate. *Anaphylaxis*, the major life threatening complication has attracted most attention, leading to developments such as prophylactic skin testing and medication regimes. Arguments about the administration of chymopapain under *general anaesthesia* or under neuroleptic analgesia appear to have been resolved in favour of the latter method. Attitudes to the use of *discography* have swung between two absolutes, either contraindication or indispensability. The real danger with the use of discography appears to be the over diagnosis of disc prolapses bearing in mind that leakage of dye into the spinal canal is not necessarily an indication of the presence of a disc prolapse into the spinal canal. Discography is essential before the injection of any neucleolytic agent into the intervertebral discs for one reason only; *if the discography gives rise to venography of the epidural veins, then this should constitute an absolute contra-indication to the injection of chymopapain,* which may then find its way into the epidural venous system and produce major neurological complications such as paraplegia, quadriplegia, or sub-arachnoid haemorrhage.

Chymopapain is still widely used in Europe particularly in France, Belgium and Germany. In the recent monograph Focus on Chemonucleolysis, Bonneville (1988), the complications of neucleolysis are discussed and the statement made on page 105 "The paraparetic and paraplegic syndromes are only found in the North American series". This suggests an immunity on the part of Europeans to these complications. This statement is difficult to accept on a scientific basis, particularly when the real mechanism of the causation of these complications has remained unexplained.

b) Technique for Surgery

i) Pre-Operative Preparation

These routines are set out in Chapter 10. X-rays of the patient's spine should always be available in the operating theatre.

ii) Anaesthesia

General anaesthesia with muscular relaxation and mechanical ventilation is most commonly employed. Cardiac monitoring is recommended.

iii) Positioning

Of all the factors which may be critical to the success of this operation, none is more important than the position in which the patient is placed before operation commences. A variety of suitable postures is shown in the following illustrations (Figs. 3.16–3.19).

Prone Position

The most versatile and easily managed is the prone position. A supporting sponge rubber U-piece is simple to construct and inexpensive. The right arm is shown dependent and supported on a well-padded arm rest which is suspended below the level of the table. Ulnar neuritis may occur unless the arm is carefully postured in this way. The left arm may rest by the patient's side. The table is angled in the centre. The surgeon's assistant and other observers will have unobstructed views of procedures throughout the course of the operation. The entire range of surgical manoeuvres that may be required for the execution of even the most complex operation, including trans-dural excision of prolapsed disc tissue, can be accomplished in comfort and without undue constraints on the duration of the operation.

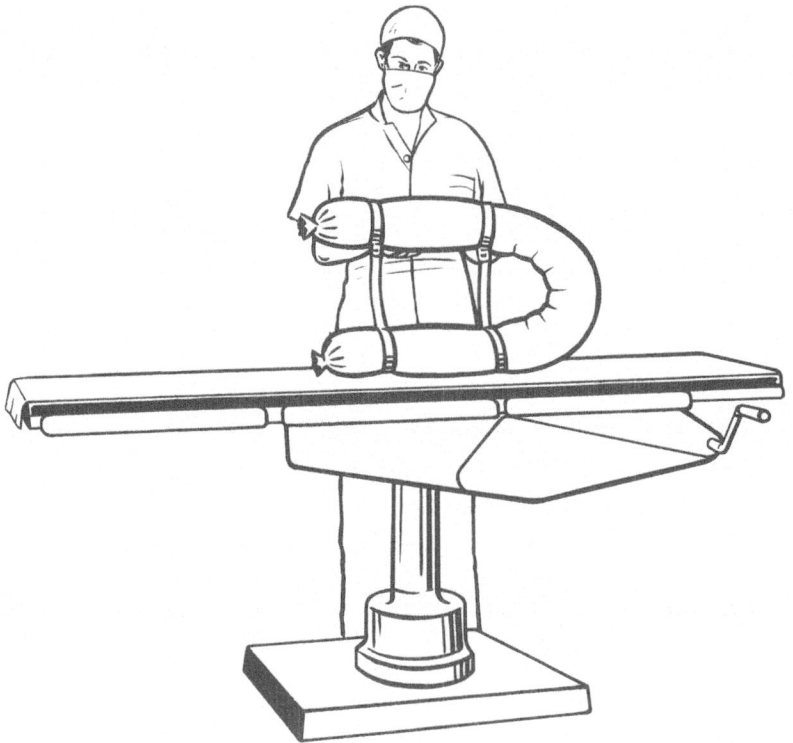

Figure 3.16. A drawing illustrating a simple supporting sponge rubber "U"-piece

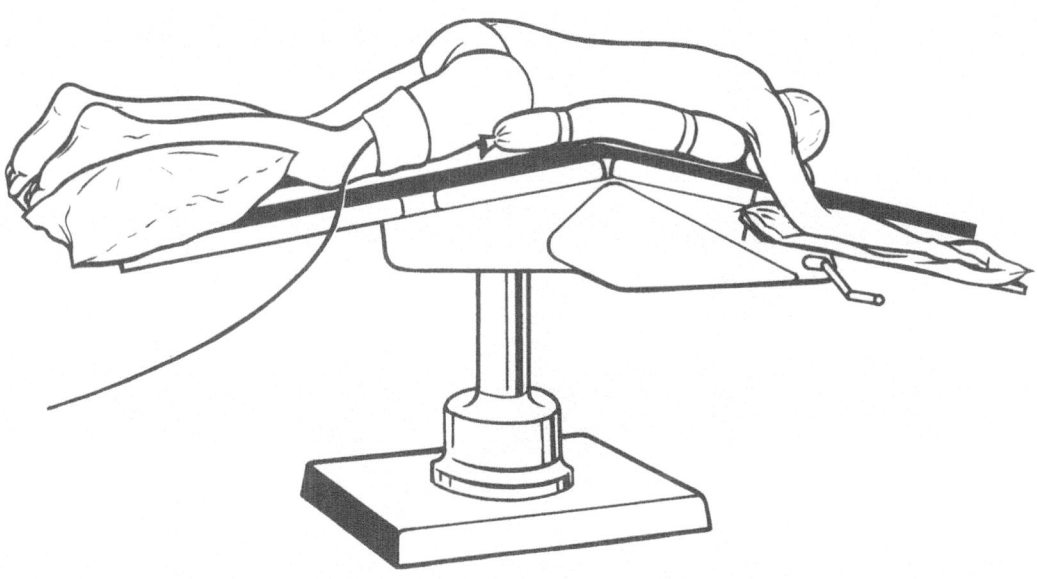

Figure 3.17. The posturing of the patient on this "U"-piece. The right arm is shown dependent and supported on a well-padded arm rest which is suspended below the level of the table. Ulnar neuritis may occur unless the arm is carefully postured in this way. The left arm may rest by the patient's side. The table is angled in the centre

Kneeling Position

In this position, with the use of a simple frame to support the buttocks, excellent operating conditions are provided. Use of this posture can only be recommended for operations of short duration. Alternatively, the patient may be placed in this position with pillows under the chest so that the abdomen is unsupported. A pillow is placed under the patient's feet and a restraining strap across the legs, though venous obstruction in the lower limbs is then likely to occur. The table is angled. The major objections to the use of this particular posture revolve around the difficulties of setting the patient in position and of dealing with emergencies, which may require the patient to be turned rapidly into a supine position. Particular attention should be paid to the ulnar nerves in this position.

Lateral Position

The use of this position can be recommended in special circumstances, for example, when the patient is extremely obese or when there are special chest problems which may complicate anaesthesia. A pillow should be placed between the patient's legs, a restraining strap crossing the iliac crest, and a sandbag placed above the dependent iliac crest. The table is angled in the centre. There are objections to the routine use of this position: (i) the assistant surgeon is rarely comfortable and has a restricted view of the operation field; (ii) lighting of the wound area may be difficult; (iii) haemorrhage control is often more difficult to obtain as is access to the nerve root canal on the dependent side of the spine.

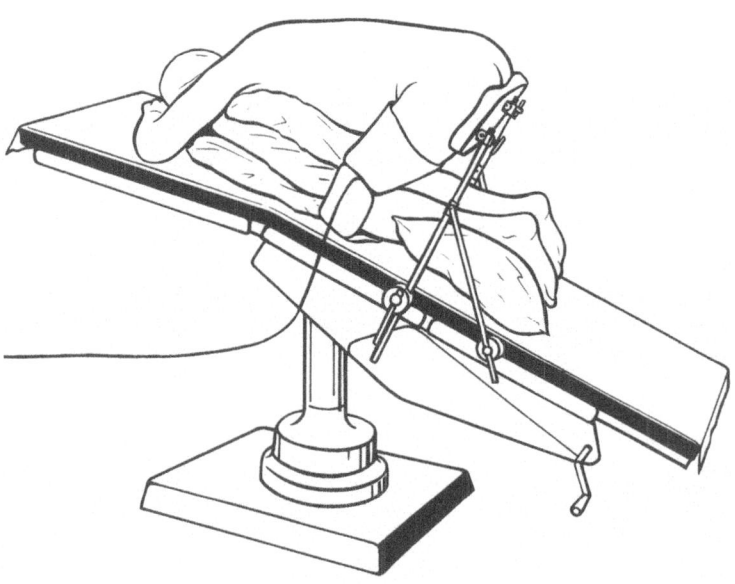

Figure 3.18. A drawing depicting the kneeling position. A simple frame is used to support the buttocks

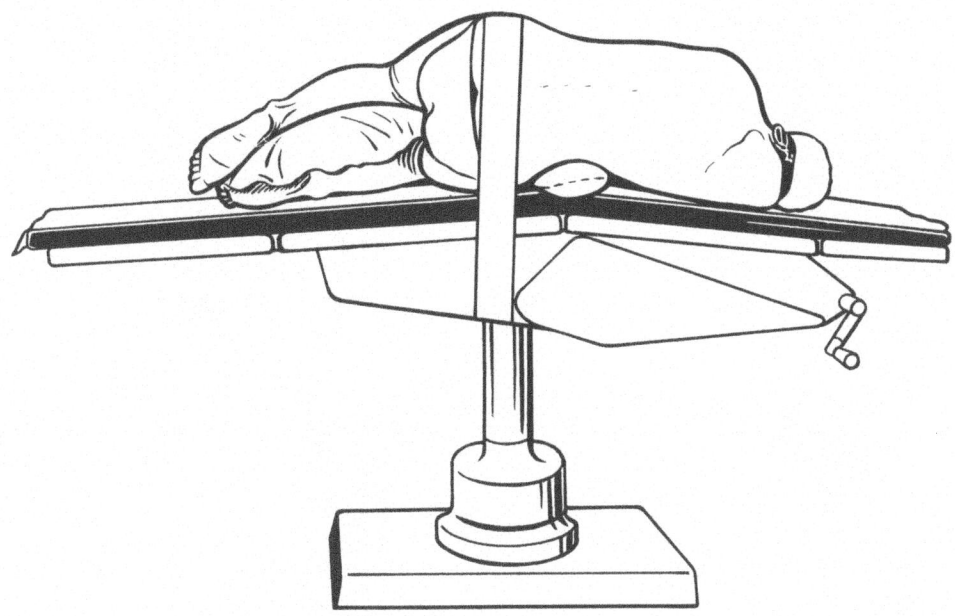

Figure 3.19. The lateral position. The use of this position can be recommended in special circumstances, for example, when the patient is extremely obese or when there are special chest problems which may complicate anaesthesia. Note the pillow between the patient's legs, the restraining strap crossing the iliac crest, the sandbag placed above the dependent iliac crest. The table is angled in the centre. There are objections to the routine use of this position: 1. the assistant surgeon is rarely comfortable and has a restricted view of the operative field; 2. lighting of the wound area may be difficult; 3. haemorrhage control is often more difficult to obtain, as is access to the nerve root canal on the dependent side of the spine

iv) Instruments (Figs. 3.20–3.21)

The recommended essential special instruments and disposable supplies are listed below:

1. Self-retaining retractors.
2. Fine sucker.
3. Bayonet forceps.
4. Long-handled carrier for size 11 or 15 blade scalpel.
5. Watson-Cheyne probe.
6. Nerve root retractor, such as a Scaglietti probe (10 inches–25 cm long).
7. A range of bone rongeurs.
8. A range of pituitary-type rongeurs, straight, angled outwards at 45 degrees and at 90 degrees with cutting tips of varying dimensions.
9. Hammer.
10. Fine osteotomes and chisels.
11. Ring curettes.
12. 6/0 suture material on fine cutting needles with a fine needle holder.
13. Patties and haemostatic gauze or sponge materials.
14. Bone wax.
15. Bi-polar coagulator.

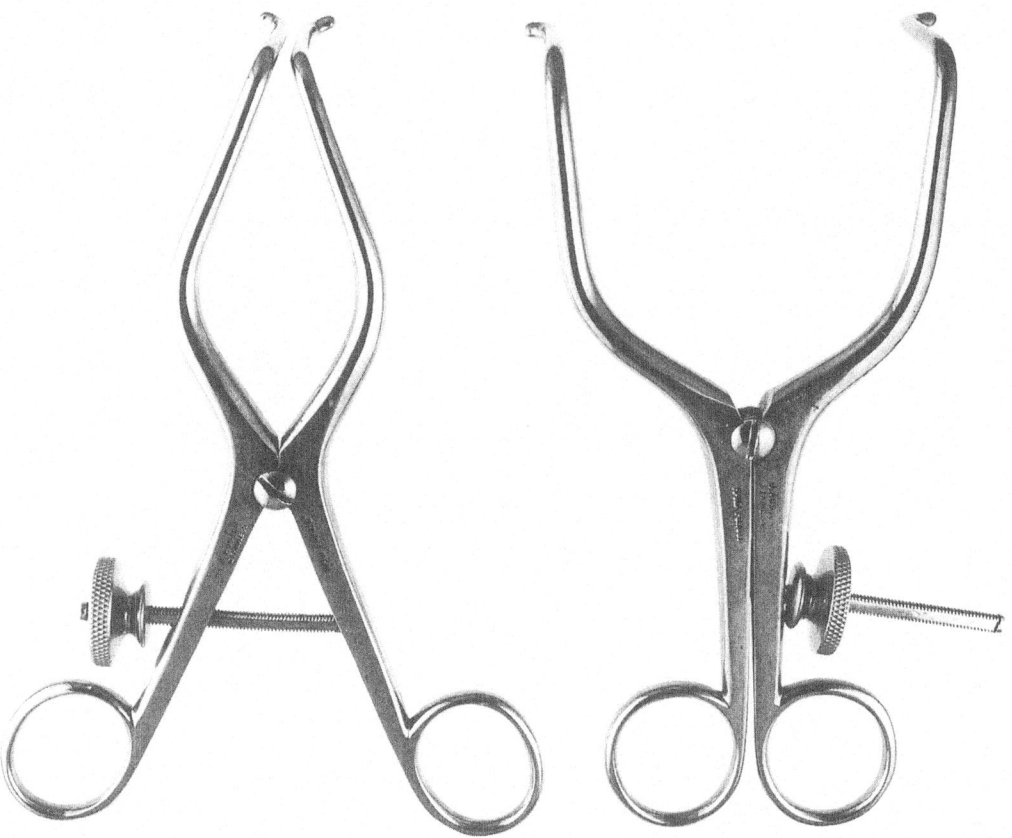

Figure 3.20. A photograph showing the modified Gelpi retractors, which are recommended for use in almost any situation where the spinal canal is to be explored

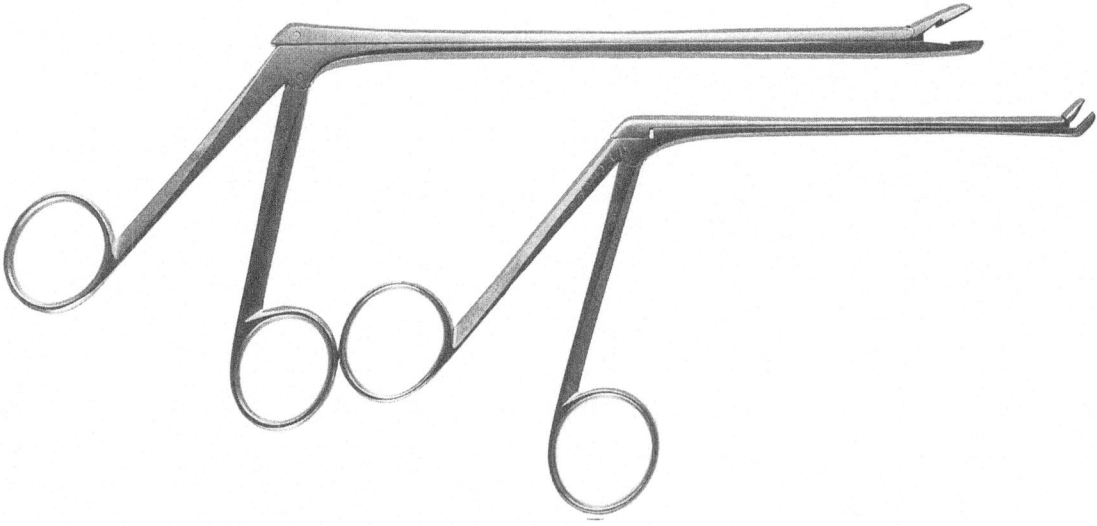

Figure 3.21. A photograph of straight and angled pituitary rongeurs which should be available in various shaft lengths and cup sizes for use in the surgery of disc prolapses

Before the skin incision is made the surgeon should once again inspect the patient's X-rays, paying attention to vertebral anomalies, such as spina bifida occulta and sacralization and noting certain lesions such as spondylolisthesis or isolated disc resorption. The level of the planned exposure of the spine should be noted.

Radiographs of the lumbar spine taken in the operating theatre are often of poor quality and cannot, therefore, be relied upon to identify a particular spinal level.

v) Incision

The skin incision is made in the mid-line or slightly to the right or left of the spinous processes, extending longitudinally a short distance above and below the vertebral interspace to be explored. It is deepened at once through the subcutaneous fat layer to the level of the lumbo-dorsal fascia. In extremely obese patients the depth of the subcutaneous fat layer between the skin and the lumbo-dorsal aponeurosis over the lumbo-sacral area may be 12 cm or more. In such cases this fatty tissue should be carefully handled, avoiding excessive burning with the coagulating diathermy (see "Wound Closure", pp. 144, 145).

vi) Separation of the Paraspinal Muscles

An incision is made in the lumbo-dorsal aponeurosis on one side of the tip of the spinous process approximately 5 mm from the mid-line using the cutting current diathermy passed through a suitable blade-shaped end. The lumbo-dorsal aponeurosis is a thin shining silvery membrane, the fibres of which are orientated largely transversely. This structure acts as an extensor mechanism in lumbar spinal movement through its attachments to the powerful latissimus dorsi and abdominal wall muscles (Fig. 3.22).

Immediately beneath it are the silvery vertically orientated fibres of the sacrospinalis aponeurosis (Fig. 3.23). The incision continues proximally and distally adjacent to the sides of the spinous processes and parallel to the interspinous ligaments. Some bleeding will occur at this stage from posterior branches of the lumbar arteries related to the middle of the side of each spinous process. The muscle mass may be retracted with a closed dissecting forceps placed into the depth of the space, so that the diathermy blade may cut the musculo-tendinous attachments from the inferior surfaces of the spinous processes and laminal margins and from the interspinous ligaments near their bases. Throughout this procedure the smoke generated by the diathermy cutting tip may be evacuated with a sucker.

The muscle mass is next separated from the outer surface of each lamina using an appropriate elevator such as the Cobb, taking care to preserve the periosteum of the lamina. *This manoeuvre should be carried out cautiously and sub-periosteal dissection avoided as this inflicts unnecessary damage to the laminal blood supply.* Following the use of the muscle elevator which raises the paraspinal muscles laterally to the level of the apophyseal joint capsule, which should be carefully preserved, further bleeding may be encountered from posterior branches of the lumbar arteries and veins in this area. Bleeding is readily controlled following insertion of cotton Raytec swabs, (bearing X-ray markers), packed into the depths of the wound along its length. When these are removed later, a few individual bleeding vessels may need to be coagulated with diathermy.

If necessary the same approach is then repeated on the opposite side of the spinous processes, preserving the interspinous ligaments until the paraspinal muscle mass has been similarly separated from the roof of the spinal canal. Cotton Raytec swabs are again inserted and a self-retaining retractor of the surgeons's choice is then prepared for insertion. When a small unilateral disc prolapse is to be removed, special retractors are available which will permit exposure of the interlaminar space on one side only. These vary from speculum shaped instruments to retractors with one narrow blade coupled with a probe-like limb. These are advocated by surgeons who practise micro-discectomy or so called minimal intervention surgery.

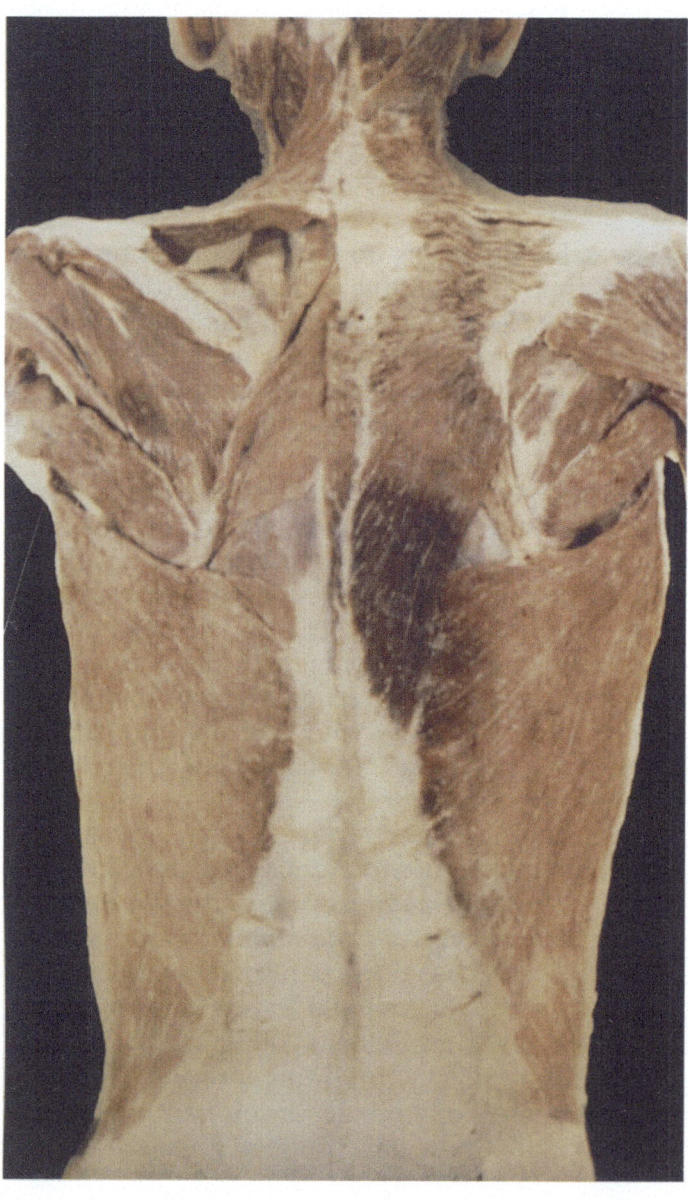

Figure 3.22

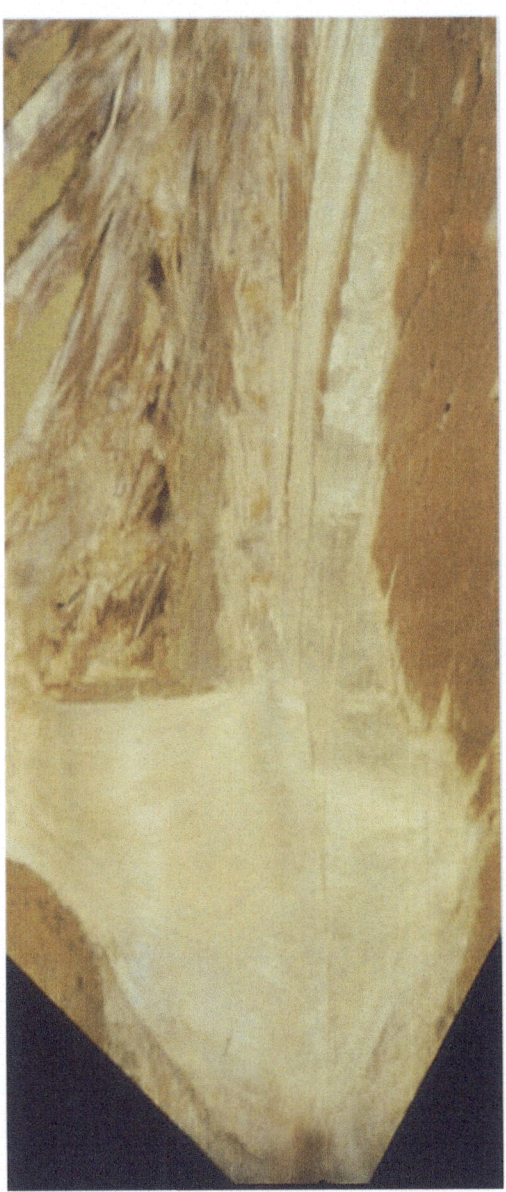

Figure 3.23. A photograph of a dissection of the lumbo-sacral spine seen from behind. In the lower half of the specimen on the left side, the intact thoraco-lumbar fascia is seen with its shining silver fibres orientated largely transversely. Above this the paraspinal muscles have been removed. On the right side the cut edge of the thoraco-lumbar fascia is visible. Beneath this thin membrane the vertically orientated aponeurotic fibres of the sacrospinalis muscles can be seen. [Reproduced with permission of the editor John E. Nixon from: Spinal Stenosis, p. 21, London: Edward Arnold, 1991]

Figure 3.22. A photograph of a dissection of the muscles of the back to show the large triangular shaped lumbo-dorsal aponeurosis, the apex of which extends up towards to the mid-thoracic spine, the base of which lies across the iliac crests inferiorly. The attachments of the latissimus dorsi and abdominal muscles to its lateral edge on both sides can be seen. (Photographed with the permission of the Dean of the Faculty of Medicine Professor Graham Ryan in the University of Melbourne)

Unless the technique described is followed carefully, considerable blood loss may occur, even during this preliminary stage of the approach to the disc prolapse (Figs. 3.24, 3.25). Presuming both sides of an intervertebral disc space are to be exposed the cotton Raytec swabs are removed from the lower end of the wound on either side of the spinous process. Hand held retractors expose the back of the sacrum allowing the first self-retaining retractor to be inserted and fixed in place. This procedure is repeated at the upper end of the wound and a second self retaining retractor inserted.

When the self-retaining retractors have been positioned, the surgeon should take note of the time of their application. *These instruments obstruct the circulation in the separated paraspinal muscles. At the end of an hour they should be removed for*

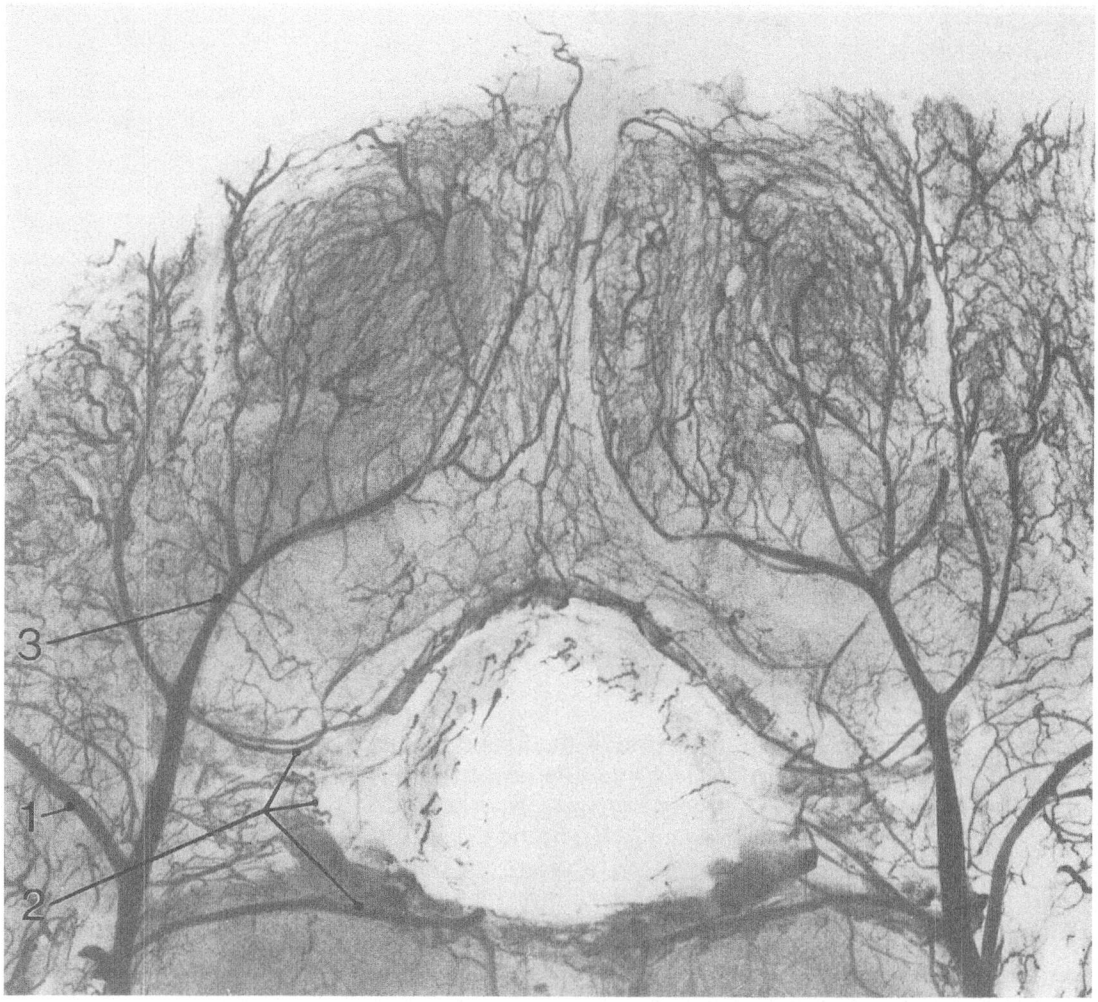

Figure 3.24. A thin transverse section to show details of the arterial distribution in relation to the spinal canal, the vertebral body in front and the lamina and spinous process behind. At the level of the intervertebral foramen, note: *1* the anterior abdominal wall branches; *2* the intermediate or spinal canal branches; and *3* posterior to the intervertebral foramen, the posterior branches in relation to the lamina and spinous process

about five minutes to prevent muscle damage. During the rest period the wound should be irrigated with Ringer's solution or normal saline.

At this stage Raytec swabs are again packed firmly along one of the paraspinal gutters while attention is focussed on the opposite side to identify the lumbo-sacral junction. Soft tissue remnants of muscle fibres and fat are then removed from the interspace which is to be opened. This cleaning up process should involve the use of the sucker through which fatty tissue can be removed. The sucker should then be used as a retractor placed inferior to the shining silvery facet joint capsule in the region of the pars interarticularis of the inferior lamina. While the sucker is being manipulated in the left hand the surgeon may then use either a curette or a straight pituitary rongeur with an appropriate sized cup to take off the muscle remnants from

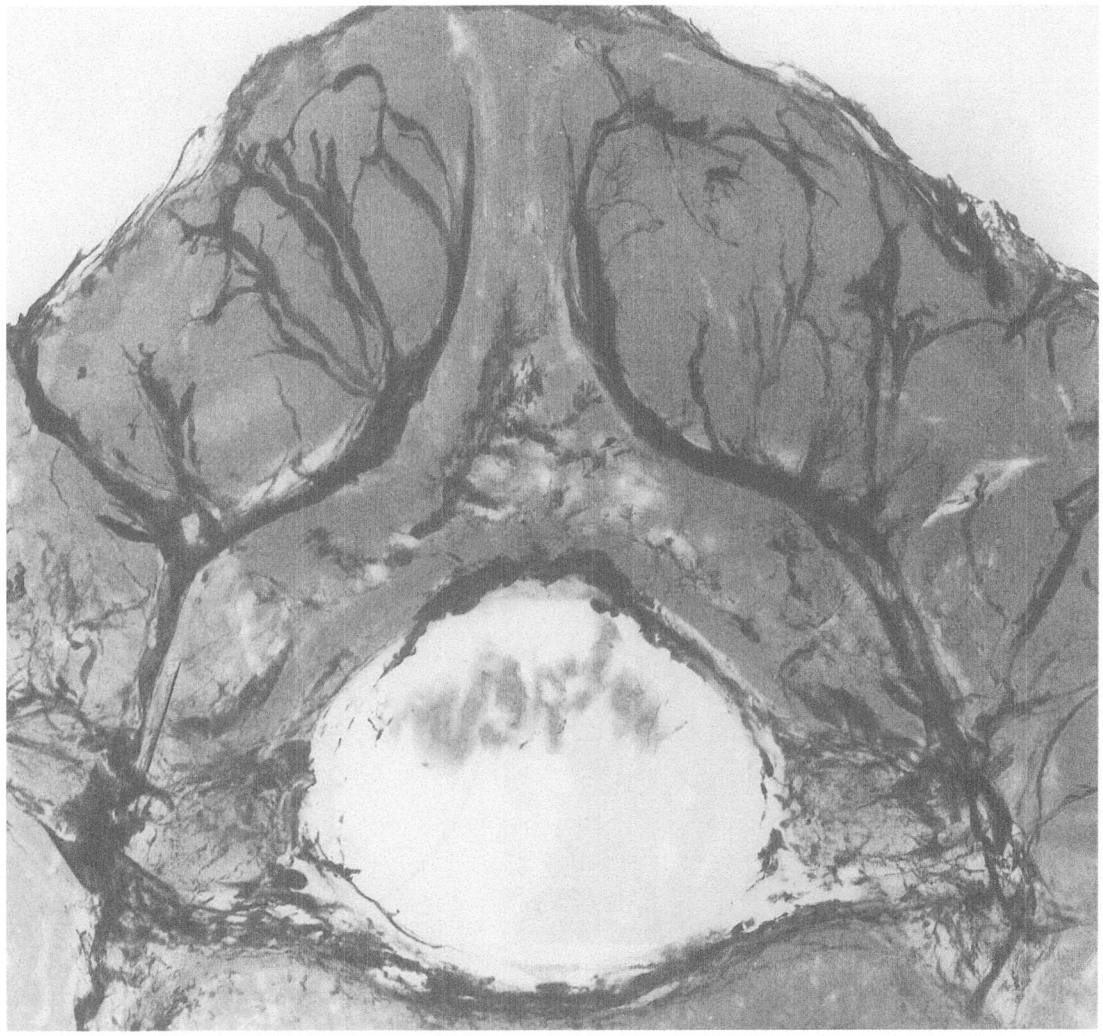

Figure 3.25. A radiograph of a transverse section of a lumbar vertebra from an adult to show the relations of the main stems of the lumbar veins (posterior external vertebral venous plexus) to the spinous process and lamina. [Reproduced by courtesy of J. B. Lippincott and Company from: Clin. Orthop. Rel. Res., No. 115 (1976)]

the interspinous ligament and the adjacent laminal margins together with remnants of soft tissues from the posterior surface of the ligamentum flavum.

Bleeding should not be a problem during these manoeuvres providing the sucker tip is used as a retractor in the manner described. On the other hand if fatty tissues and muscle remnants are *removed inferior and lateral to the facet joints* at individual interspaces profuse haemorrhage may be precipitated and the resultant efforts to control it with diathermy have the potential to inflict serious damage not only on the blood supply of the muscle but on the blood supply of the nerve root in the intervertebral foramen.

The main stem of the posterior branch of the lumbar artery is found constantly at the middle of the outer edge of the pars interarticularis. From it, arcuate branches pass upwards and downwards towards the capsules of the apophyseal joints (Figs. 3.26 a, b, 3.27). Haemorrhage points are easily identified although care must be

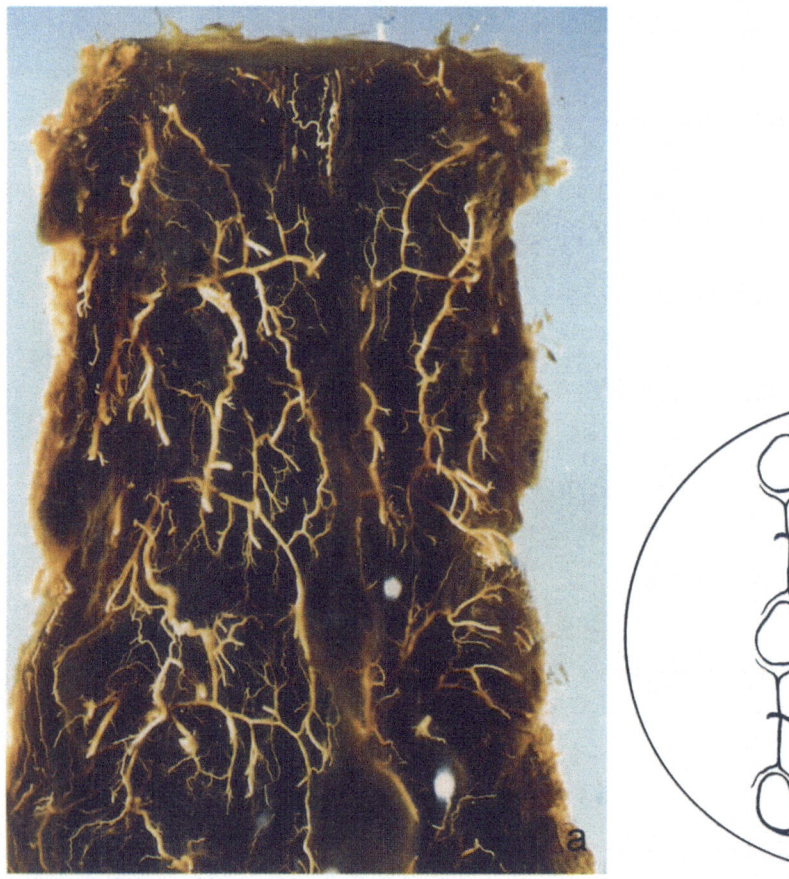
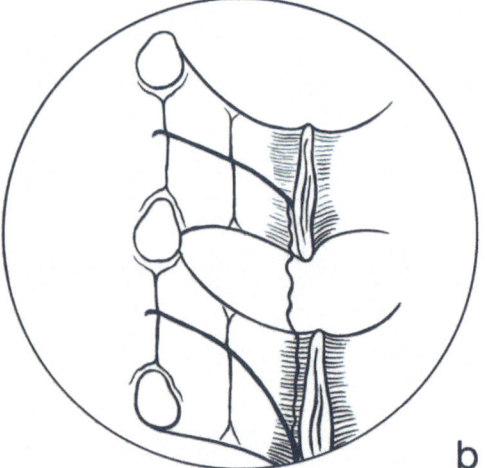

Figures 3.26 a, b. A photograph of the posterior aspect of the upper lumbar spine of an adult prepared by the Spalteholz method, following injection of the lumbar aorta. The specimen is slightly tilted to the right side to provide a clear view of the posterior spinal branches of three adjacent lumbar arteries. An explanatory diagram is shown alongside, in which the main course of each lumbar artery across the back of the lamina and up the middle of the spinous process is shown with its ascending and descending vertical muscular branches and the arcuate systems formed around the facet joints

taken not to diathermy the main stem far anterior to the anterior margin of the pars interarticularis. Damage to entrant neural arteries at the intervertebral foramen is thereby avoided. The main stem of the posterior branch of each lumbar artery is accompanied by the corresponding and somewhat larger vein (Crock and Yoshizawa, 1977).

In cases where exposure of both sides of the interspace may be required, the detailed clearing process just described is completed on the opposite side. At this stage, it will be noted that there are some silvery *capsular fibres* extending medially on to the yellow *ligamentum flavum* for some distance at its upper margin where it passes beneath the inferior margin of the superior lamina of the interspace (Fig. 3.28). These fibres should be incised at their inferior laminal attachment and then removed with a straight pituitary rongeur from below, the jaws of which should be directed beneath the superior laminal margin, parallel to its anterior surface.

Portions of the inferior surface of the superior lamina at the interspace may need to be excised using an outward-angled rongeur. Some surgeons favour the use of chisels or gouges for this particular manoeuvre. Bone wax may be applied to the cut surface of the cancellous bone to control bleeding (Fig. 3.29).

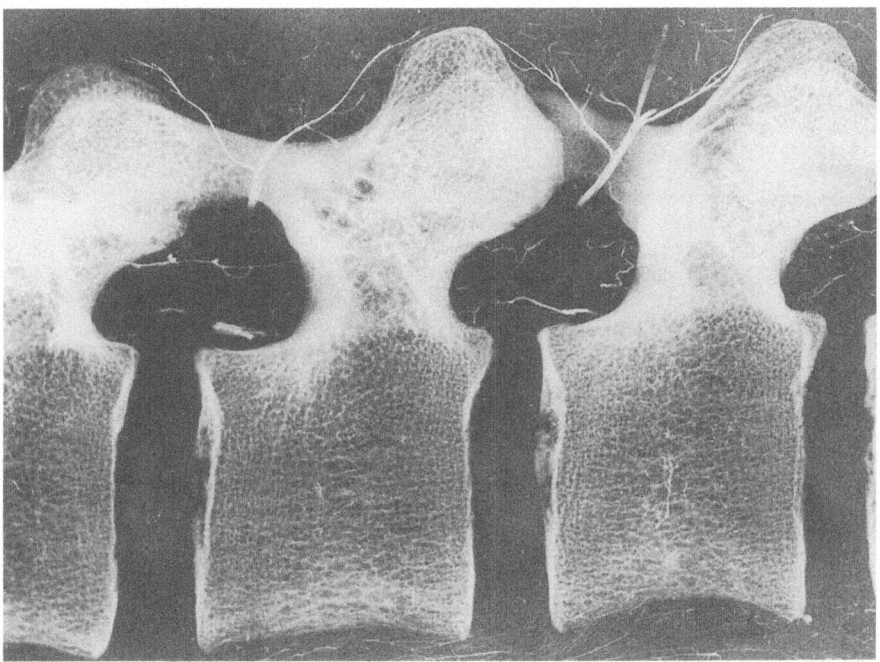

Figure 3.27. A radiograph of a thin sagittal section of the lumbar spine, showing the relations of the posterior branches of two lumbar arteries as they course backwards behind the intervertebral foramina. These arteries are constant lateral relations of the pars interarticularis of each lamina. In the intervertebral foramen shown on the left, the anterior and posterior spinal canal branches of the lumbar artery can be seen, separated by a clear band, this area being occupied by the nerve root at that level. Note also the branches which encircle the facet joint system and supply it. [Reproduced by courtesy of J. B. Lippincott and Company from: Clin. Orthop. Rel. Res., No. 115 (1976)]

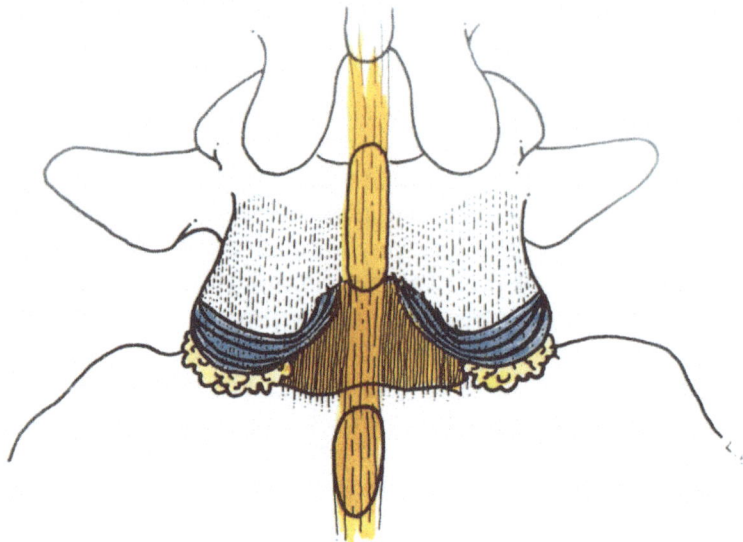

Figure 3.28. A drawing depicting the relations of the ligamentum flavum. The extra-synovial fat pads are shown in exaggerated form. Note the extension of capsular fibres on to the posterior surface of the ligamentum flavum and adjacent inferior laminal margins

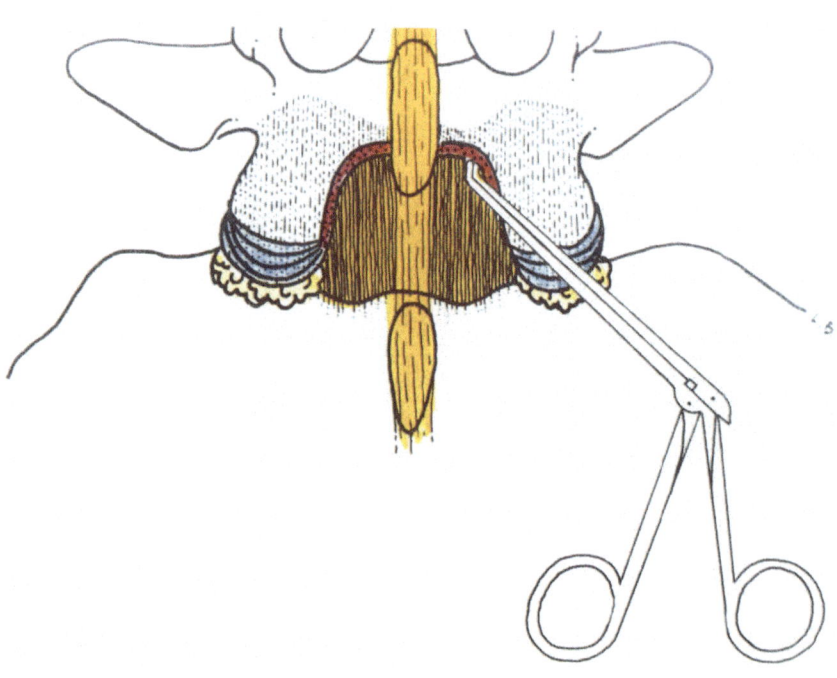

Figure 3.29. A drawing showing the method of removal of portions of the inferior surface of the superior lamina at the interspace, using an outward-angled rongeur. In some cases the interspinous ligament may be removed along with a portion of the inferior surface of the spinous process at the upper level of the interspace

vii) Opening of Spinal Canal

This can be performed in a number of ways. Two techniques will be described, one using a fine toothed forceps and small scalpel blade such as a number 11 or number 15, the other combining the use of a 45 degree forward-angled curette with a 2 mm cup with the use of a fine toothed forceps and scalpel of appropriate size.

a)

The ligamentum flavum may be incised vertically in the mid line. The cut edge is picked up with a fine toothed forceps and the incision deepened until either epidural fat or the dura itself is exposed. The blunt end of a Watson Cheyne dissector may then be used to widen the opening into the spinal canal. Through the vertical split in the ligamentum flavum thus created a small moistened cotton patty is inserted between it and the epidural fat using the curved end of the dissector. The ligamentum flavum is then cut in a lateral direction, first at the lower edge of the interspace, until a flap is raised and turned out laterally and then along the upper edge of the interspace.

Even at this early stage of opening the spinal canal, the presence of a large prolapse can be suspected if the insertion of the patty or patties is difficult as they are pushed laterally under the ligamentum flavum.

When the ligamentum flavum has been turned laterally as a flap to the level of the apophyseal joint, a fourth incision is then commonly made in it, again in a vertical direction to excise the flap. Some surgeons simply raise a flap of ligamentum flavum and retract it laterally during the procedure allowing it to fall back into place at the end of the operation.

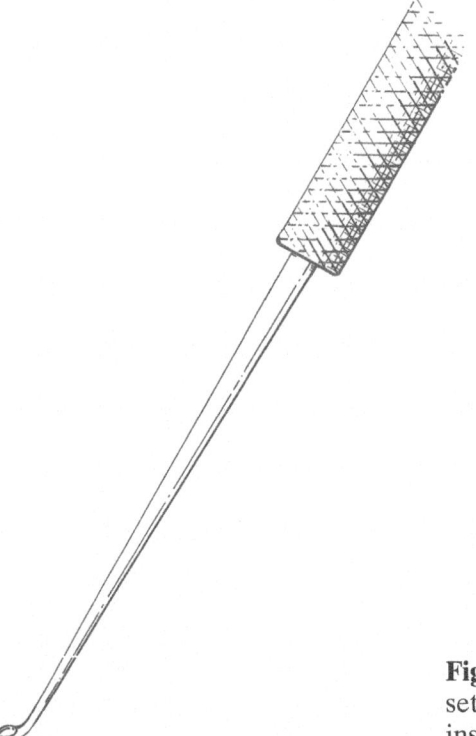

Figure 3.30. A drawing to show the 2 mm cupped curette set at an angle of about 45 degrees to the shaft of the instrument

b)

Using a 45 degree angled curette with a 2mm cup the thin inferior fibres of the ligamentum flavum which overlap the superior margin of the inferior lamina can be scraped off defining the superior margin of this lamina. The angle of the curette is then changed so that the curette is passed into the spinal canal immediately to the anterior surface of the lamina and moved from lateral to medial side until the inferior attachment of the ligamentum flavum lies free. This done, a 45 degree angled rongeur may be inserted allowing removal of a small portion of the upper margin of the inferior lamina (Figs. 3.31,3.32).

The free edge of the ligamentum flavum can then be grasped with a fine toothed forceps and the blunt end of a Watson Cheyne dissector inserted with a small patty allowing the safe dissection of the ligamentum flavum and its removal either with the use of a fine scalpel or piece-meal with an angled pituitary rongeur, the epidural fat and dura being held out of the way with a patty and sucker. This second method of removal of the ligamentum flavum is particularly applicable in cases of spinal stenosis where gross pathological changes have occurred in the ligamentum flavum,

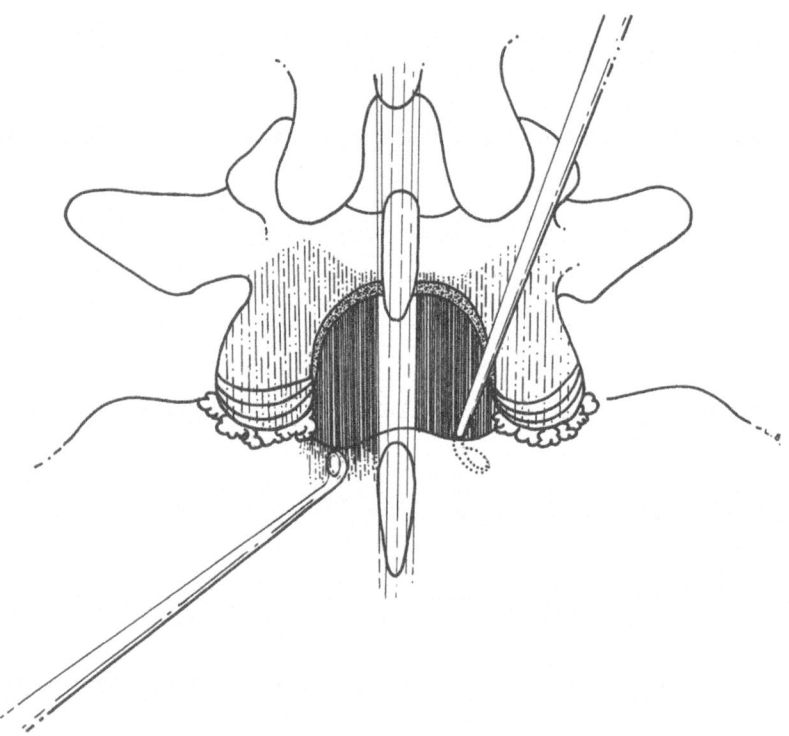

Figure 3.31. A drawing depicting on the left side the method of using the curette to remove the superficial fibres of the ligamentum flavum which pass on to the dorsal surface of S1 lamina just beyond its superior margin. On the right side following removal of these loosened fragments of ligamentum flavum the curette is introduced cautiously beneath the superior margin of the S1 lamina and manipulated from medial to lateral side to free the attachment of the ligamentum flavum from the bone

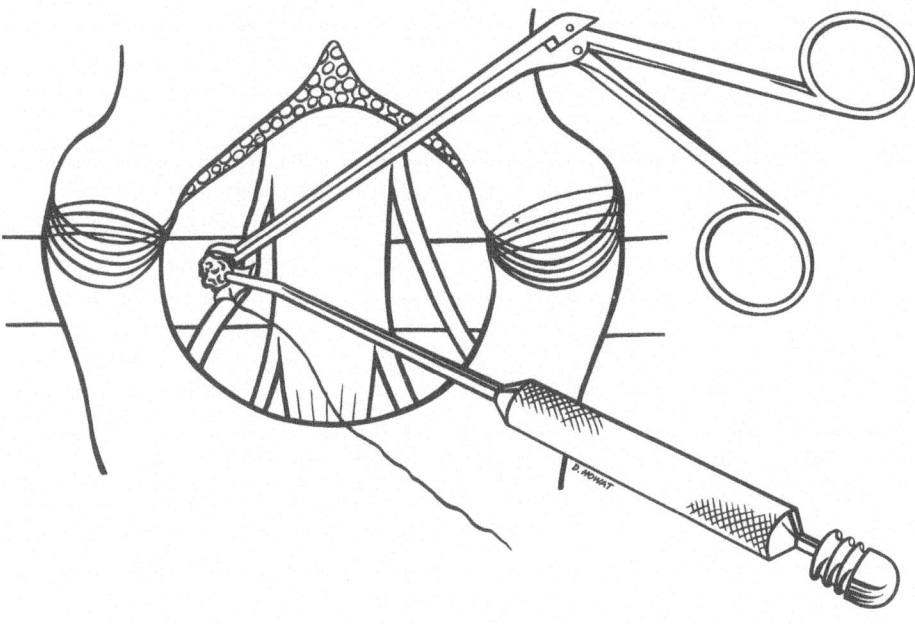

Figure 3.32. A drawing depicting the disposition of the sucker and patty and straight pituitary rongeur at the time of removal of a fragment of prolapsed tissue

rendering it thickened, atrophic or calcified. In such circumstances dural injury is less likely to occur with the use of this technique.

Following this initial opening into the spinal canal, the surgeon must then identify certain landmarks. The Watson-Cheyne probe is invaluable for this purpose. Either the blunt or curved end may be inserted depending on the size of the protrusion at the affected level. If the prolapse is small, then the blunt end may be inserted laterally so that the pedicle on the inferior side of the intervertebral disc space may be palpated. The regional nerve root is then palpated. Moving upwards, the posterior surface of the disc may be felt and the disposition of a prolapse assessed.

viii) Extending Exposure

Wider exposure may be required and this is usually most easily achieved with a 45 degree outward-angled rongeur. Assuming, for example, that it is necessary to remove more of the outer edge of the ligamentum flavum, then the sucker with a moistened patty on its tip may be used to retract the dura and nerve roots towards the mid-line, while the rongeur is inserted beneath the edge of the ligamentum flavum under direct vision. Depending on the size of the prolapse, it may or may not be possible to insert the angled rongeur. If attempts are made to force the foot-plate of the rongeur between the ligamentum flavum and the nerve root which is being pressed backwards by a large disc prolapse, the root may be bruised or crushed. On occasions, even a thin rongeur cannot be inserted. The interspace will then need to be enlarged, either superiorly or inferiorly or in both directions, until sufficient space has been created to allow identification of the nerve root as it traverses the interspace.

With a large sub-rhizal prolapse at the L5/S1 level, for example, it may be necessary to enlarge the interspace by removal of part of the superior border of the lamina of S1, commencing initially in the mid-line and passing laterally, and to perform a decompression of the S1 nerve root canal by removing the medial portion of the S1 facet flush with the inner margin of the S1 pedicle. In the operation of nerve root canal decompression, the apex of the facet also needs to be removed (see p. 35).

ix) Management of Venous Haemorrhage

During the more complicated manoeuvres of this type, haemorrhage from the internal vertebral venous plexus surrounding the nerve root and lateral to it may occur. This haemorrhage is usually not troublesome when the patient is in the prone position. On occasions, however, the internal vertebral venous plexus may be distended and brisk venous haemorrhage may occur following damage to some of the radicular branches of this system of veins. The detailed anatomy of the anterior internal vertebral venous plexus in the lumbar region is described on pp. 19, 20. Venous haemorrhage is always readily controlled with the gentle use of a patty and sucker as illustrated in Fig. 3.32. Occasionally, bleeding from one of the large venous radicles can be troublesome and it may be necessary to identify this using the sucker and a patty. The bleeding points are grasped with the bayonet forceps and coagulated with low-voltage or bipolar coagulating currents.

At other times, bleeding from several points of the plexiform system of veins can be controlled by light packing with a haemostatic substance held in place with a moistened patty.

Bleeding should be minimal, and good exposure of the field obtained before any attempt is made to retract the nerve root for the final exposure of prolapsed disc material.

x) Excision of Disc Tissue

For the sake of clarity and brevity, special points of technique will be described in relation to individual types of disc prolapse.

Small Sub-Rhizal Prolapse

Partial excision of the ligamentum flavum on one side will afford satisfactory access to the canal. Initially, identification of the landmarks of pedicle, disc and affected nerve root is made using the sucker and patty as a medial retractor and the blunt end of the Watson-Cheyne dissector in the lateral part of the canal.

Blunt dissection will separate the epidural fat, and the nerve root can usually be easily retracted medially. The discrete rounded prolapse with intact annular fibres is then outlined and a suitable root retractor inserted. The surgeon may use the sucker with a moist patty on its tip as a retractor laterally in the interspace while the assistant holds the nerve root medially. In a dry field it should then be possible to incise the annular fibres over the prolapse in a cruciate fashion using a No. 11 or 15 blade scalpel. The prolapsed tissue then begins to emerge spontaneously and it may be picked out with a straight pituitary rongeur of appropriate dimension varying from 1 to 4 mm bite.

Only a small volume of disc tissue can be removed in such cases and curettage of the interspace is not recommended.

Large Sub-Rhizal Prolapse

In such cases, adequate exposure on the side of the prolapse is essential. Technical details for the enlargement both superiorly and inferiorly have been outlined above. Identification of the affected root may be a problem, because in such circumstances the root is often flattened and its lateral margin not easily identified, being of the same colour as the disc prolapse beneath it. Use of an operating loop may be helpful, as it is essential under such circumstances to identify the nerve root sleeve at its junction with the dura above or to identify the main stem of the nerve root at the level of the inferior pedicle. By either method, with the use of an appropriate nerve root dissector, the outer edge of the nerve root can be identified and retracted medially. Very fine straight and curved pituitary rongeurs will be required in such a case to *remove the first of the fragments* of prolapsed tissue, possibly through a minute incision in intact annular fibres. Only after the initial removal of fragments with small instruments will it become possible to complete the dissection and retraction of the nerve root medially from the bulk of the prolapse.

As the tension on the nerve root is released, its retraction becomes easier. The opening in the annular fibres may be enlarged under vision and rongeurs of increasing cup size inserted for removal of free disc fragments from the interspace. The sucker with a patty on the end of it may be used as a retractor held by the surgeon in his left hand, while with the rongeur in his right hand, the fragments are lifted out from the interspace (Fig. 3.30). In such cases, quite large amounts of the disc material may be removed, but the risk of penetration of rongeurs deep into the interspace with the possibility of damage to intra-abdominal structures is high (Fig. 3.33 a, b). The use of ring curettes is recommended in such cases for curettage of loose disc fragments and vertebral end-plate material. *When large amounts of disc material have been removed, of the order of several grams of tissue, then it is wise to perform nerve root canal and foraminal decompressions on both sides of the interspace,* completing removal of ligamentum flavum far laterally and of the inner margins of the superior articular facets of the inferior vertebra, to the level of the inner margins of the pedicles. In addition, with angled rongeurs it may be necessary to remove the apices of both the superior facets on the inferior side of the interspace. *Excision of the whole facet joint in the course of this operation must be avoided.*

The Management of Sequestrated Disc Fragments

Free fragments of disc tissue in the spinal canal may pose specific problems at operation. If, for example, free fragments of disc tissue are found at the lumbo-sacral level, yet the posterior annular fibres of the L5/S1 disc space are found to be normal, exploration of the higher interspace is essential. In these circumstances careful palpation of the L5/S1 disc with the blunt end of the Watson Cheyne dissector, beneath the dural sac towards the mid-line, will be necessary before it can be safely assumed that the disc tissue has not prolapsed from that interspace. If, on the other hand, the L4/5 interspace has been exposed and a rather adherent nerve root re-

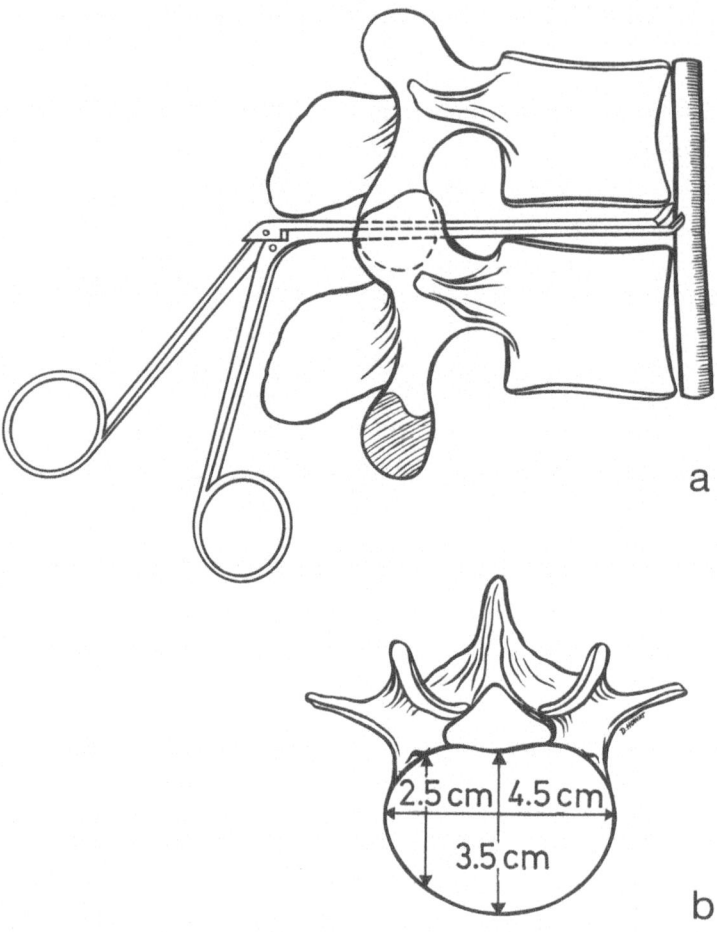

Figures 3.33a,b. a A drawing to highlight the potential danger of penetration of a rongeur through the disc space into the abdominal cavity where great vessels or other intra-abdominal structures may be injured. **b** A drawing to illustrate the dimensions of a lumbar vertebral body in an adult of average size

tracted from the back of the disc to reveal a circumscribed rounded defect in the annulus, then free sequestrated disc material may be found at the lower interspace. Identification of the orientation of sequestrated disc fragments has been greatly aided by MRI with gadolinium enhancement (Figs. 3.7a,b, 3.8a,b, 3.9).

Central Disc Prolapse

The presence of a central disc prolapse is usually, though not always, suspected in the early stages of opening of the spinal canal. For example, it may be opened on one side and the nerve root which comes into view cannot be retracted towards the midline, though the disc beneath and lateral to it appears normal. In such a case, digital palpation of the dural sac is essential and will lead the surgeon to establish this diagnosis. Wide exposure is then required even involving excision of the whole of the spinous process and central part of the arch of the lamina on the superior side of the interspace.

Trans-Dural Approach

Having determined to remove the fragments by a trans-dural approach, then the special instruments listed above must be available, especially the fine sutures and needle holders which will be required to repair the dural opening. In addition long lintine strips with attached threads should be available, as these may need to be placed along each edge of the dural sac to prevent seepage of blood into the sub-arachnoid space after the dura has been opened.

The dura is incised in the mid-line with a No. 15 blade scalpel and a protective probe or a bistoury introduced beneath the dura so that the incision in it can be completed over the desired length. *The use of low vacuum suction is essential,* the sucker tip being guarded by a small patty. Filaments of the cauda equina can be retracted easily to either side using smooth rounded instruments. *At no stage should an unguarded sucker be placed within the dural sac itself as a nerve root may be avulsed up the sucker.* The actual process of removal of disc tissue is usually easy and can be rapidly accomplished by the trans-dural route following separate incision of the dura and the posterior longitudinal ligament over the disc space. *The prolapsed tissue often emerges on one side of this ligament.*

Cerebrospinal fluid is allowed to escape. It should be aspirated from the wound, but at all times the sucker should now be covered with a patty. An inexperienced surgeon or an inexperienced assistant may, from any point onwards in this operation, inflict irreversible damage on filaments of the cauda equina. Remembering that the vessels of the cauda equina are minute, only smooth rounded instruments should be used to retract the filaments from the mid-line laterally on each side (Fig. 3.34).

Bearing these hazards in mind, the actual process of removal of disc tissue is easily and rapidly accomplished by the trans-dural route following separate incision of the dura and the posterior longitudinal ligament over the disc space. *It is likely, however, that the prolapse will have emerged on one side of this ligament.*

Depending on the volume of disc material that can be removed with straight or angled pituitary rongeurs of varying sizes, so the question of curettage of the disc

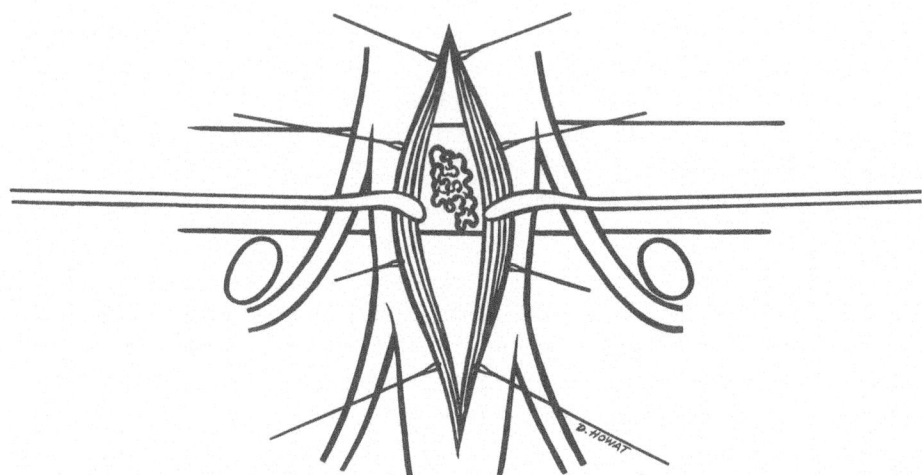

Figure 3.34. A drawing to illustrate exposure of a central disc prolapse trans-durally, filaments of the cauda equina being retracted from the mid-line laterally on each side with smooth rounded instruments

space may arise. If large quantities of disc material can be removed easily, it is wise to use a ring curette to clear other remnants, recalling once again the risk of instruments penetrating into the abdominal cavity.

Although some authors recommend closure of the anterior layer of the dural sac following this procedure, this is not always necessary. However, careful closure of the posterior layer should be effected using a continuous 6/0 dural stitch. The retaining sutures which were earlier inserted, are used to retract the dura in the final stages of closure and care is taken at all times to avoid transfixion of any of the cauda equina filaments in the closing suture.

In cases of this type, especially when many fragments of intervertebral disc tissue have been removed from the interspace, it is wise to perform bilateral nerve root canal decompression to complete the procedure, to prevent recurrence of sciatica later following reduction in height of the disc space.

xi) Disc Prolapses Associated with Other Special Problems

Spinal Canal Stenosis

This situation should be recognized pre-operatively in most instances, especially if myelography has been performed. The disc prolapses found in these cases are often small. It is essential to perform an adequate spinal or nerve root canal decompression on both sides in such cases.

Nerve Root and Other Anomalies

The recognition of nerve root and vascular anomalies requires excellent technique during the exposure. A lower lumbar nerve root sometimes arises from the dural sac at right angles, passing directly laterally through the intervertebral foramen across the posterior surface of the disc. Mistaken easily for a prolapse at operation, it may be incised, excised or avulsed in error.

Isolated Disc Resorption

Unilateral sciatica in cases of isolated disc resorption is not common (Crock, 1976). The most important part of the surgery for this condition is the nerve root canal decompression and "foraminotomy" which can usually be performed with preservation of the relevant laminal arch. The "disc prolapse" in such instances usually consists of a small fragment of vertebral end-plate cartilage, which may be adherent to the under-surface of the nerve root. Careful dissection is required to remove it, as the root may be flattened in these circumstances.

Spondylolisthesis

Disc prolapse may occur at the level of a spondylolisthesis or above it. Excision of the prolapsed disc fragments is essential, but questions of complete spinal canal and nerve root canal decompression including removal of the loose lamina, together with decisions on the use of spinal fusion techniques then arise.

xii) Upper Lumbar Disc Prolapse

Upper lumbar disc prolapses may occur in the L1/2, L2/3 area in association with the conus medullaris in some cases. Operations in this area carry hazards of spinal cord injury, and retraction of the dural sac must be performed with great care at all times. Similarly, the introduction of large-jawed rongeurs or large ring curettes may be hazardous. Extra-peritoneal approaches to these anterior prolapses can be recommended with confidence.

Microdiscectomy and Percutaneous Lumbar Discectomy

As indicated in the introductory paragraph in this chapter the use of minimal invasive procedures for disc surgery is increasing. Interested readers are referred to "The Principles of Microsurgery for Lumbar Disc Disease", McCulloch J., 1989, and to "Percutaneous Lumbar Discectomy" edited by Mayer M. H. and Broch M., 1989, listed in the bibliography.

xiii) Extra-Foraminal Disc Prolapse

This type of disc prolapse is uncommon, although it can be readily identified with CT scanning, CT discography, or MRI examination of the spine (Fig. 3.10).

The level of disc prolapse should be confirmed with control radiographs in the operating theatre. A short skin incision is made over the middle of the appropriate sacro-spinalis muscle mass. The thoraco-lumbar fascia is then split in the line of the skin incision and the muscle fibres beneath it separated by blunt dissection. Microsurgical type retractors can be inserted to expose the vertically orientated fibres of the intertransverse muscle. The medial border of this muscle is identified between the two transverse processes at their junctions with the pedicles. The fibres are separated from the upper surface of the inferior transverse process and retracted laterally. The nerve root is then seen where it lies outside the intervertebral foramen. An operating microscope is useful in deep dissection of this type, but it is not essential. With careful blunt dissection, the nerve root may be separated from the disc prolapse, which is removed in the usual manner, under vision. The main branches of the lumbar artery and its accompanying veins are intimately related to the lateral aspect of the emerging nerve root. They should be identified carefully with blunt dissection. Haemorrhage from them should not be a problem. However, in this situation diathermy should be used with extreme caution if bleeding becomes troublesome (see Figs. 1.19, 1.20 in Chapter 1).

xiv) Preserving the Bony Canal

In the past it has been common practice to cut a narrow channel in a lamina, between the two ligamenta flava related to it, while seeking an elusive disc prolapse. This interference with the roofing apparatus of the spinal canal is to be avoided, particularly in cases with spinal canal or nerve root canal stenosis, because it may lead to the development of stenosis of the canal following growth of new bone into the area of the laminal defect (see Chapter 9, pp. 302, 307). Exploration of an intervertebral disc space can be accurately and competently performed through a limited inter-laminar exposure, carried out along the lines recommended above. If no lesion is found at one level, due to error, then it is better to look at the next level upwards or downwards from the primary exploration without disturbing the integrity of the lamina. This problem should not arise if investigations of good quality have been obtained before surgery.

xv) Wound Closure

Haemostasis must be obtained before wound closure. Venous bleeding from the spinal canal can always be controlled with small pledgets of gelfoam or equivalent substances applied to the bleeding sites. Bleeding from the cut surfaces of bone is occasionally troublesome. It is readily stopped by applying bone wax to the oozing surfaces. When the self-retaining retractors are removed some bleeding points, arterial, venous or both, may be identified in the paraspinal muscles. These should be coagulated with diathermy.

Undue haste, poor haemorrhage control and careless handling of rongeurs or root retractors may lead to serious dural injuries. Indeed, dural tears may be inflicted even before the ligamentum flavum has been opened if rongeurs "slip" into the spinal canal.

Dural tears are most likely to occur in complicated cases, for example, where there is associated spinal canal stenosis and opening of the canal proves difficult, or again, in the course of separating an adherent root from a disc prolapse. These defects should be identified carefully and repaired with fine sutures. Extensile exposure of the dural sac and nerve roots may be required, involving removal of adjacent spinous processes and excision of the centre of one or more laminae. The partes interarticulares must always be preserved and facet joint capsules left intact.

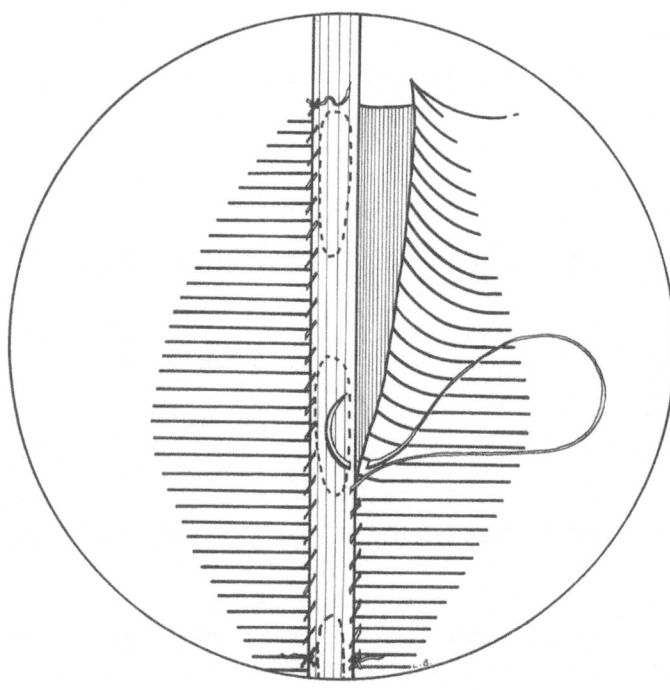

Figure 3.35. A drawing to show the recommended method of re-attachment of the lumbo-dorsal aponeurosis to the supraspinous ligaments using a continuous fine suture first on one side then on the other

Deep sutures should not be used to approximate the paraspinal muscles. The lumbo-dorsal aponeuroses should be sutured to the mid-line supra-spinous ligaments as shown in Fig. 3.35. Providing the spinous processes and the integrity of the interspinous ligaments has been preserved, drain tubes are not required.

The skin is best closed with fine absorbable subcuticular sutures such as 3-0 Dexon.

In extremely obese patients with thick layers of subcutaneous fat, the use of multiple sutures in this tissue should be avoided. Rough handling of it with forceps or retractors and the excessive use of diathermy to control bleeding from it will likely result in leakage of liquified fat from the wound post-operatively. Infection of this tissue plane may subsequently become troublesome. These problems can be prevented by closing the wound with a few widely separated tension sutures of heavy grade nylon mounted on long curved needles. A length of plastic or rubber tubing is threaded on to each suture so that the nylon having passed through the skin and full thickness of the fatty layer four centimetres on either side of the wound edge can be tied on one side of the tubing. The skin edges can then be brought together either with a subcuticular suture or with Steristrips[1]. Even with this special care, the dressings may become soaked with oedema fluid for several days after operation. The volume of this fluid leaking from such a wound can be surprisingly large and may raise the fear of a cerebrospinal fluid fistula. The wet dressings should be changed regularly, using aseptic technique, until the wound becomes dry.

---

[1] 3M Health Care Limited, 3M House, Morley Street, Loughborough, Leicestershire LE11 1EP.

4

Intervertebral Disc Calcification

4.1. Introduction

Although calcification of the nucleus pulposus is not a common pathological finding in intervertebral discs, it warrants discussion for a number of reasons.

4.2. Clinical Features

First of all, it is one of the few causes of acute excruciating spinal pain, the most common being pathological fractures, acute inflammatory lesions, some tumours and the vascular catastrophe of dissecting aortic aneurysm.

Secondly, paraplegia of sudden onset may complicate prolapse of calcified nuclear material into the thoracic spinal canal. This cause of paraplegia may go unrecognized if the calcified nuclear material is dispersed into the spinal canal where it may be difficult to see on plain X-rays. An erroneous diagnosis, such as acute ascending polyneuritis or vascular accident to the cord may then be made.

Thirdly, while Köhler and Zimmer (1968) have stated that it is relatively common in adults, the belief is widespread that it is of little clinical significance. Indeed, Nachemson (1976) included intervertebral disc calcification in a list of radiological findings in the lumbar spine which, in his view, have no significance as causes of low back pain.

Surgeons in consultant practice should beware of generalizations about disease processes which may lead them to think that certain pathological changes cannot be related to a patient's symptoms.

While it is clear that nucleus pulposus calcification may be associated with localized spinal pain of moderate severity and that the pain usually responds to simple conservative methods of treatment, it is equally clear that this disc disorder may have serious consequences for individual patients and that surgical operations may be required in the course of treatment.

Plain X-rays, and C.T. images in axial, coronal and sagittal planes provide excellent outlines of these lesions. MRI is not useful, unless the thoracic cord is compressed.

4.3. Patterns in Children

Clinical syndromes associated with nucleus pulposus calcification in children are well recognized, though rare. Bouts of acute painful wry neck or severe spinal pain of sudden onset, with fever, moderate elevation of the erythrocyte sedimentation rate and occasional increase in white cell counts, subside rapidly with rest. Typically, widespread calcification of variable density outlines the area of one or more of the nuclei pulposi. This calcification usually disappears within a few weeks of its first recognition on the X-ray examination of the spine (Fig. 4.1).

The natural history of symptomatic paediatric intervertebral disc calcification has been defined recently by Sonnabend *et al.* (1982), following a review of 35 papers on the subject. Most of these cases occur in the cervical discs. Trauma seems to play a part, at least as a precipitating factor. In children, the disorder is usually asymptomatic in the thoracic spine.

In this review of 89 children with symptoms attributed to the lesion, the sex ratio boys:girls was 1.5:1, but in children who were asymptomatic, it was 0.5:1.

Crock (1982) reported twelve cases of intervertebral disc calcification in adults, ten of whom required surgical treatment for the relief of severe intractable pain, not responsive to conservative measures of treatment. Only two of these patients were males.

The sites of disc calcification also differed markedly from that seen in children (Table 4.1).

In dogs with disc calcification, involvement of the sacral intervertebral discs occurs in about 4 or 5%. Apparently not previously reported in man, I have observed a female patient with the condition in the first sacral intervertebral disc, where it had caused troublesome sacral pain for a number of years (Figs. 4.2 a, b).

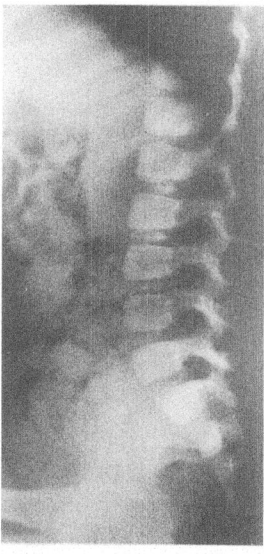

Figure 4.1. A lateral X-ray of the thoraco-lumbar spine in a child aged 11, showing nucleus pulposus calcification at multiple levels. Note the straight lumbar spine due to muscle spasm

Table 4.1

Age	Sex	Site
54	F	L 3/4
46	M	T 10/11
42	F	T 11/12
46	F	L 3/4
45	F	L 5/S 1
51	F	T 9/10, T 10/11
33	F	T 12/L 1
38	F	L 1/2
57	F	L 4/5, L 5/S 1
47	F	L 1/2
56	M	L 1/2
60	F	T 8/9

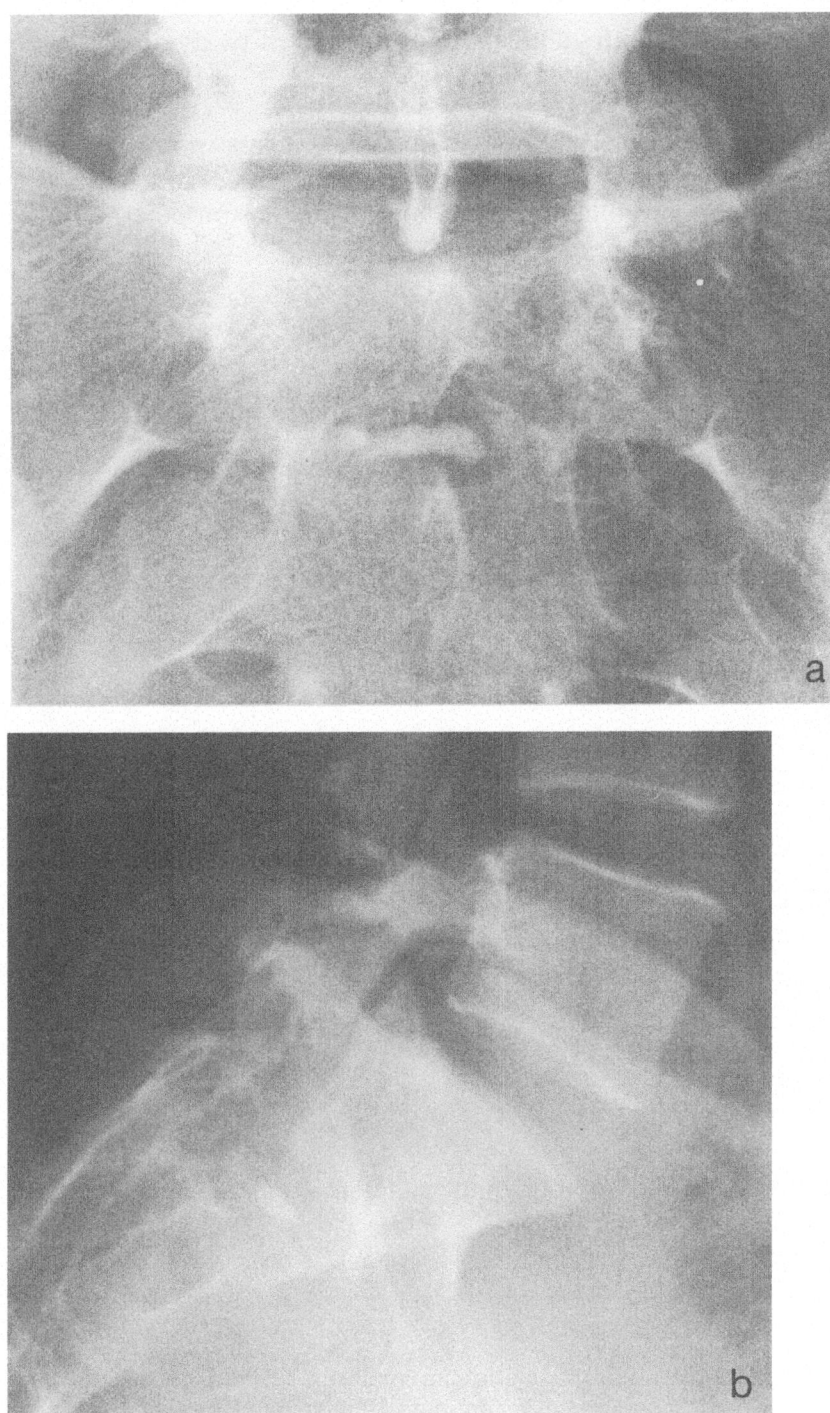

Figures 4.2. Antero-posterior (**a**) and lateral views (**b**) of the sacrum in a female aged 36, showing nucleus pulposus calcification in a rudimentary sacral intervertebral disc

4.4. *Patterns in Adults*

The radiological appearances of calcific deposits in this series of twelve cases were classified into four groups.

1. Small discrete irregularly opaque shadows within the nucleus pulposus lying nearer the posterior than the anterior boundary (Figs. 4.3 a, b, 4.4).
2. Widespread calcification of variable density giving the nucleus pulposus a fluffy outline (Figs. 4.5, 4.6).

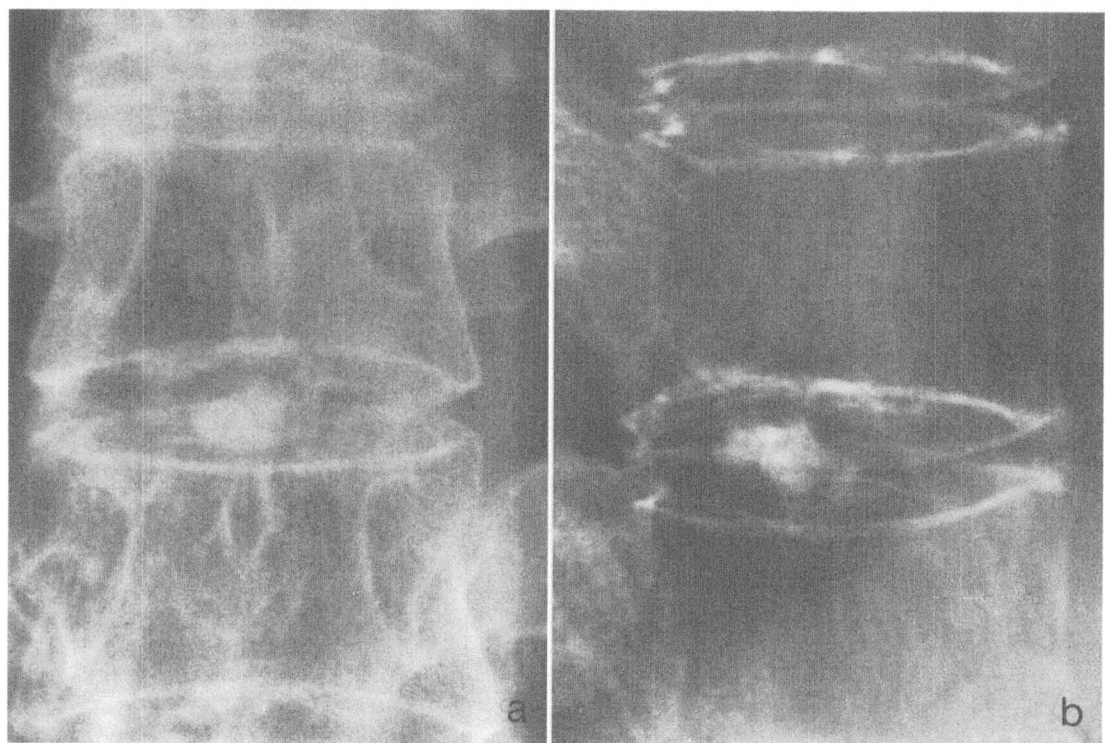

Figures 4.3 a, b. Antero-posterior and lateral X-rays of the mid-dorsal spine in a female patient aged 60 showing *type 1* nucleus pulposus calcification

Figure 4.4. Lateral X-ray of the thoraco-lumbar junction in a male aged 56 years showing *type 1* nucleus pulposus calcification. This X-ray appearance remained unchanged in eight years

Figure 4.5. Lateral X-ray of the thoracic spine showing type 2 nucleus pulposus calcification at the T11/12 intervertebral disc space in a female patient aged 42

Figure 4.6. Lateral tomogram of the L4/5 and L5/S1 area of the spine in a female patient aged 45 years showing *type 2* nucleus pulposus calcification at L5/S1

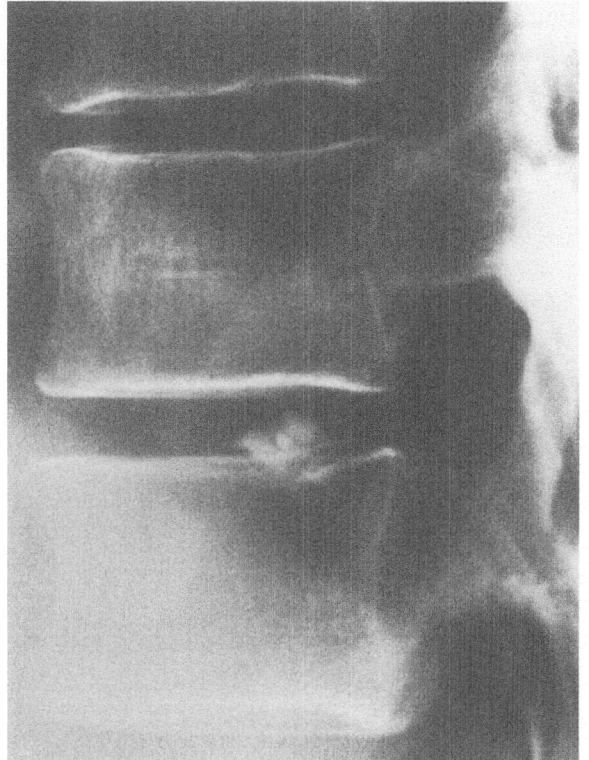

Figure 4.4

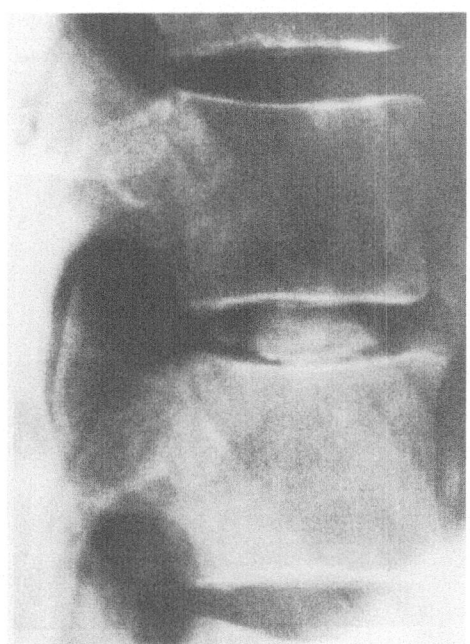

Figure 4.5

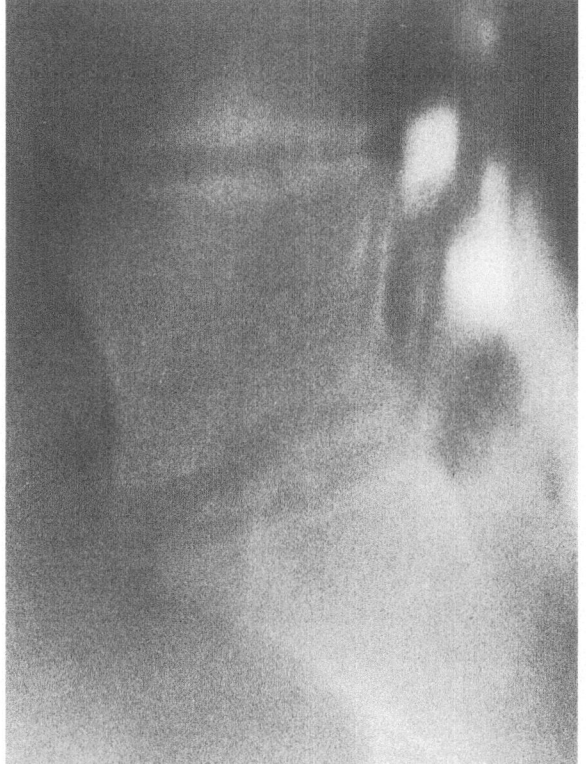

Figure 4.6

3. Small discretely outlined zones of calcification lying adjacent to one vertebral end-plate but peripherally located in the nucleus pulposus (Figs. 4.7 a, b).
4. Discrete aggregates of densely calcified material confined to the area of the nucleus pulposus (Figs. 4.8–4.10).

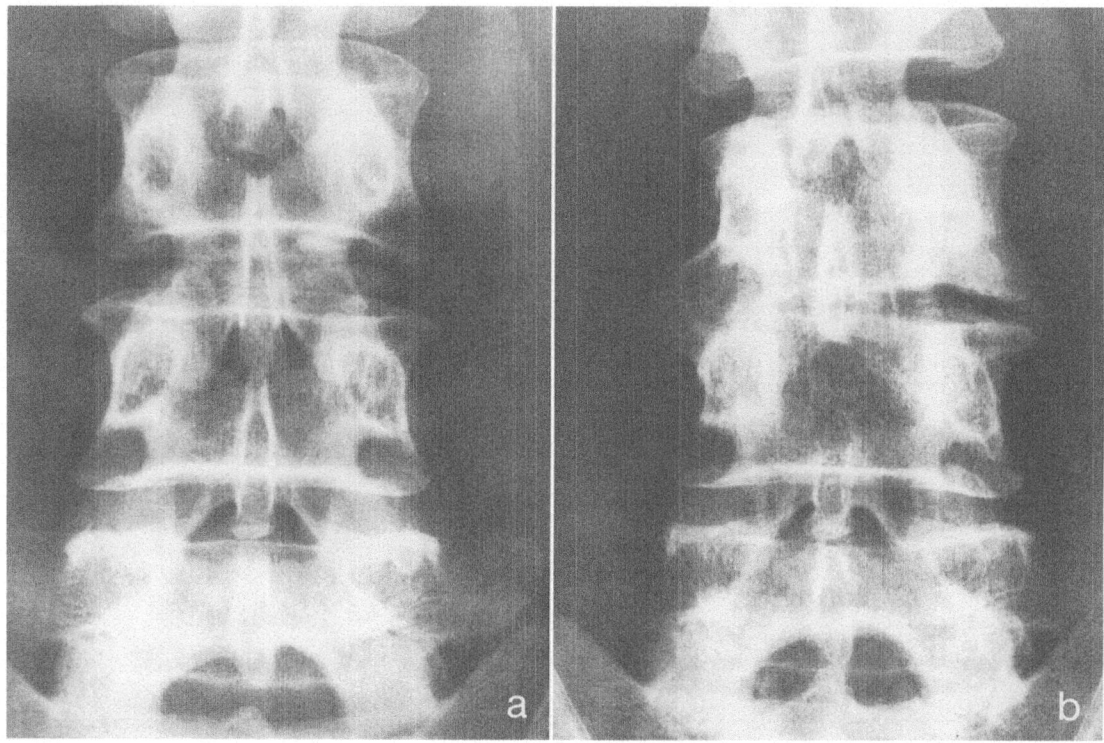

Figures 4.7. a Antero-posterior view of the lumbar spine in a female patient aged 54 years showing *type 3* nucleus pulposus calcification at the L3/4 level on the right side of the photograph. **b** Antero-posterior photograph of the lumbar spine showing spontaneous interbody fusion at the L3/4 level six years after partial disc excision

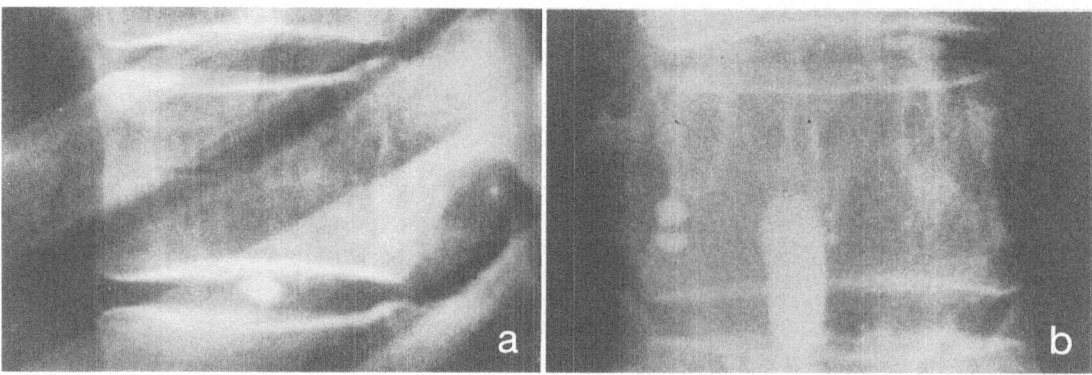

Figures 4.8 a, b. Lateral and antero-posterior radiographs of the thoracic spine in a female patient aged 47 years showing *type 4* nucleus pulposus calcification at the T 8/9 inter-vertebral disc level. The middle lobe of the right lung was adherent to this disc in the paravertebral gutter, the remainder of the pleural cavity being free of adhesions

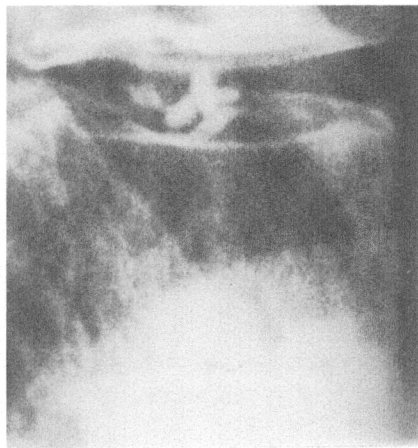

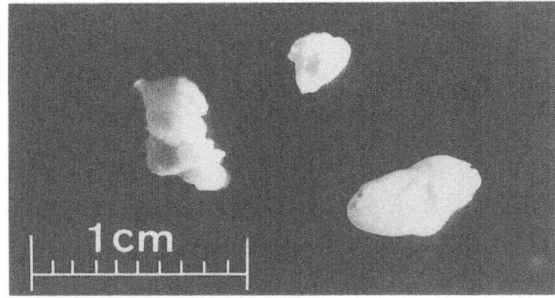

Figure 4.9   **Figure 4.10**

Figure 4.9. A lateral radiograph of the thoracic spine showing *type 4* nucleus pulposus calcification at the T 10/11 intervertebral disc space in a male patient aged 46

Figure 4.10. A photograph of the calcium calculi removed at operation from the disc shown in Fig. 4.9

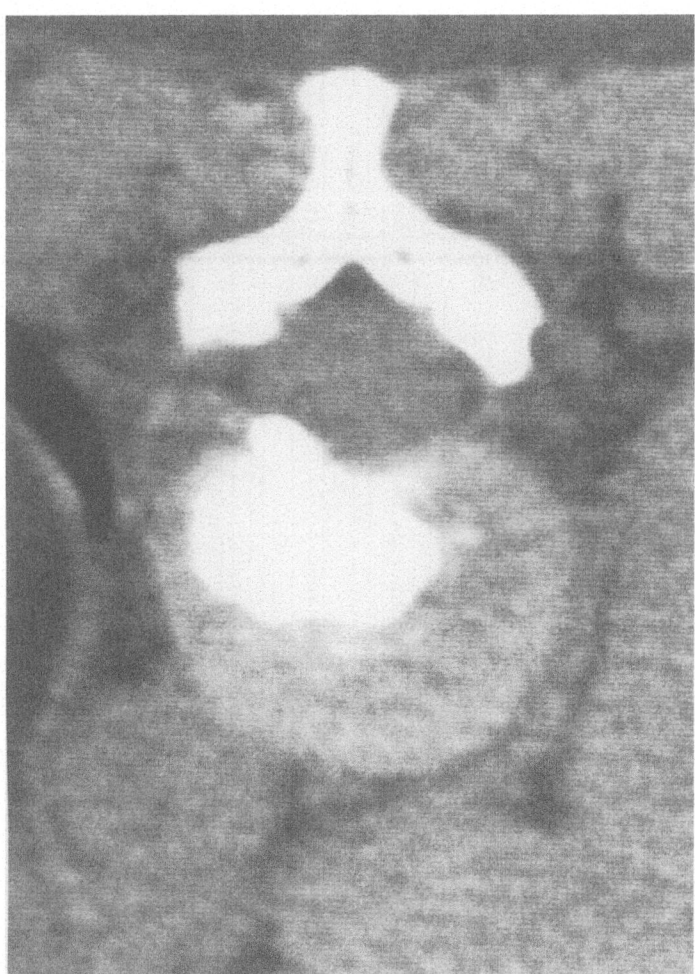

Figure 4.11. A computerised tomograph showing the pattern of calcification of disc tissues at the disc between the vertebrae T 11/12, in a female, aged 49 years. The calcification (type 2) is shown extending postero-laterally into the spinal canal where it is related to the antero-lateral aspect of the spinal cord on the left side

Table 4.2. Protocols

	Case 1	Case 2	Case 3
Sex	Female	Male	Female
Age	54	46	42
Occupation	Home duties	Workman	Home duties and nurse
X-ray	L3/4	T10/11	T11/12
Type of lesion	3	4	2
Date of presentation	May, 1970	February, 1971	October, 1973
Date of operation	October, 1970	1976	September, 1974
Trauma	None	Heavy blow to trunk	Heavy lifting
Major symptoms	Excruciating lumbar back pain with referred leg pain	Lower thoracic pain, weakness of legs	Severe low thoracic spinal pain, radiating around lower ribs
Intra-disc hydro-cortisone injection	Not administered	Not administered	Not administered
Previous surgery	None	Lumbar spine fusion - 8 years earlier for tuberculous disease, T11 to L1	Nil
Type of operation	Trans-lumbar canal partial disc excision	Interbody fusion	Interbody fusion
Result	Improved. Spontaneous interbody fusion observed in X-rays several years after operation	Improved	Improved

	Case 4	Case 5	Case 6
Sex	Female	Female	Female
Age	46	45	51
Occupation	Home duties and factory worker	Home duties	Home duties and telephonist
X-ray	L3/4	L5/S1	T9/10, T10/11
Type of lesion	3	2	3
Date of presentation	August, 1975	1976	1977
Date of operation	September, 1975	1976	1977
Trauma	Lifting	None	None
Major symptoms	Excruciating mid-lumbar pain, (R) hip flexed	Severe low back pain – marked lumbar spasm	Severe thoraco-lumbar junction pain
Intra-disc hydro-cortisone injection	No help	No help	No help
Previous surgery	None	Lumbar spinal fusion L4/5 for degenerative disc disease	Multiple operations including lumbar fusion for lumbar spondylosis and degenerative spondylolisthesis at L4/5 level
Type of operation	Trans-lumbar canal partial disc excision	Interbody fusion	Extra-pleural partial disc excisions
Result	Improved	Fair	Fair

	Case 7	Case 8	Case 9
Sex	Female	Female	Female
Age	33	38	57
Occupation	Home duties and nurse	Home duties and nurse	Home duties
X-ray	T12/L1	L1/2	L4/5, L5/S1
Type of lesion	3	3	2
Date of presentation	December, 1976	1973	1978
Date of operation	March, 1978	1978	March, 1979
Trauma	None	Heavy lifting	Back pain persisted following motor vehicle accident
Major symptoms	Severe mid- to upper lumbar pain, occasional (L) thigh pain	Severe upper lumbar back pain	Severe lumbar back pain, buttock pain. Marked muscle spasm
Intra-disc hydro-cortisone injection	No help	No help	No help
Previous surgery	Cervical fusion	Intercostal neurectomy	Lumbar laminectomy
Type of operation	Extra-pleural interbody fusion	Extra-peritoneal disc excision	Extra-peritoneal partial disc excisions
Result	Fair	Improved	Improved

	Case 10	Case 11	Case 12
Sex	Female	Male	Female
Age	47	56	60
Occupation	Home duties and factory worker	School teacher	Home duties
X-ray	T 8/9	L 1/2	T 8/9
Type of lesion	4	1	1
Date of presentation	July, 1979	February, 1972	1976
Date of operation	October, 1979	No operation	No operation
Trauma	Lifting and twisting	Digging	None
Major symptoms	Severe thoracic pain, aggravated by deep breathing, radiating around chest wall	Upper lumbar back pain	Mid-thoracic back pain
Intra-disc hydro-cortisone injection	Not administered	Not administered	Not administered
Previous surgery	Lumbar laminectomy	None	None
Type of operation	Trans-pleural disc excision	No operation	No operation
Result	Improved	Improved with brace and analgesics	Improved with brace and analgesics

Computerised tomography may provide valuable information on the spatial distribution of calcified disc tissue with particular reference to its relation to the spinal canal and its neural contents (Fig. 4.11).

a) Clinical Features

Examples of type 1 nucleus pulposus calcification are illustrated in Figs. 4.3, a, b, 4.4. These patients, one female (Figs. 4.3 a, b) and the other male (Fig. 4.4), presented with spinal pain of sudden onset, localized respectively to the mid-thoracic spine and to the upper lumbar zone. In both, symptoms were controlled promptly with simple measures including the use of spinal supports for some months. The radiological appearance of the calcification shown in Fig. 4.4 remained unchanged in X-rays taken at follow-up eight years later. There were no outstanding clinical features characterizing these cases.

By contrast, more serious problems were seen in the ten patients whose details are shown in Table 4.2. Eventually all were treated surgically.

In four of the patients in the surgical group, nucleus pulposus calcification was found in the mid- and low lumbar discs. These patients presented with severe low back pain and paraspinal muscle spasm. One had a unilateral psoas muscle spasm preventing hip extension. The severity of the pain was such that family members complained bitterly that conservative treatment was ineffective, and they insisted that their relative should be admitted to hospital.

In the other six patients in the surgical group, nucleus pulposus calcifications were localized in the upper lumbar and lower thoracic discs. Again, *the pain of which they complained was intense in character,* localized in the upper lumbar and upper abdominal regions, and in the thoracic spine and radiating to one or both sides of the thoracic cage. Deep breathing, coughing and sneezing aggravated the pain. Paraspinal muscle spasm was also marked. One patient, the only male in the series, presented with low thoracic pain and weakness of his legs. There were no specific abnormal neurological findings in any of these patients.

b) Pathological Findings

There were two striking observations made at operation. One concerned the local inflammatory response apparently induced by the nucleus pulposus calcification in the region of affected discs. The other related to the appearance and texture of the calcified material removed.

Within the spinal canal, in the retro-peritoneal space and between the parietal and visceral pleura, adhesions were found related to the affected discs. The most remarkable evidence of this pathology was seen in the right hemi-thorax (case 10) where well-formed filmy adhesions had to be divided between the visceral pleura of the middle lobe of the lung in the paravertebral gutter and the antero-lateral surface of the disc between T 8 and T 9, immediately adjacent to the nucleus pulposus calcification (Figs. 4.8 a, b) on the right side of the disc space.

The calcified material removed from the intervertebral discs at operation was either white in appearance, with the consistency of soft paste, or in the shape of irregular calculi, slightly yellowish in colour.

Histological examination was carried out on tissue removed in five cases. In each case degenerative fibro-cartilage was found associated with calcification.

Table 4.3. Patterns of nucleus pulposus calcification

	Female	Male
Type 1	1	1
Type 2	3	–
Type 3	5	–
Type 4	1	1

Chemical analysis confirmed the presence of calcium in the tissues. No abnormal cartilaginous proliferation was found in any case, nor was there any evidence of specific inflammation.

c) *Surgical Treatment*

The types of operation carried out in the ten patients reported by Crock (1982), are set out in Table 4.2.

Summary

While calcification of the nucleus pulposus is a rare disorder of thoracic and lumbar discs in adults, it seems reasonable to draw attention to a number of observations made in this series of ten patients who underwent surgical operations for this problem.

Nine out of ten of the patients were female and in eight out of the ten there was some history of trauma.

Six of the patients had had some form of spinal surgery performed prior to the onset of their nucleus pulposus calcification.

While the pathological changes induced within the disc itself include some features of non-specific inflammation, it is interesting to note the capacity of this lesion to induce non-specific inflammatory changes at the surface of an affected disc.

Observations of retro-peritoneal fibrosis, perineural fibrosis in the spinal canal and localized pleural reactions have been reported in this series.

The pain in certain cases of nucleus pulposus calcification is acute in onset, intense in character and frequently unrelieved by conservative measures. In particular, intra-disc injections of hydrocortisone appear to be ineffective, whereas in cases of acute supraspinatus tendonitis they often relieve patients of pain.

Analysis of the findings in the ten patients presented in this chapter suggests that acute nucleus pulposus calcification deserves more serious consideration in clinical practice than is normally accorded to it.

In the past five years I have treated a further four women with lesions in the thoracic spine, only two of whom required operations, while the one male, with a lesion at T 12/L 1 intervertebral disc, responded to conservative care.

5

Spondylolisthesis

5.1. Planning of Treatment

Spondylolisthesis is a condition in which one vertebral body slips forward on the one below it. Associated with the forward displacement of the vertebral body there is either a laminal defect or degenerative arthritis of the inferior laminal facet joints.

The most common type of spondylolisthesis requiring surgical treatment is that seen with pseudarthroses in the lamina, so-called spondylolytic spondylolisthesis. Pseudarthroses occur in the pars interarticularis on each side. These take the form of asymmetrical false joints with false capsules and synovial linings in which osseous loose bodies may be found.

In degenerative spondylolisthesis the slip of the vertebral body is associated with degenerative arthritis of the inferior facet joints of the lamina; this condition is seen most commonly in women after the menopause.

Spondylolisthesis usually occurs at one level in the lumbar region, though rarely two or more adjacent levels may be involved (Fig. 5.1). Spondylolisthesis is one of the academic subjects that has appealed to orthopaedic surgeons for many years. It has been classified in various ways, five clinical groups being widely recognised: congenital, isthmic, degenerative, traumatic, and pathological. The academic aspects of this subject will not be dealt with in depth in this chapter. Readers may refer to the published work of Newman, Wiltse, McNab, and Louis, listed in the short bibliography which is found at the end of this book.

Frederickson and colleagues (1984 and 1990) have published important observations on the natural history of spondylolysis and spondylolisthesis. They suggest that a child with spondylolysis or spondylolisthesis can be permitted to enjoy a normal childhood and adolescence without restriction of activities and without fear of progressive listhesis or disabling pain. Slipping may increase up to the age of 16 but does so rarely. Development of the pars interarticularis defect, with or without spondylolisthesis, does not cause pain in most patients. Knowledge of these important observations is therefore extremely important in advising patients who present with these conditions causing symptoms. The majority of them are likely to respond to conservative treatment.

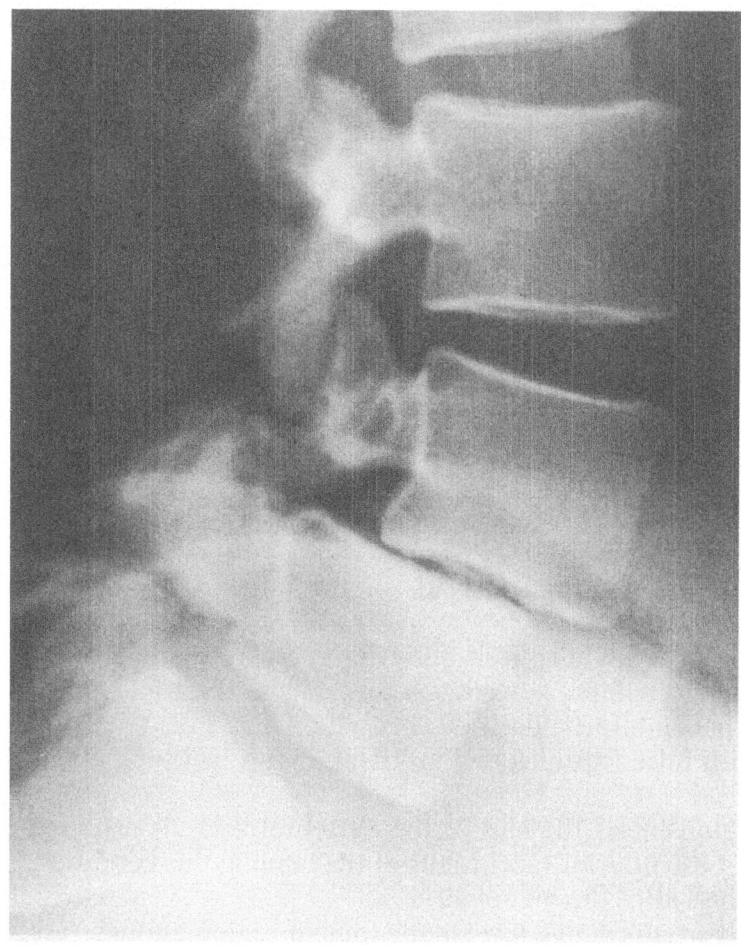

Figure 5.1. A lateral radiograph of the lumbar spine of a woman aged 45 years showing spondylolytic spondylolisthesis, Grade 1, at L5/S1 with a normal intervertebral disc, and Grade 2 at L4/5 with disc resorption at that level. This patient only required conservative treatment for low back pain

a) History

Patients may develop a wide range of symptoms and signs, including back pain, referred leg pain, a combination of back and leg pain, or in severe cases, evidence of lower cauda equina dysfunction with impairment of bladder function and impotence in the male. In the extreme example of vertebral body slip, described as spondyloptosis, the pelvic outlet may become obstructed during labour, rendering Caesarean section essential (Fig. 5.2).

In practice, no single operation will necessarily produce a cure in symptomatic patients with spondylolisthesis. Hence it is necessary to make a careful analysis of each case, attempting to introduce some rationale to the planning of surgical treatment (Figs. 5.3 a–c).

In assessing individual patients with a view to selecting a particular type of operation, one must first take account of the outstanding features in the clinical history. Careful analysis of individual symptom patterns may indicate, for example, that decompression of the spinal canal alone may be the operation of choice. This will be the case where the patient's dominant symptoms are of bilateral buttock and leg pain.

Where the symptom pattern combines the complaints of back and leg pain, then both decompression of the spinal canal and combined spinal fusion may be indicated. For the treatment of back pain alone, spinal fusion may be indicated.

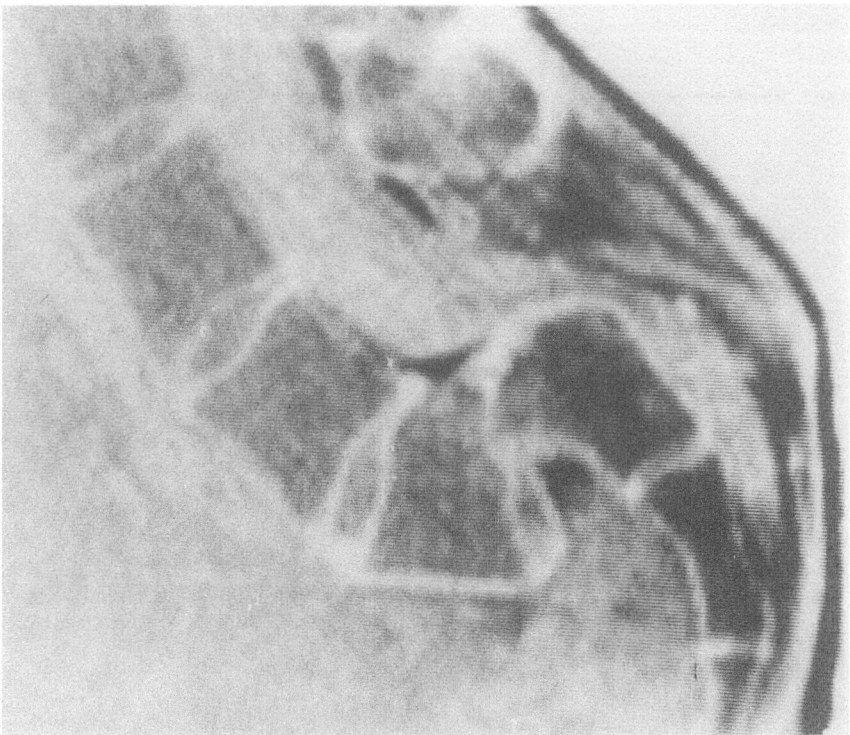

Figure 5.2. A mid-sagittal MR image showing the spondyloptosis at L5/S1 in a 16 year old girl whose photographs appear in Figures 5.13 and 5.16

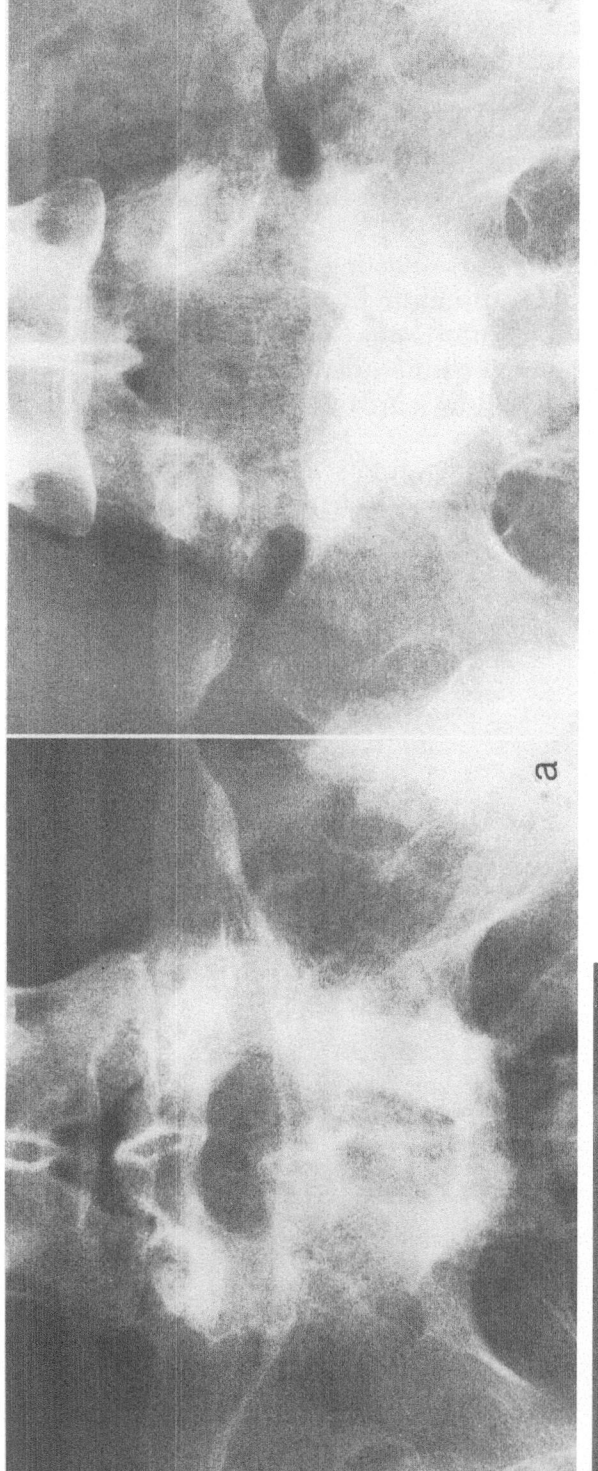

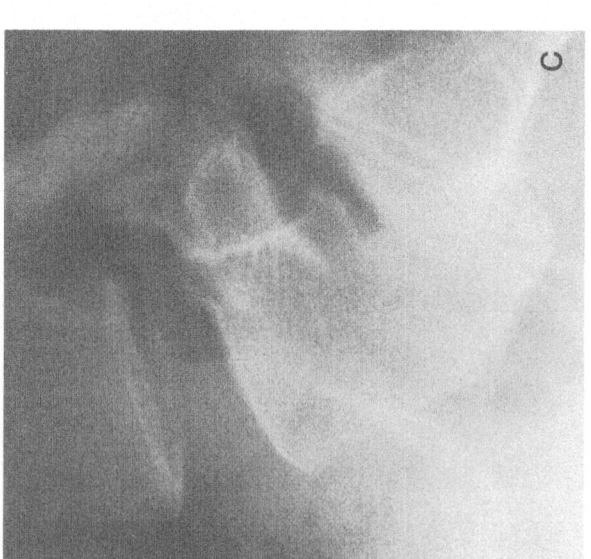

Figures 5.3a–c. a Antero-posterior view of the lumbo-sacral junction in a patient with spondylolisthesis which has been treated by anterior interbody fusion. **b** A radiograph following decompression laminectomy for persistent leg pain after successful anterior fusion. Note the appearance of the pedicles and refer to Fig. 5.7 (4). **c** A lateral radiograph showing the anterior interbody fusion and the extent of the spinal canal decompression

b) *Physical Parameters*

Having considered the history, four physical parameters should be analyzed in each case before the definitive decision can be taken on the type of surgical procedure required.

i) Role of the Laminal Pseudarthroses in Symptom Production

The first of these is the role of the laminal pseudarthroses in symptom production. The structure of the pseudarthroses varies considerably. Defects in the pars interarticularis are usually bilateral, though rarely symmetrical. They are often associated with bulky false joints from which recognizable synovial tissue may be extracted and in which a number of loose bodies may be found. These pseudarthroses are immediate posterior relations of the emerging nerve roots at the intervertebral foramina on both sides. Their obtrusions into the intervertebral foramina and nerve root canals may be the sole cause of referred leg pain in patients with spondylolytic spondylolisthesis, or in rare cases of spondylolysis (Figs. 5.4a,b). Before any surgical treatment is considered, infiltration of the pseudarthroses under bi-planar X-ray control, with the installation of local anaesthetic and hydrocortisone should be considered. Many patients become asymptomatic following this simple measure.

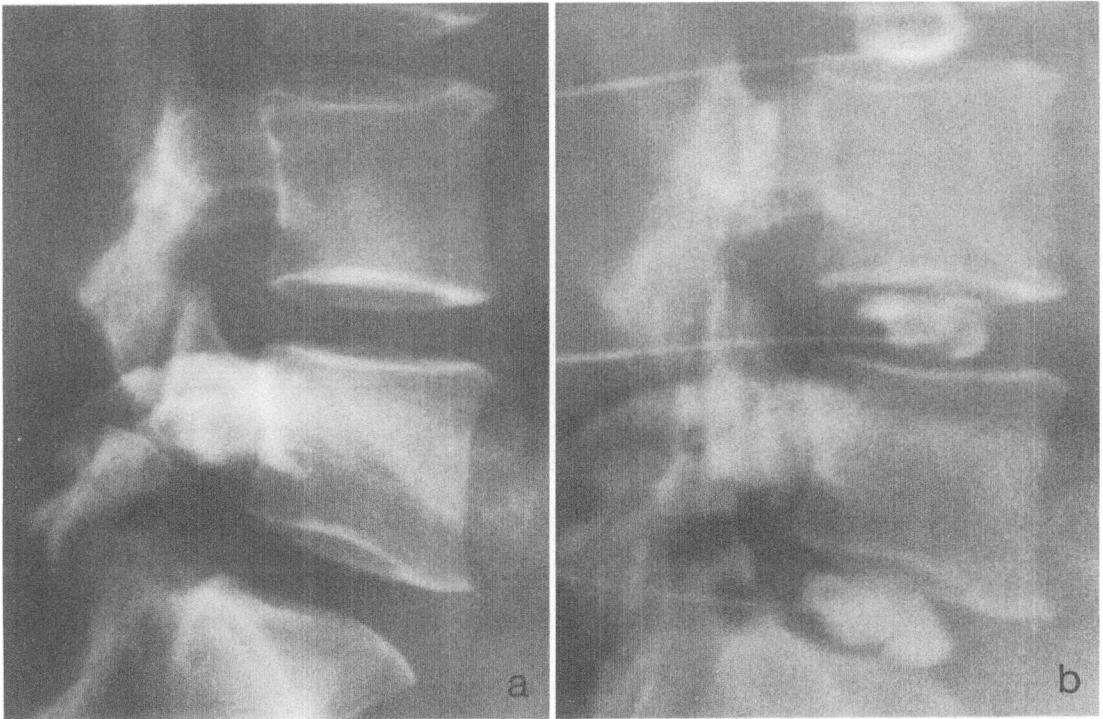

Figures 5.4a,b. a A lateral radiograph of the lower lumbar spine showing a spondylolytic defect in the lamina of L5. **b** Normal discograms at L3/4, L4/5 and L5/S1 in this case

In the usual case with bilateral laminal defects, the spinous process, lamina and inferior articular processes remain as a single unit which is loose in the vertebral column. When the spinous process is grasped with an instrument during operation, this whole unit can be moved freely. It has been described as the "rattler". Removal of the "rattler" is said to relieve nerve root pressure. However, if only the "rattler" is removed, the proximal portions of the pseudarthroses which remain attached to the pars interarticularis on each side, leading up to the superior articular facets, remain in the spine where they continue to compress the emerging nerve roots. The related nerve roots cannot be seen throughout their courses unless these proximal segments of the pseudarthroses are also removed, thereby completing the nerve root decompressions. Simple removal of the "rattler", therefore, is always inadequate (Figs. 5.5–7).

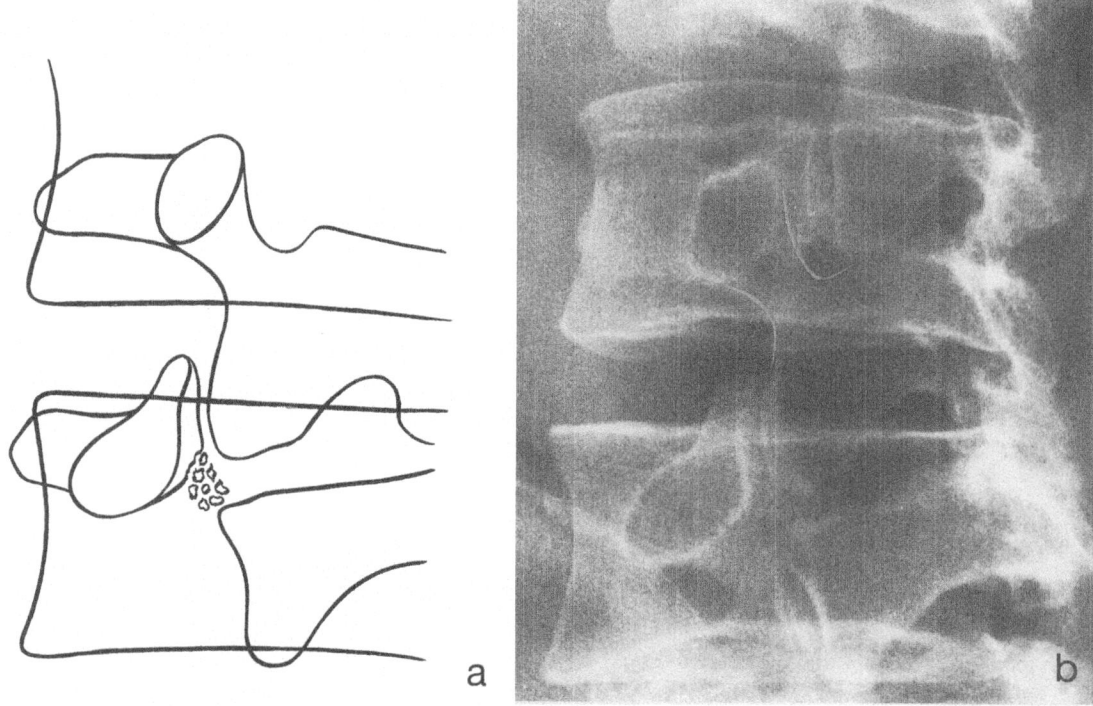

Figures 5.5a,b. **a** A drawing to illustrate a spondylolytic defect in the lower of two laminae which are viewed obliquely. **b** An oblique radiograph of the lower lumbar spine showing a normal lamina with the pars interarticularis outlined in the middle of the photograph and the spondylolytic defect involving the lowest lamina shown on the film. Loose bodies in the pseudarthrosis are clearly visible

---

Figures 5.7. **1** and **2** show the relationship of the laminal pseudarthroses to the spinal nerves. The soft tissues such as ligamentum flavum, false capsule and synovium are not depicted. **3** and **4** show the nerve root relations after removal of the "rattler" of spondylolysis, and the correct method of decompression (**4**) of the root canal and intervertebral foramen on the left side of the drawing

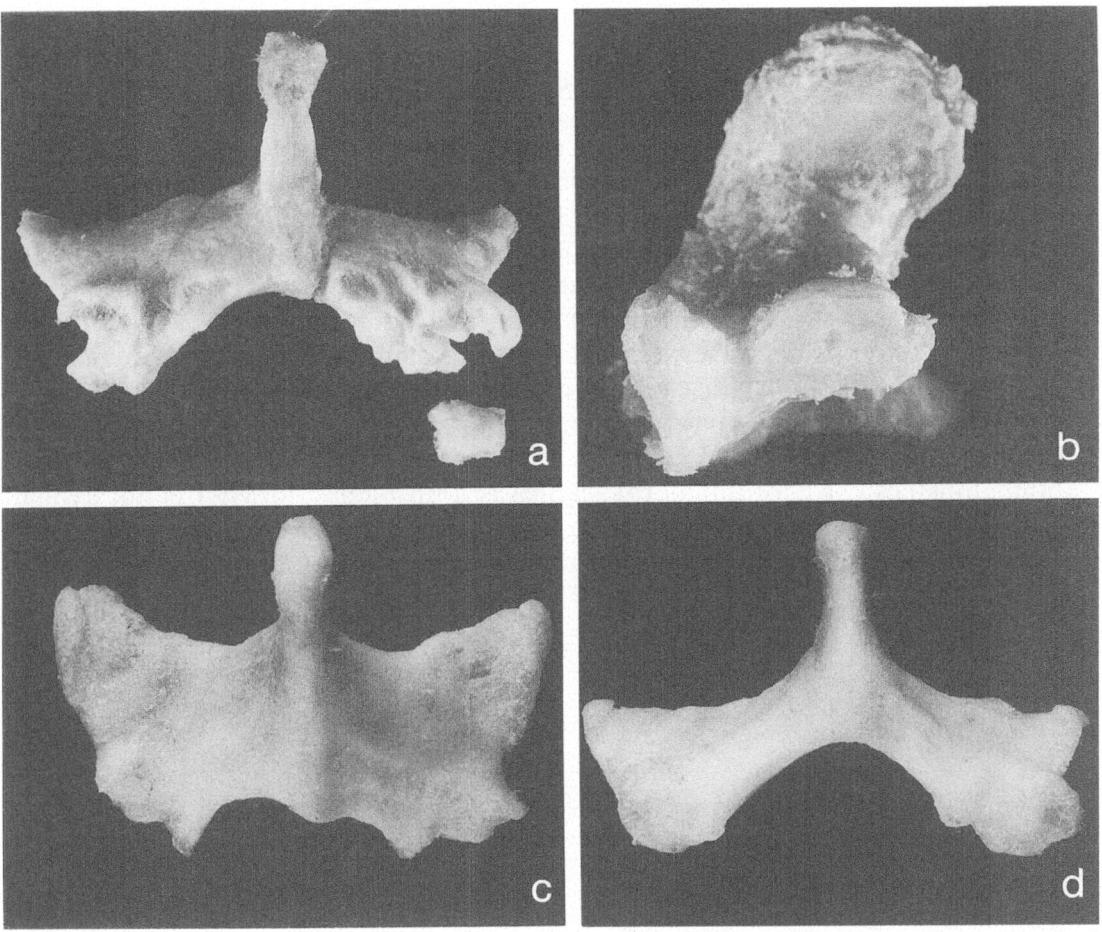

Figures 5.6 a–d. Photographs of loose laminae ("rattlers") removed at operations from patients with spondylolytic spondylolisthesis. The specimens have been photographed from above except **b**, which is a lateral photograph. In **a**, note the complex nature of the pseudarthroses with the loose body on the right side of the photograph. In **b**, the large pseudarthrosis is visible in profile and the inferior facet of the lamina is visible on the bottom right of the photograph. The views of the specimens in **c** and **d** show the asymmetrical nature of the pseudarthroses on either side of the lamina

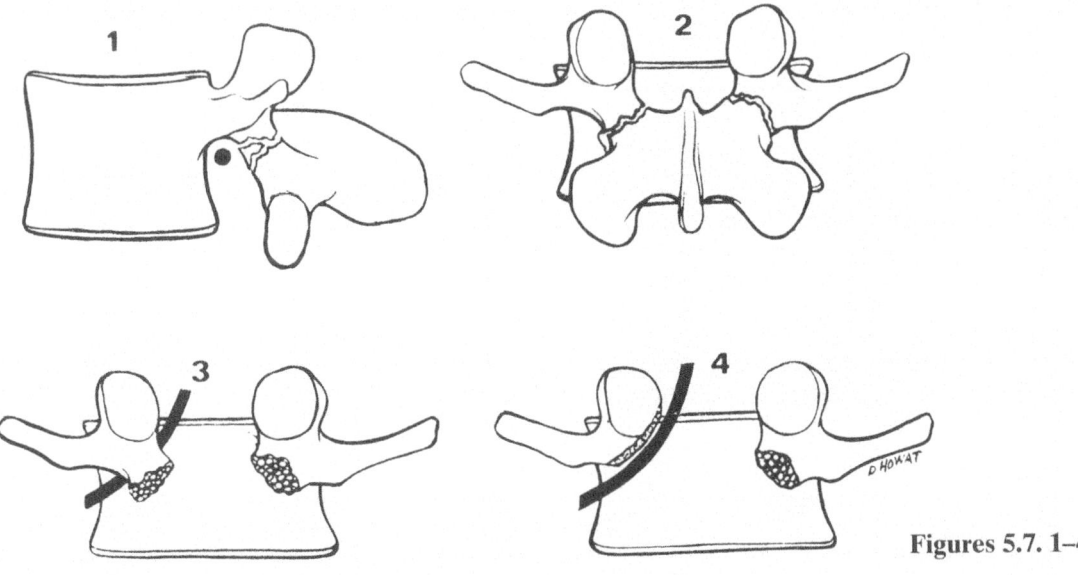

Figures 5.7. 1–4

ii) State of the Disc Adjacent to Slip

The second parameter to be considered concerns the state of discs adjacent to the vertebral slip, both above and below it. MRI alone usually suffices to provide this information (Fig. 5.8). Where this technology is not available, discography may be an essential special investigation when the symptom pattern is characterized by a mixture of back and leg pain. For example, in the case of spondylolisthesis at L4/5, if the discograms at L3/4 and L5/S1 are normal, then operative treatment should be restricted to the L4/5 segment alone (Figs. 5.9a,b). In other circumstances, the presence of disruptive disc lesions demonstrated by discography above the level of the spondylolisthesis may help in planning the extent of the spinal fusion procedure (Figs. 5.10a,b). Finally, in assessing the state of the discs in cases of spondylolisthesis, where unilateral sciatica is a problem and MRI is not available, lumbar radiculography may be used to exclude the diagnosis of disc prolapse, either at the level of the vertebral slip or at some adjacent disc space.

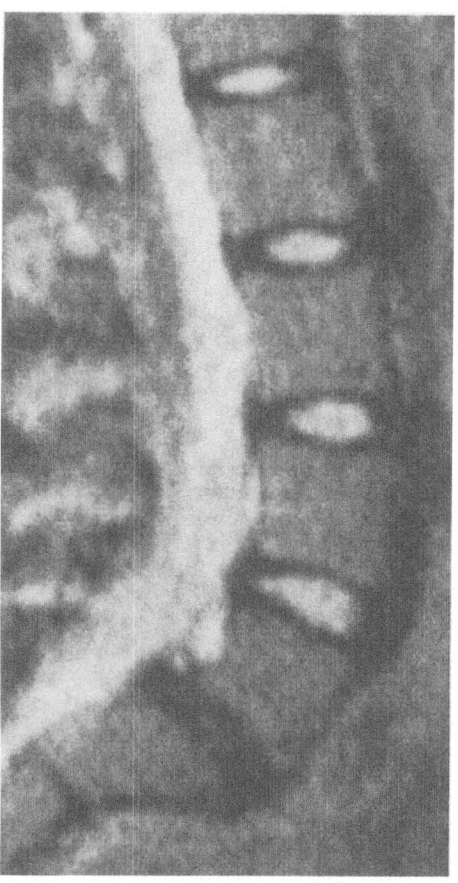

Figure 5.8. The mid-sagittal T2 weighted sequence MRI from a 20 year old female with Grade 1 spondylolisthesis at L5/S1

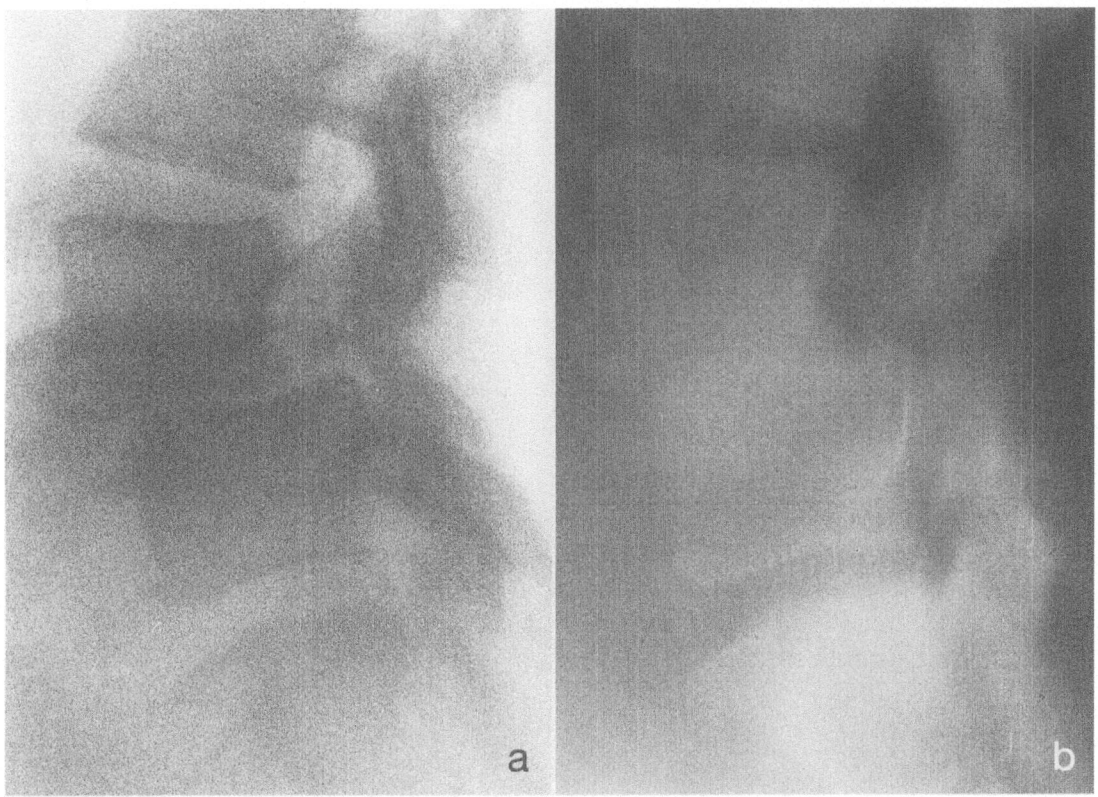

Figures 5.9a,b. **a** A lateral radiograph of the lumbar spine in a 45 year old man showing Grade 2 spondylolisthesis at L4/5. **b** Interbody grafts have been inserted transversely. The tomogram shows the appearance one year after operation

iii) Shape of the Spinal Canal

The third parameter to be considered is the shape of the spinal canal. When a patient with spondylolisthesis is found to have laminal abnormalities, then again, myelography may be necessary if the symptoms include referred leg pain (Figs. 5.11a,b). In such cases, associated spinal canal stenosis may be found. CT or MRI examinations if available may render myelography unnecessary. In the presence of spinal stenosis in these cases it is probably safer to perform spinal fusion concomitantly with decompression of the spinal canal.

iv) Degree of the Vertebral Slip

The fourth parameter for consideration is the degree of vertebral slip. Increase in the degree of slip usually occurs gradually over a number of years, in association with progressive narrowing of the related intervertebral disc (Figs. 5.12a,b). In the presence of Grade I or Grade II spondylolisthesis, anterior interbody fusion may be satisfactory. However, this method should be reserved for thin patients who have had neither previous abdominal surgery, nor antecedent histories of venous thrombosis. For cases with higher grades of slip, in which spinal fusion is being considered, standard methods of posterior fusion or intertransverse alar fusion may be consid-

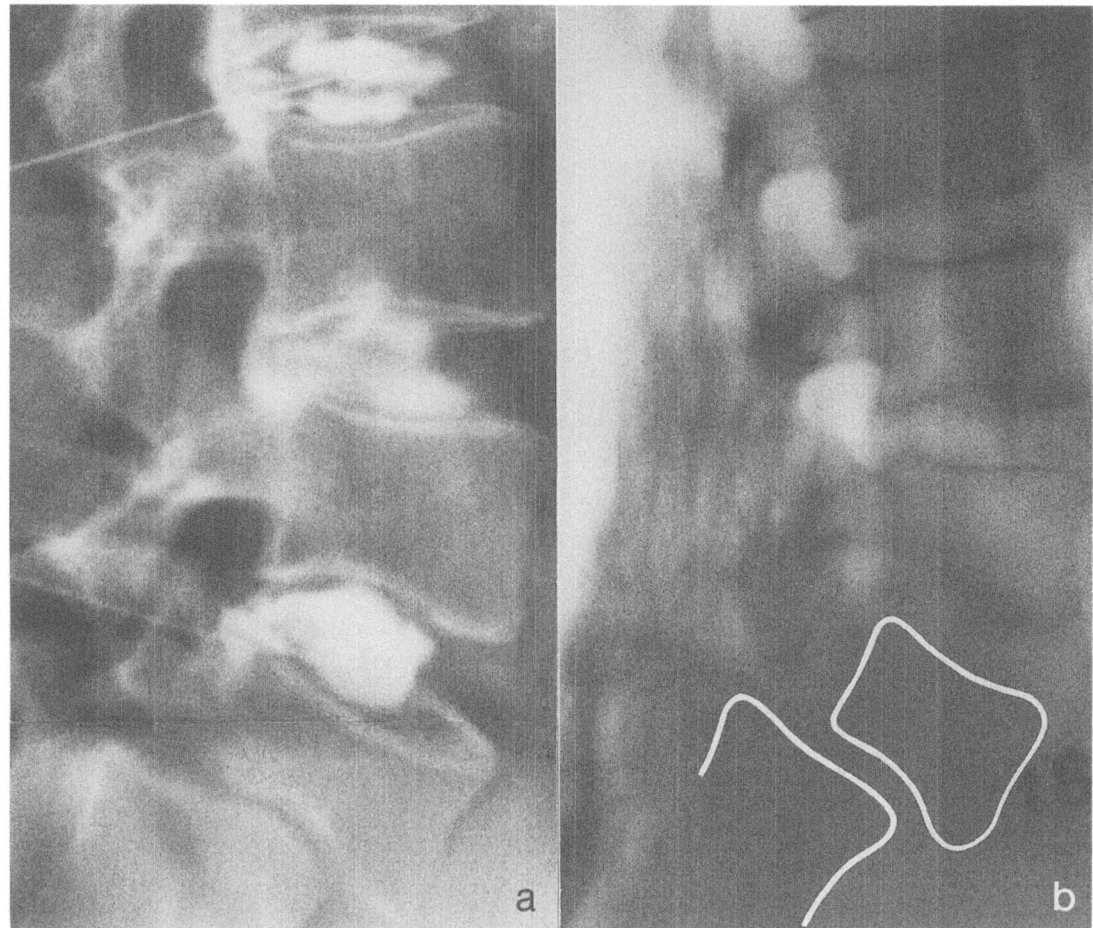

Figures 5.10a,b. a A lateral radiograph of the lumbar spine of a man aged 45, showing Grade 2 spondylolisthesis at L5/S1, with discograms at L2/3, L3/4 and L4/5. Post-traumatic disc disruptions are shown at each level, causing severe back pain. The patient had fallen from a height of 25 feet (8 metres). **b** A lateral tomogram of the same patient's spine taken 9 months after an extensive multi-level posterior spinal fusion, which was planned after the discography shown in Fig. 5.10 a

ered. Freebody (1971) has described a method for anterior lumbar interbody fusion applicable even in advanced grades of spondylolisthesis. This method calls for special training and even then its success rests on the surgeon having above average skill. In extreme cases the upper vertebral body may slip and roll off the lower vertebral end-plate, the condition being described as spondyloptosis.

Spondyloptosis is rare so that even experienced spinal surgeons may have dealt with only a few cases. Patients may present in early adolescence with grotesque deformity (Fig. 5.13). Following a period of bed rest muscle spasm often subsides and the scoliotic element of the deformity will decrease.

Wiltse (1990) has published a long term review of more than thirty cases treated satisfactorily by in-situ intertransverse alar fusion. In some of these patients neurological deficits resolved without spinal canal decompression and excellent ranges of spinal motion were regained after fusion.

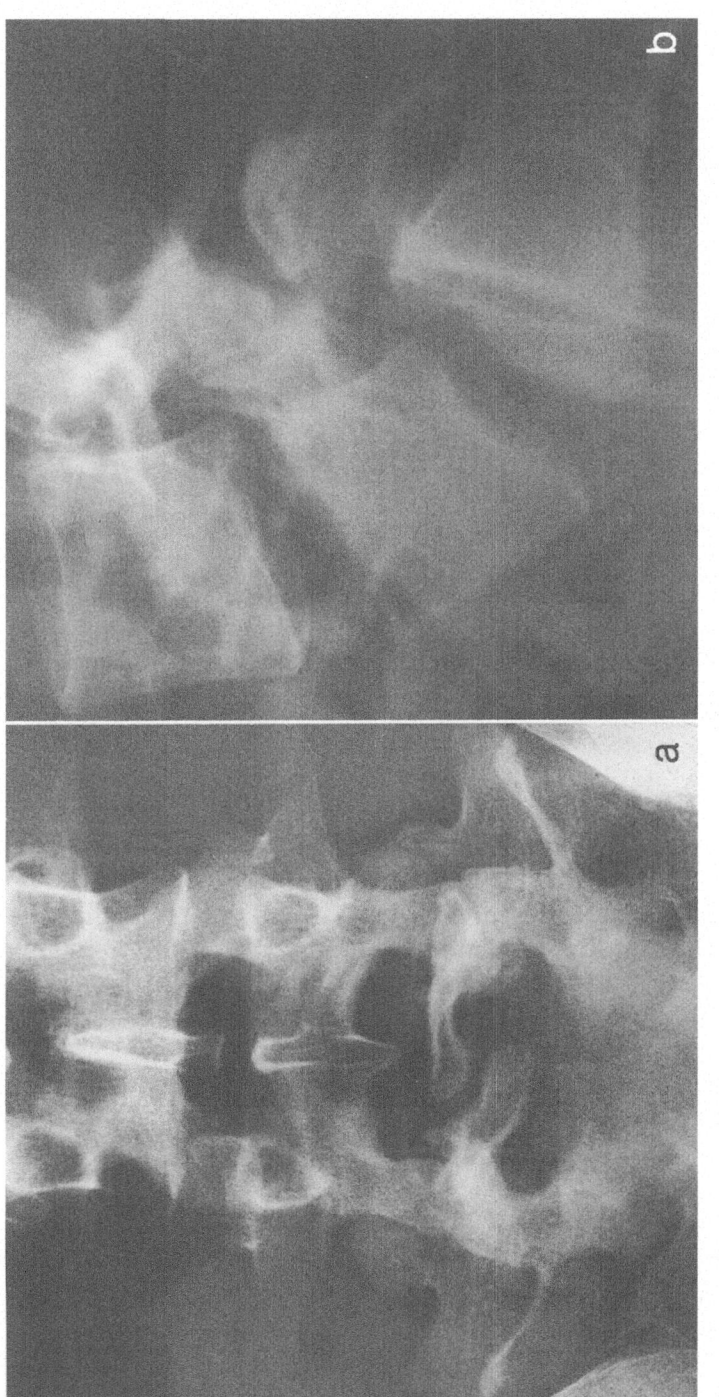

Figures 5.11a,b. a Antero-posterior and **b** lateral radiographs of the lower lumbar spine in a 21 year old male with Grade 1 spondylolisthesis. Spondylolytic defects are visible at L5/S1 but the lamina is grossly abnormal with spina bifida occulta

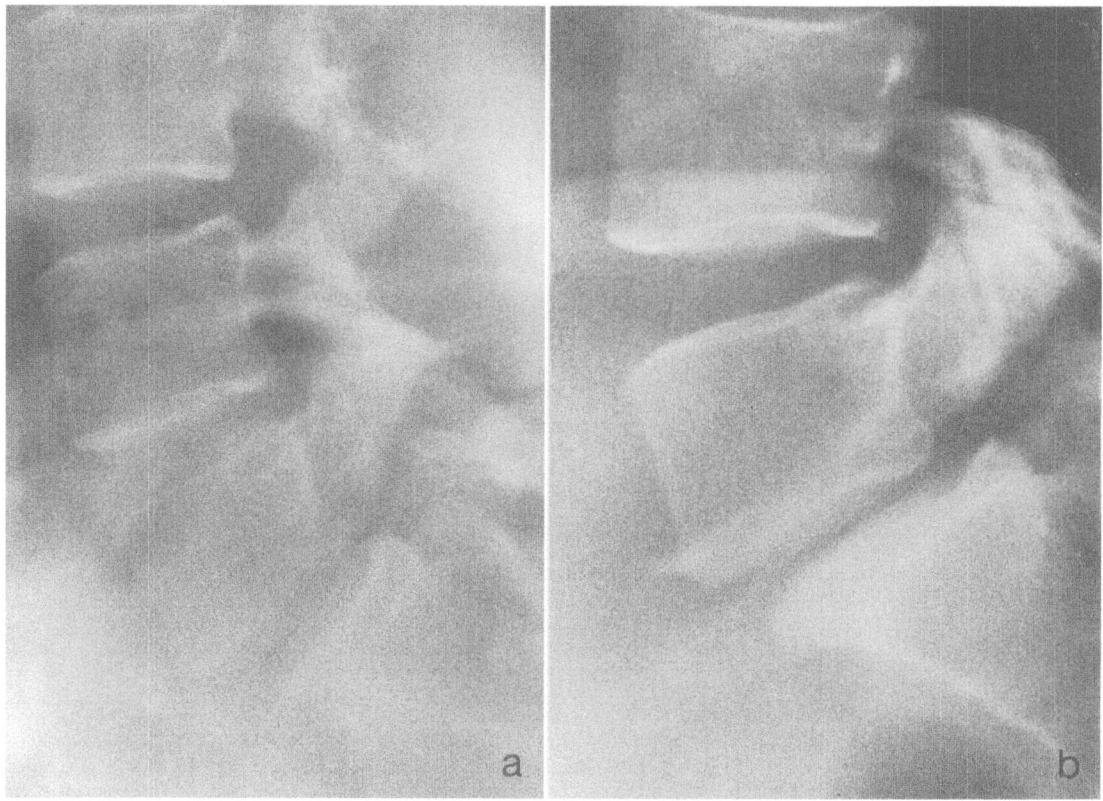

Figures 5.12 a, b. Lateral radiographs of the lumbar spine in an adult showing in (**a**) spondylolytic spondylolisthesis Grade 1 at L5/S1 with a normal intervertebral disc. The same spine five years later (**b**) showing disc resorption and increase in slip to Grade 2

Interest in the surgical treatment of high grade vertebral slipping has increased since pedicle screw fixation devices have become widely available in the past five years.

Attempts have been made to reduce the deformities of slip and roll by manipulation or traction prior to anterior interbody fusion with internal fixation.

Olerud (1988) has developed versatile instruments based on pedicle screws which may be inserted percutaneously, with which over a period of weeks the deformities can be reduced before spinal fusion is performed.

Treatment involving reduction and spinal fusion with internal fixation is always difficult and carries high risks of neurological damage, graft failure and recurrence of deformity (Figs. 5.14 a–c). Roy Camille *et al.* (1991).

In the presence of gross deformity such as that illustrated in Fig. 5.13, plain radiographs can be difficult to interpret whilst MRI provides excellent detail (Fig. 5.2). The pedicles of L 5 in this girl's spine were atrophic and unsuitable for placing pedicle screws percutaneously. The patient was placed prone on a Wilson frame with her legs resting on a canvas sling attached to a lifting device to allow hyperextension of the pelvis as an aid to reduction following spinal canal decompression.

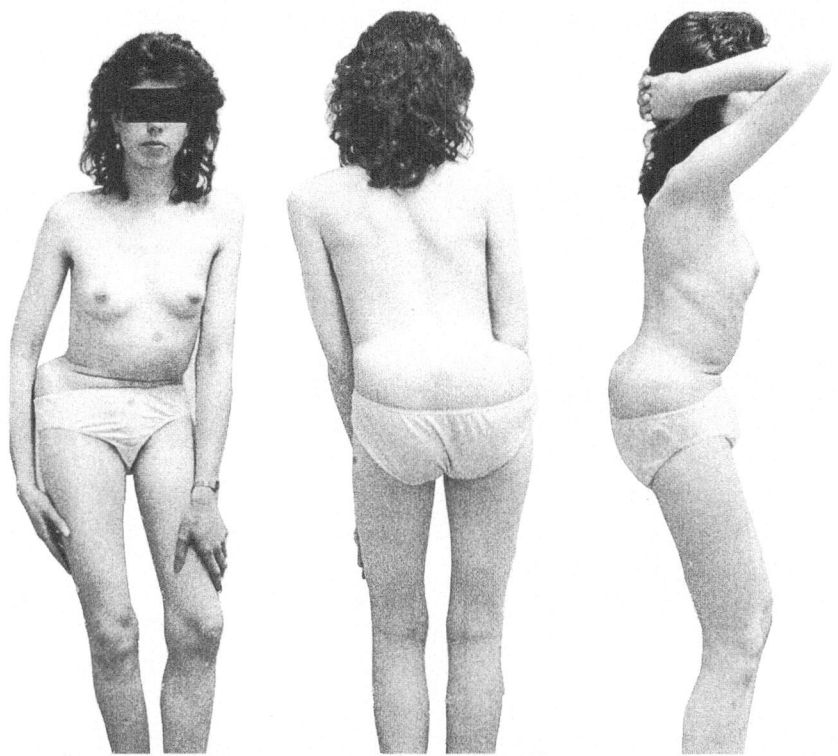

Figure 5.13. Pre-operative photographs of a 16 year old girl presenting with severe spinal deformity of acute onset associated with spondyloptosis of L5 on S1

The fifth lumbar lamina was removed in toto. The S1 nerve roots were thin and tightly stretched over the posterior border of the superior end-plate of the S1 vertebral body. The intervertebral disc was excised in part and a stout probe inserted in to the disc space as the legs were elevated thus aiding in reduction of the vertebral slip of L5 on S1.

The pedicles of L5 were then carefully identified and pedicle screws inserted into both L5 and S1. Satisfactory reduction of the deformity was then fixed with the application of the pedicle screw fixation device illustrated in Fig. 5.15. The wound was then closed and the patient returned to the ward.

She was nursed, log-rolling, for one week and then an anterior lumbar interbody fusion operation performed using autogenous grafts cut from the left iliac crest. Difficulties should be anticipated at each stage of these operations because of regional anatomical distortions. Even exposure of the anterior surface of the lumbosacral disc following the first stage reduction proved difficult in this case.

Following the second stage operation the patient was fitted with a half spica.

The end result in this case was excellent with interbody fusion and pedicle screw fixation involving L5/S1 alone, without supplementary intertransverse alar fusion (Fig. 5.16).

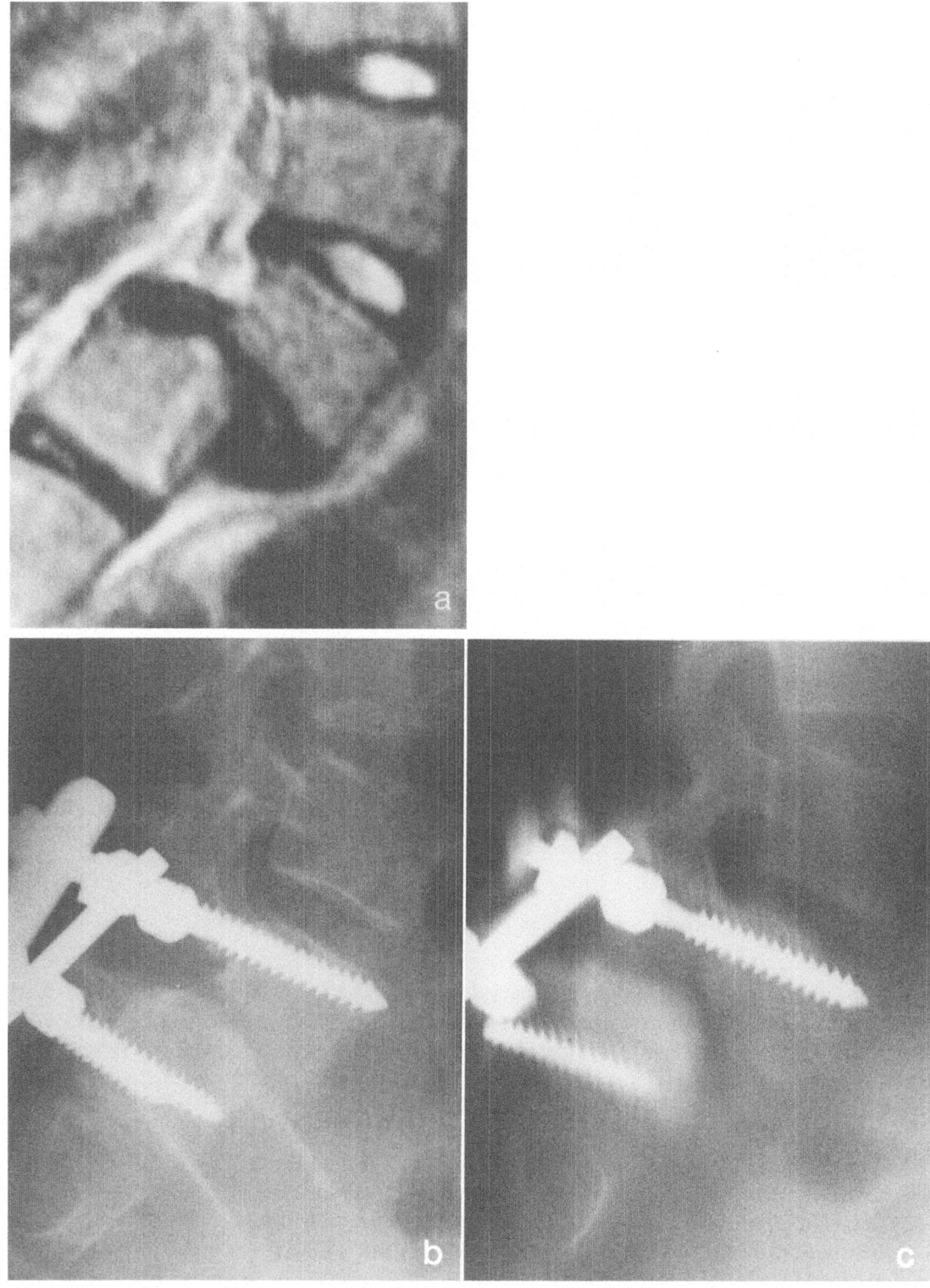

Figures 5.14a–c. **a** A mid-sagittal MR image showing spondyloptosis in an 11 year old girl at the L5/S1 level with normal discs above at L3/4 and L4/5. **b** A post-operative lateral view of the lower lumbar spine showing reduction of the spondyloptosis, fixation with Steffee pedicle screws and plates and an anterior interbody graft in situ. **c** A lateral radiogram two months after operation showing failure of the sacral pedicle screws with recurrence of the deformity. The device was removed and the deformity accepted. Fusion eventually occurred with slight further loss of position

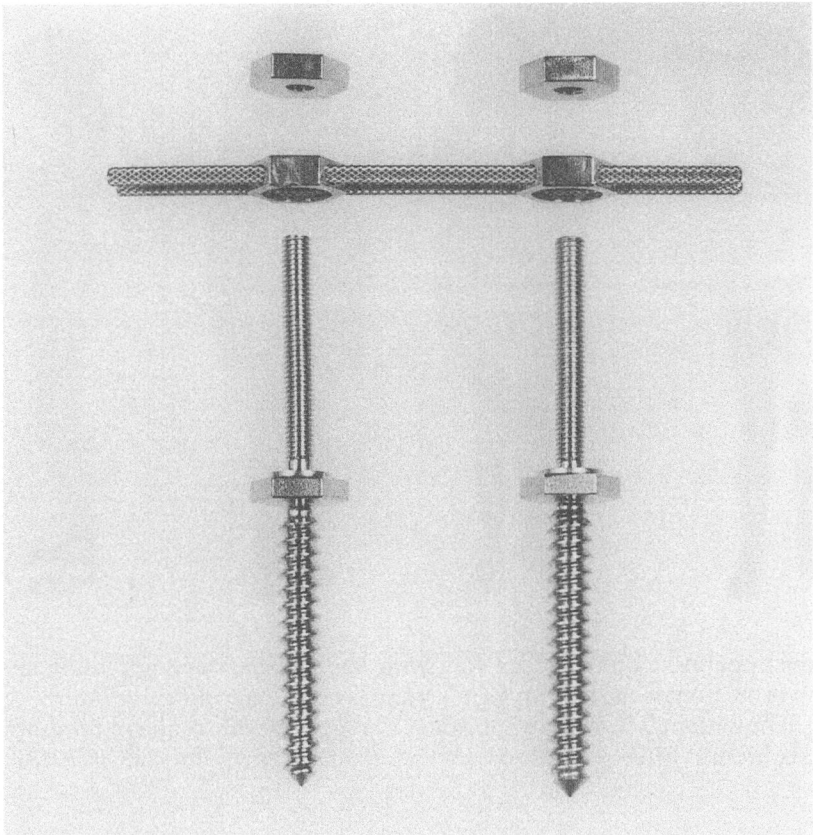

Figure 5.15. Photograph of the Crock Pericic pedicle screw fixation system which was used successfully in the treatment of the patient whose photographs appear in Figs. 5.13, 16. This spinal fixation system is manufactured by the Yufu Itonaga Co., Ltd., No. 31-20, 2-chome, Yushima Bunkyo-ku, Tokyo 113, Japan

In summary spondyloptosis can be treated successfully by in-situ intertransverse alar fusion. Its treatment by reduction and spinal fusion is far more complex, more time consuming and potentially more hazardous to the patient although the end result in successfully treated cases is clearly optimal.

In children, symptomatic spondylolisthesis may require surgical treatment and this should be undertaken early if there is any fear of increase in the degree of the vertebral slip. Bilateral intertransverse alar fusion is usually effective.

The choice of treatment in patients with symptomatic degenerative spondylolisthesis follows the same general lines outlined above. Conservative spinal canal decompression with bilateral foraminotomies and nerve root canal decompression, preserving the midline structures and re-attaching the lumbo-dorsal fascia to the supraspinous and interspinous ligaments at the end of the procedure, gives good results in many cases. This type of spinal canal decompression may be combined with intertransverse fusion. Some surgeons favour reduction of these deformities with pedicle screws and either posterior interbody fusion or intertransverse fusion. In older patients with marked osteoporosis the simpler surgical procedures outlined above are often safer for the patient and provide satisfactory relief of symptoms.

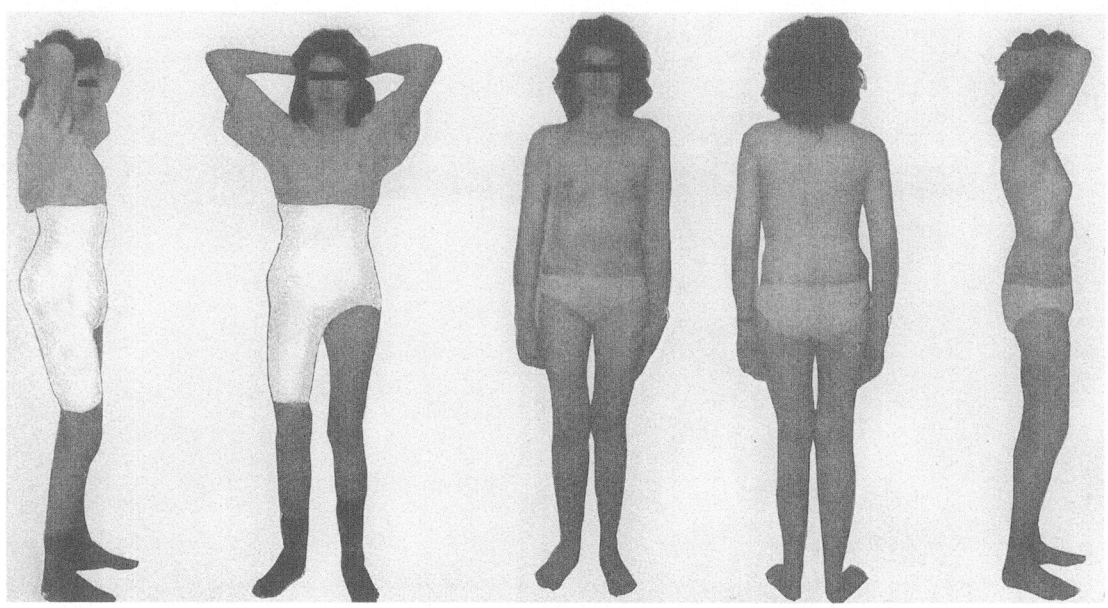

Figure 5.16. On the left post-operative photographs following spinal canal decompression and pedicle screw fixation with reduction of the spondyloptosis and second stage anterior interbody fusion between L5 and S1. The patient is wearing a half spica. On the right side of the photograph her appearance is shown six months after operation by which time she was symptom-free. (See Fig. 5.2)

5.2. *Technique of Postero-Lateral Inter-Transverse Alar Spinal Fusion*

a) *Indications*

This operation has virtually replaced the older methods of posterior spinal fusion introduced by Hibbs and Albee earlier this century, along with many variants such as "H" grafts and screw fixation with facet grafts.

When the transverse processes are sturdy this method of spinal fusion can be recommended for the treatment of:

1. spondylolisthesis, especially in children;
2. lumbar spondylosis causing back pain;
3. failed anterior interbody fusions.

b) *Preliminary Preparation*

Blood loss is often considerable so that blood transfusion facilities must be available. The patient's spinal X-rays and MRI must be displayed in the operating room.

c) Positioning

Patients should be placed prone on a suitable frame to avoid compression of the abdominal cavity (see pp. 122–124).

d) Incisions

In children a long mid-line incision is recommended, extending from L2 to the lower sacrum.

In adults, a midline skin incision is made and the skin flaps can be retracted to either side to allow parallel vertical incisions to be made in the lumbo-dorsal fascia for the paraspinal sacrospinalis splitting approach to the transverse processes and alar of the sacrum advocated by Wiltse (1978) (Figs. 5.17 a–c).

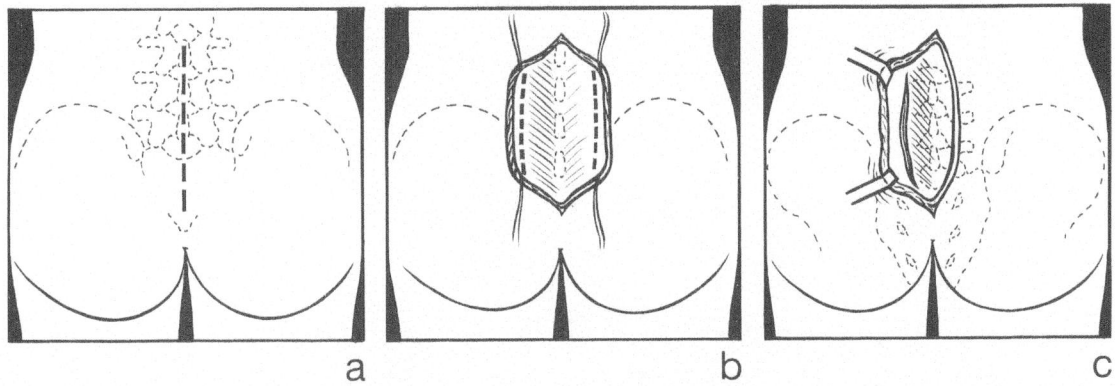

Figures 5.17 a–c. Drawings to illustrate the mid-line skin incision and the laterally placed incisions in the lumbo-dorsal fascia for the paraspinal sacrospinalis splitting approach recommended by Wiltse

e) Exposure of the Graft Bed

If the mid-line incision is used, the paraspinal muscles are separated as described on pp. 127–133. Their dissection is carried laterally beyond the facet joints until the posterior surfaces of the transverse processes and the alae of the sacrum on both sides can be palpated. The bulky paraspinal muscle mass is then retracted backwards and laterally to the level of the tips of the transverse processes. Blood loss may be considerable during this stage of the operation and it is often difficult to see the transverse processes of L5 in the depth of the wound unless the paraspinal muscles have been separated from as high as the lamina of L2.

Using the lateral paraspinal muscle splitting incision of Wiltse (1978), less extensive longitudinal dissection of these muscles is required to gain good exposure of the bony structures to be "fused". Modified Gelpi retractors inserted between the separated muscle fibres aid in obtaining a clear view (Fig. 5.18).

Preparation of the bed for the graft requires meticulous attention to detail. The intertransverse ligaments and muscles should be preserved. For fusions at L5/S1 level the capsules of the lumbo-sacral facet joints should be excised allowing access to the joint surfaces for excision of their articular cartilages and sub-chondral bone plates. The facet joint capsules between the superior facets of L5 and the inferior facets of L4 should be preserved intact. All remnants of soft tissues must be removed from the sacral alae, from the inferior facets of L5, from the lateral aspects of the partes interarticulares on both sides, from the outer aspects of the pedicles of L5 and cephalad from the outer aspects of the superior facets of L5, and then from the posterior surfaces of the transverse processes of L5.

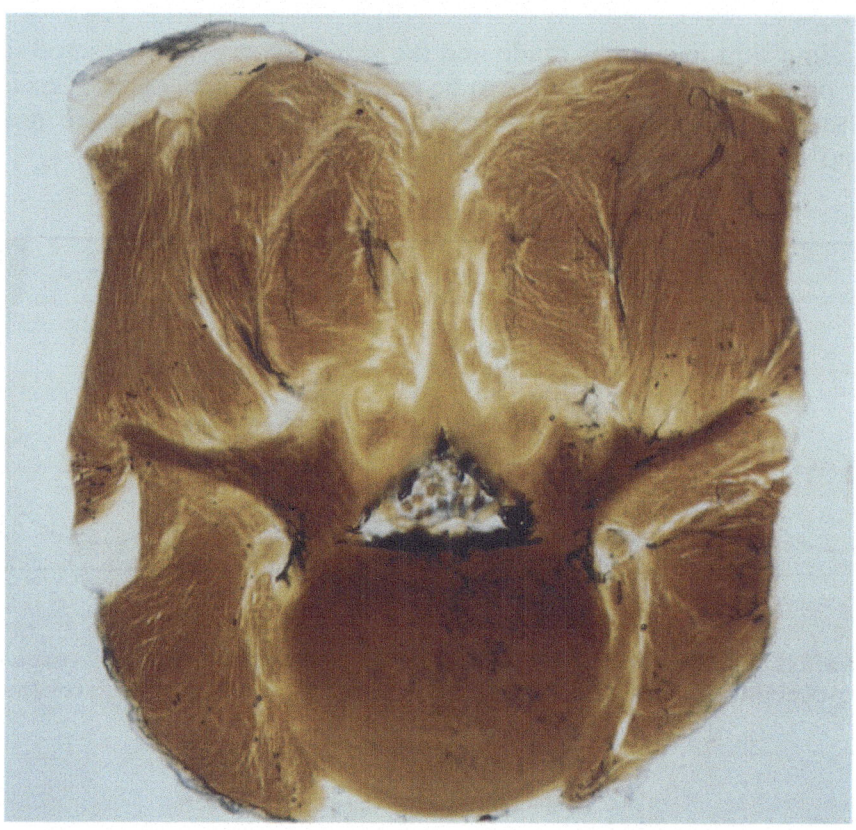

Figure 5.18.   A photograph of a transverse section of a mid-lumbar vertebra, with the paraspinal muscles intact. The specimen has been cleared by the Spalteholz technique. Note the arrangements of the paraspinal muscles posteriorly, with a plane of cleavage clearly visible between the muscle bundles related to the posterior aspects of the transverse processes at their junctions with the superior articular facets. This is the plane of cleavage recommended for use in inter-transverse-alar fusions

Figures 5.19 a–c.   a A drawing of the lower lumbar spine seen from behind to show the inter-transverse ligaments between L4, L5 and S1. On the right side note the preparation of the graft bed for an inter-transverse-alar fusion. The arrow indicates an upturned segment of bone cut from the ala of the sacrum and turned up towards the transverse process of L5. **b** A drawing to depict the preparation of the graft bed for an inter-transverse-alar fusion. Note the use of a curette to roughen the surface of the outer aspect of the superior facet of L5, leaving intact the capsule of the joint at that level. A chisel is shown turning up the flap of cortico-cancellous bone from the ala of the sacrum towards the transverse process of L5. **c** A photograph of a dissection of the lumbar spine viewed from the side to show the siting of inter-transverse grafts in relation to the spine as a whole (see arrows)

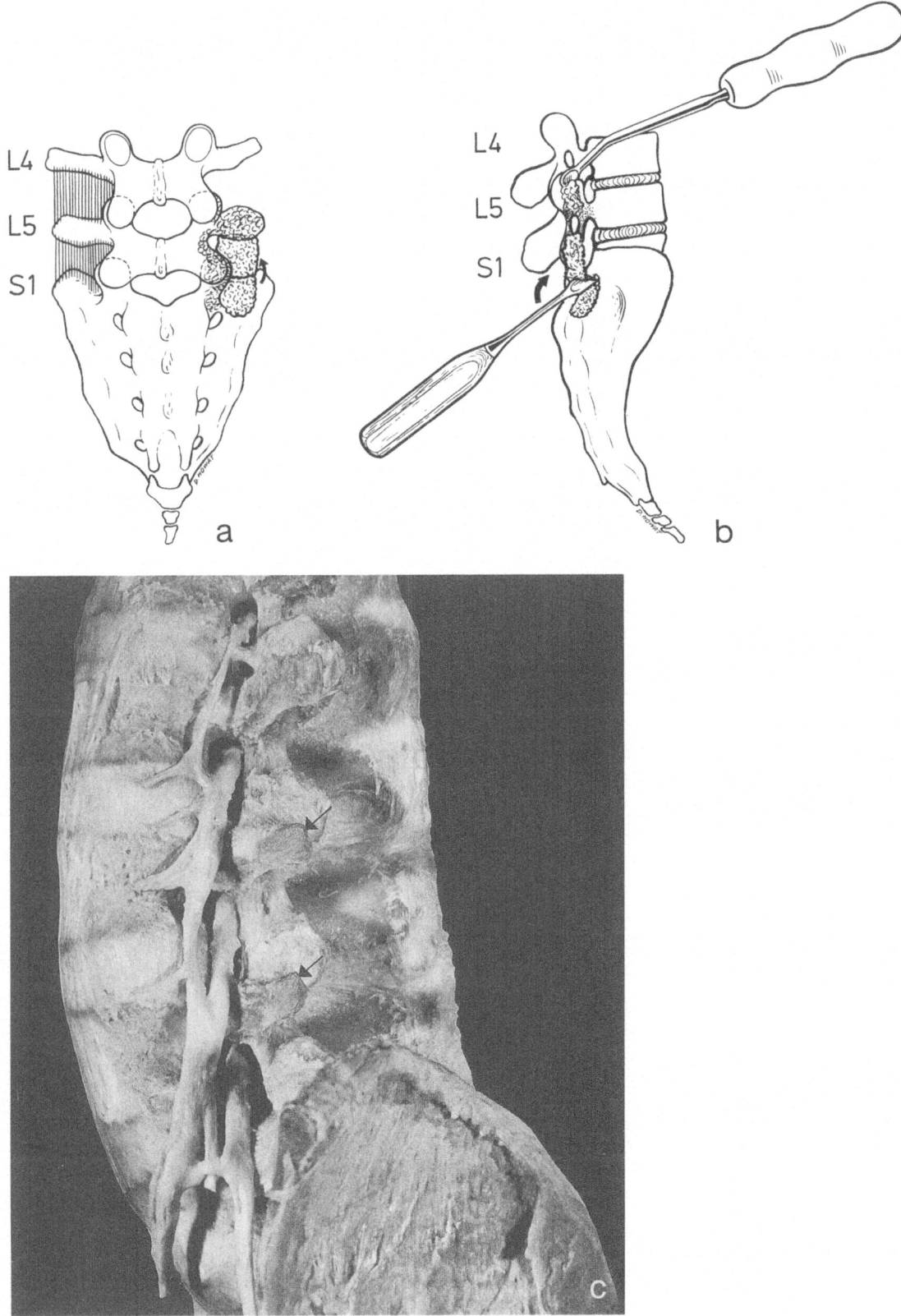

Figures 5.19 a–c

The exposed surfaces of the transverse processes of L5 should then be decorticated carefully, using a gouge and hammer or Leksell type rongeur. Then, with a stout curved curette the cortical bone on the outer sides of the L5 pedicles and superior facets of L5 should be broached to expose bleeding cancellous bone. The lateral aspect of the pars interarticularis of L5 lamina on both sides should also be roughened (Figs. 5.19 a–c).

Cortico-cancellous flaps cut from the postero-superior surface of the alae of the sacrum on both sides should be turned upwards to lie on the intertransverse ligaments, adjacent to the transverse processes of L5.

f) Preparation of Graft Bone

Autogenous grafts should be cut from the postero-lateral aspect of the iliac crest, access to this being obtained usually by undercutting the tissues between the lumbo-dorsal fascia and the iliac crest on one side.

Thin strips of cortico-cancellous bone, with other slivers of cancellous bone can be obtained usually in sufficient bulk from one side of the pelvis.

g) Placement of the Grafts

Thin strips of cancellous graft should be packed into the facet joints of L5/S1 and other strips should be placed accurately along the length of the spine extending upwards to the upper edges of the decorticated transverse processes. Cortico-cancellous strips, with the cortical surfaces directed outwards to lie facing the paraspinal muscles, should be packed in carefully. If chips of graft are pushed in roughly beneath the paraspinal muscles at the upper extremity of the fusion mass, they may come to lie above the decorticated transverse processes to which they were supposed to relate. The subsequent growth of "unwanted graft" is likely to occur, thereby setting the scene for late complications.

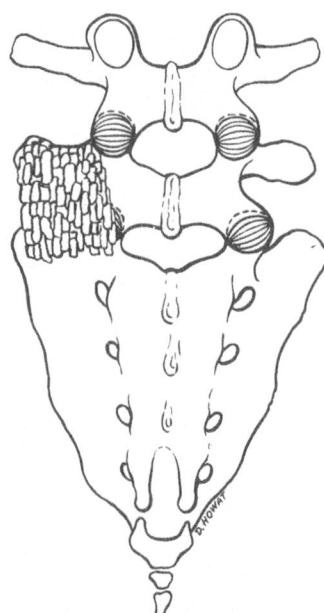

Figure 5.20. A drawing depicting the inter-transverse-alar graft mass on the left side

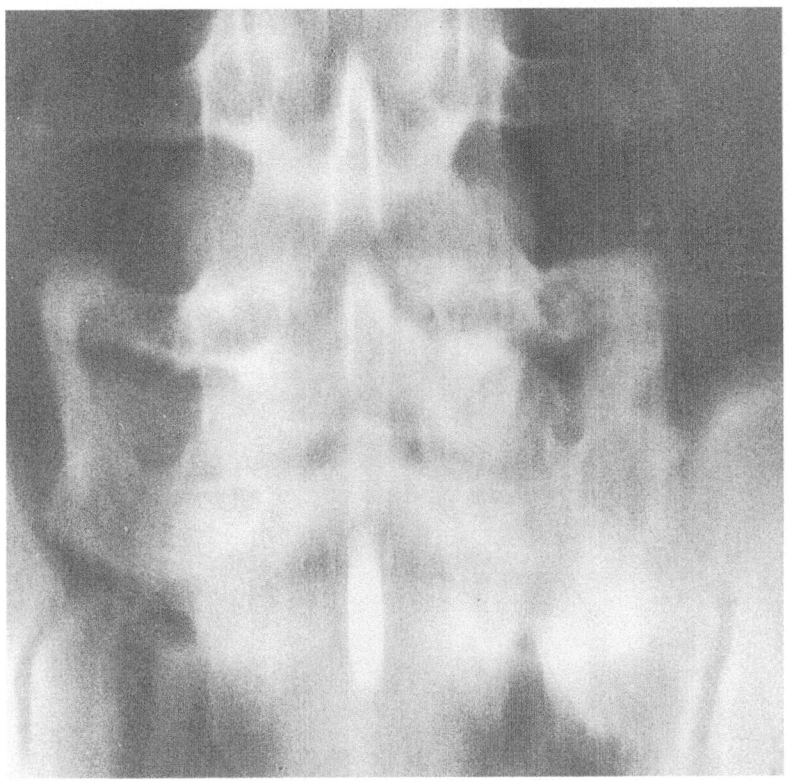

Figure 5.21. An antero-posterior tomogram showing satisfactory inter-transverse grafts at L4/5 in a patient with sacralization of the last lumbar vertebra (Mr. Chris Haw's case). Note the accurate termination of grafts at the L4 transverse processes

After placing the graft chips with equal care on both sides of the spine, the wounds should be closed with suction drainage (Figs. 5.20, 5.21, 5.23 a, b).

Where multi-level fusions have been performed, some surgeons have used screw fixation of the facet joints to aid in stability until fusion has occurred (Fig. 5.22).

h) Post-Operative Care

Retention of urine is common. It should be managed as recommended on p. 94. The routine use of catheters is best avoided especially in female patients.

Following multi-level spinal fusions, the use of surgical corsets or braces for 2–3 months after operation is recommended. Patients are encouraged to get out of bed early and to walk short distances within a few days of their operation.

i) Complications

Unless this operation is performed with the attention to detail outlined above, failure rates from non-union will be high. In cases of failure, when examining X-rays taken months after operation, it is often difficult to identify any grafted bone on one

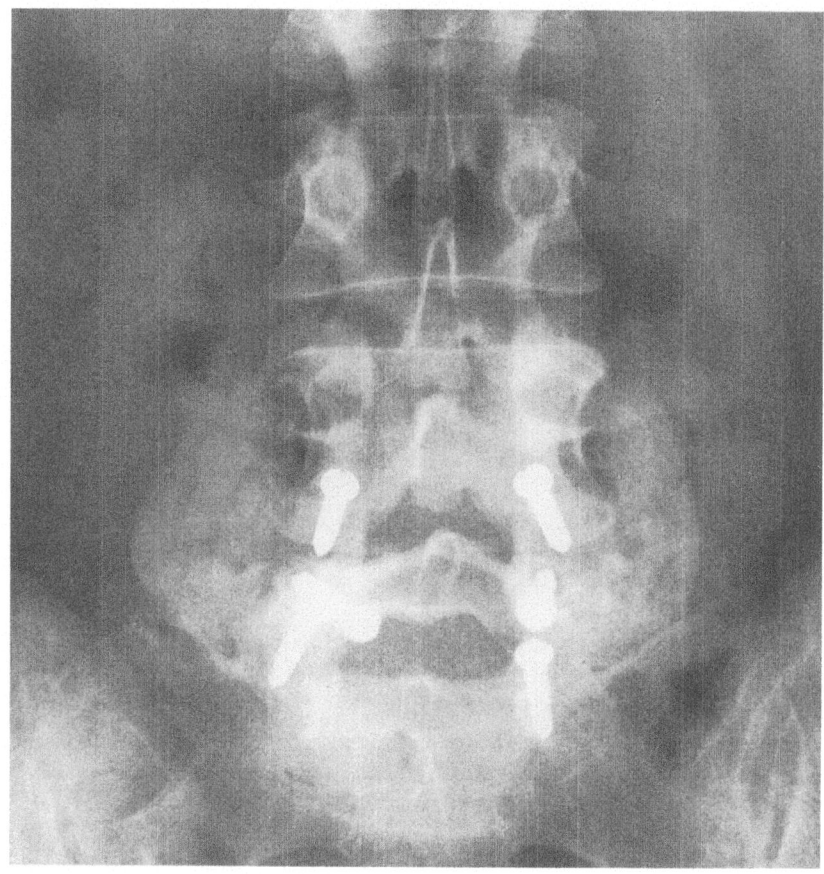

Figure 5.22. An antero-posterior radiograph of the lower lumbar spine showing a multi-level inter-transverse-alar fusion with supplementary screw fixation of the facets in the fused area (Mr. John Cloke's case)

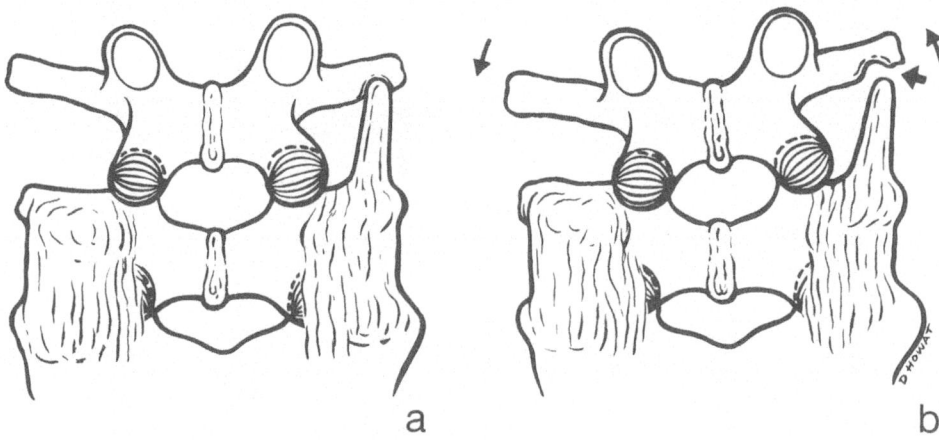

Figures 5.23 a, b. a A drawing showing inter-transverse-alar grafts with an "unwanted segment" of graft extending up on the right side producing a pseudarthrosis between the tip of the grafted bone and the transverse process above, **b** visible when the patient flexes to the opposite side. This is a cause of local chronic back pain easily relieved by excision of the "unwanted segment" of graft

or other side of the spine. Conversely, in other cases, grafted bone may hypertrophy and extend upwards in the spine 2 or 3 vertebral levels higher than planned. Segments of this "unwanted graft" may impinge on adjacent mobile posterior elements of the spine causing recurring problems such as back pain, muscle spasms and chronic spinal deformity (Figs. 5.23 a, b).

In addition, if grafted bone breaches the intertransverse muscles and ligaments, it may hypertrophy, producing nerve root irritation and foraminal stenosis. This problem has been recognised by Kirkaldy-Willis (1980) in C.T. scans of the lumbar spine taken after inter-transverse-alar fusion operations.

j) Infections

See pp. 286, 310, 314.

k) Graft Site Problems

Wiltse (1978) has warned of the risk of damaging cuneal nerves as they cross the posterior iliac crest, leading to chronic pain at the donor site.

Major complications may occur during or after the removal of large quantities of bone from the region of the posterior ilium. Attention should be focussed on the potential problems of severe haemorrhage during graft removal, sacro-iliac joint injury, lumbar hernia formation, pelvic dislocation and deep-seated infection of the pelvic bones (Figs. 5.24 a–e).

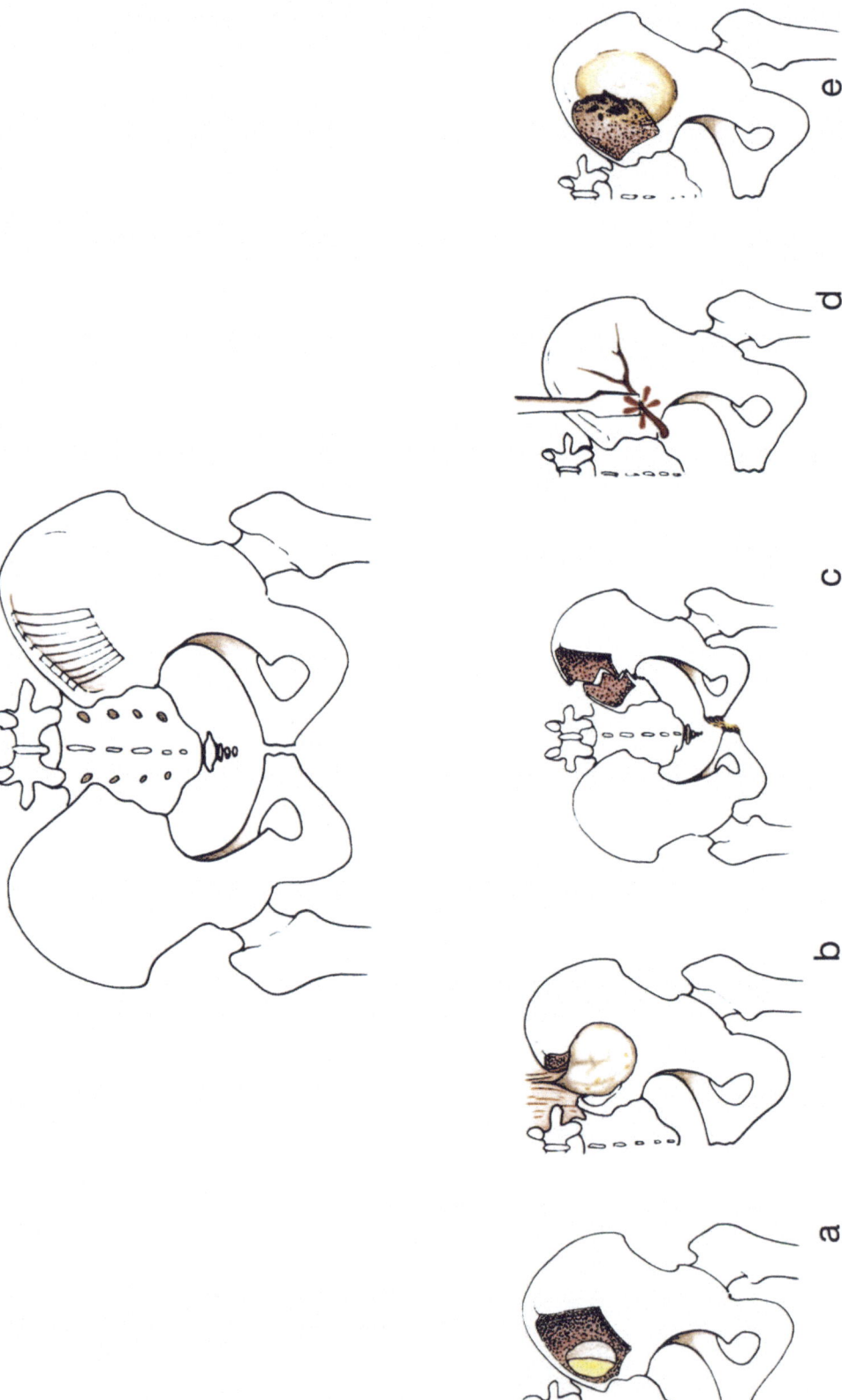

Figures 5.24a–e. Drawings depicting the potential hazards at the donor site after removing cortico-cancellous grafts from the posterior third of the iliac crest. **a** Shows penetration of the sacro-iliac joint. **b** Lumbar hernia. **c** Dislocation of the sacro-iliac joint and symphysis pubis. **d** Potential for haemorrhage from the superior gluteal artery. **e** Gross local sepsis

5.3. Spinal Canal and Nerve Root Canal Decompression with Foraminal Enlargement

a) The Gill and White Operation

After the initial exposure of the affected area of the spine (pp. 127–133), the interspinous ligaments should be excised from the superior and inferior aspects of the spinous process of the "rattler", that hyper-mobile segment of the roof of the spinal canal found in spondylolysis and spondylolytic spondylolisthesis which consists of the spinous process, the inferior articular facets and the lamina, split across its pars interarticularis on both sides and carrying the two distal surfaces of the pseudarthroses. The false joint capsules of these pseudarthroses, along with any loose bodies from within them, should then be removed with straight pituitary rongeurs. If the pseudarthroses have complex bulky opposing bony surfaces, it will not be possible to remove the "rattler" intact after excising the ligamentum flavum from both its superior margin and anterior surface. In such cases, the lamina is best divided along one side of the spinous process with a forward-angled rongeur. The spinous process is then grasped with a large bone nibbler and with the dura under constant vision, one half of the "rattler" may be rotated carefully and twisted slowly until it separates from the deep soft tissues which bind it to the proximal portion of the pseudarthrosis. The opposite segment of the "rattler" is then removed in like manner (Fig. 5.6a). This done, assuming that it is the L5 lamina which has been removed, the L5 nerve roots on both sides remain obstructed by the proximal portions of the laminal pseudarthroses and their soft tissue coverings. Removal of all these tissues on both sides is necessary to leave the pedicles of L5 clearly defined, the L5 nerve roots decompressed and the joints between the superior facets of L5 and the inferior facets of L4 essentially intact (Fig. 5.7 (3, 4)). Brisk venous haemorrhage sometimes occurs when the infero-medial cortical margin of the pedicle is breached during the decompression. This is readily stopped by applying bone wax to the bleeding area of the pedicle.

b) Simple Excision of the Laminal Pseudarthroses

Conservative excision of the laminal pseudarthroses is a satisfactory alternative to the radical decompression of the Gill and White procedure (Fig. 5.25). This operation is based on the recognition of the importance of maintaining the integrity of the spinous processes and interspinous ligaments to allow for the re-attachment of the lumbo-dorsal aponeurosis at the end of the decompression, thereby more effectively preserving its extensor function in spinal motion. It is applicable in cases where the laminal pseudarthroses are particularly bulky (Figs. 5.6a, b).

In the case of an L5/S1 spondylolysis, the lumbo-dorsal fascia is incised about 5 mm on either side of the spinous processes of L4 and L5. The paraspinal muscles are then retracted laterally to the outer margins of the L4/5 and L5/S1 facet joints. The spinous process of L5 is then grasped with a towel clip and moved upwards and downwards to identify the laminal pseudarthroses. These may be obstructed by the inferior margins of the inferior facets of the lamina of L4. Portions of the tips of these facets with surrounding capsular fibres may need to be excised before the

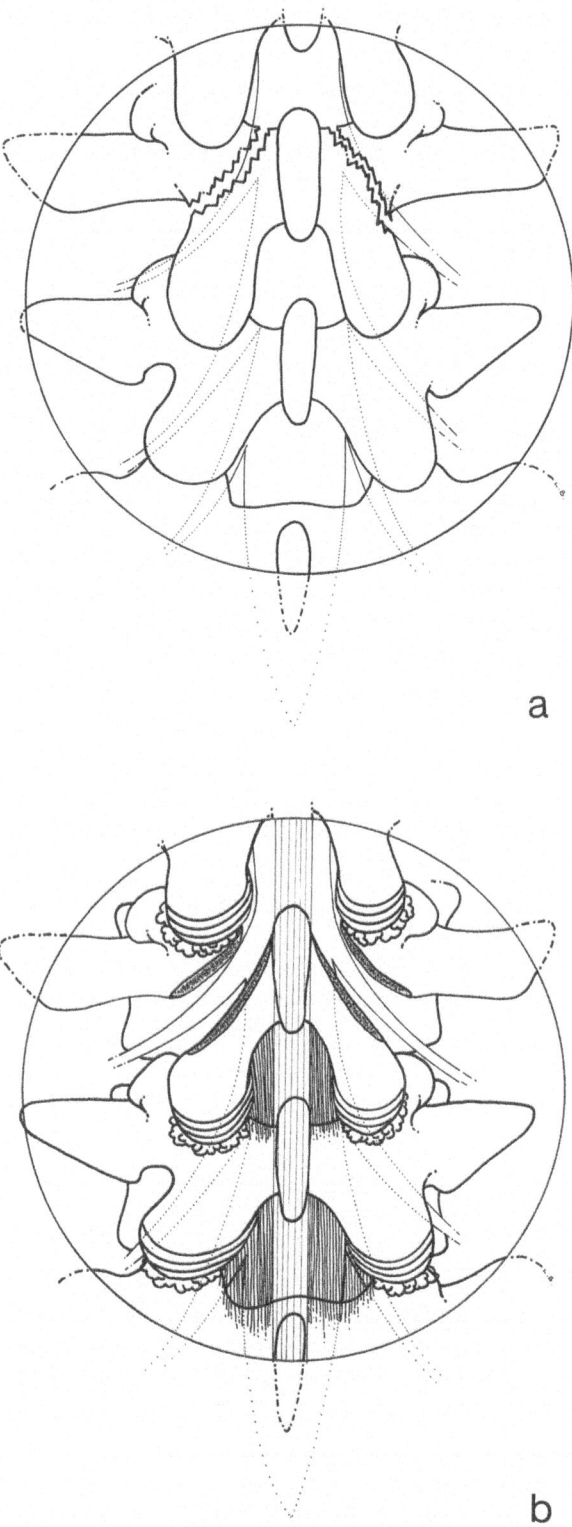

a

b

Figures 5.25. **a** A drawing showing bilateral spondylolytic defects in the lamina of L4 vertebra. **b** A drawing to show the appearances following excision of the pseudarthroses in a case of L4 spondylolysis. The "rattler" remains in situ with its ligamentum flavum undisturbed at L4/5. The interspinous ligaments are intact. The lumbo-dorsal aponeurosis is then re-attached to both sides of these ligaments at the end of the operation "false joints" in the L5 lamina can be identified. The ligamentum flavum between L4 and L5 laminae should be excised, allowing access to the pseudarthroses which should be removed with the use of appropriate instruments so that no damage is inflicted on the underlying nerve roots or the dural sac. Venous haemorrhage occurring from tributaries of the internal vertebral venous plexus surrounding the nerve roots should be controlled only with gelfoam or equivalent haemostatic agents, while pedicle vein bleeding will require the application of bone wax. Having completed the decompressions of the intervertebral foramina, the lumbo-dorsal fascia should be reattached on each side of the supraspinous and interspinous ligaments. Drainage of the wound is not required (Figs. 5.25 a,b).

5.4. Direct Repair of the Bony Defects in Spondylolysis and Spondylolisthesis

While the Gill and White procedure has been shown to give good long-term relief of leg pains in adults, there is a place for the conservation of the "rattler" in young patients in whom spinal fusion may be deemed unnecessary. Direct bone grafting of the laminal pseudoarthroses, with internal fixation using screws, has been recommended by Buck (1979). Scott (1987) has described an alternative method of grafting and fixation with tension band wires passed around the transverse processes.

6

The Surgical Management of Spinal Canal Stenosis

6.1. Introduction

With the phenomenal growth of interest in spinal disorders that has occurred in the past ten years, the various syndromes that arise in spinal stenosis are now more widely recognised. Although the range of conditions that may mimic it is broad, the differential diagnosis in the lumbar region has been largely centred around the distinctions between aortic vascular disorders and spinal stenosis. Peripherally for example, bilateral hip disease may give rise to symptoms similar to those of cauda equina claudication, while, centrally, cerebral atrophy may be attributed as the cause of unsteadiness of gait, with weakness sufficiently severe to cause the patient affected merely with lumbar canal stenosis to fall to the ground while walking.

Cervical canal stenosis is discussed in Chapter 7.

Because of its rarity in the thoracic spine, this condition as a cause of unsteadiness of gait is frequently overlooked or, if it is recognised, there is usually a prolonged delay between the time of the patient first presenting for advice and the time of establishment of the diagnosis.

Understanding of the mechanisms of the neurological symptoms and signs which arise in cases of spinal stenosis at any level is still incomplete. There has tended to be a preoccupation with the importance of vertebral canal dimensions. While these are important, particularly in the cervical and thoracic regions of the spine, it seems likely that vascular obstruction in the intervertebral foramina in the lumbar region, affecting predominantly the tributaries of the internal vertebral venous plexus, is primarily responsible for many of the symptoms in patients with lumbar canal stenosis. Professor Ooi has pioneered the use of myeloscopy and has persisted with its investigation for 20 years. He and his colleagues have been able to produce incontrovertible evidence supporting the theory that retrograde venous distension of radicular veins occurs in patients with cauda equina claudication. Swedish investigators have been able to demonstrate experimentally that persistent chronic venous obstruction of the cauda equina may lead eventually to the development of arachnoiditis of the cauda equina, Olmarker (1990). Patients who develop this problem usually have paralytic manifestations, becoming excessively weak if not paraparetic after walking. Quite clearly in some cases, there are mixed contributions from both arterial and venous obstructions in the cauda equina.

Relevant aspects of the anatomy of the arterial and venous circulation of the cauda equina are shown in the accompanying illustrations (Figs. 6.1–3).

The arteries of the cauda equina arise from branches of the lumbar arteries just outside the foramina. Each nerve root carries an anterior and posterior radicular artery which runs uninterrupted from its origin to the major channels respectively on

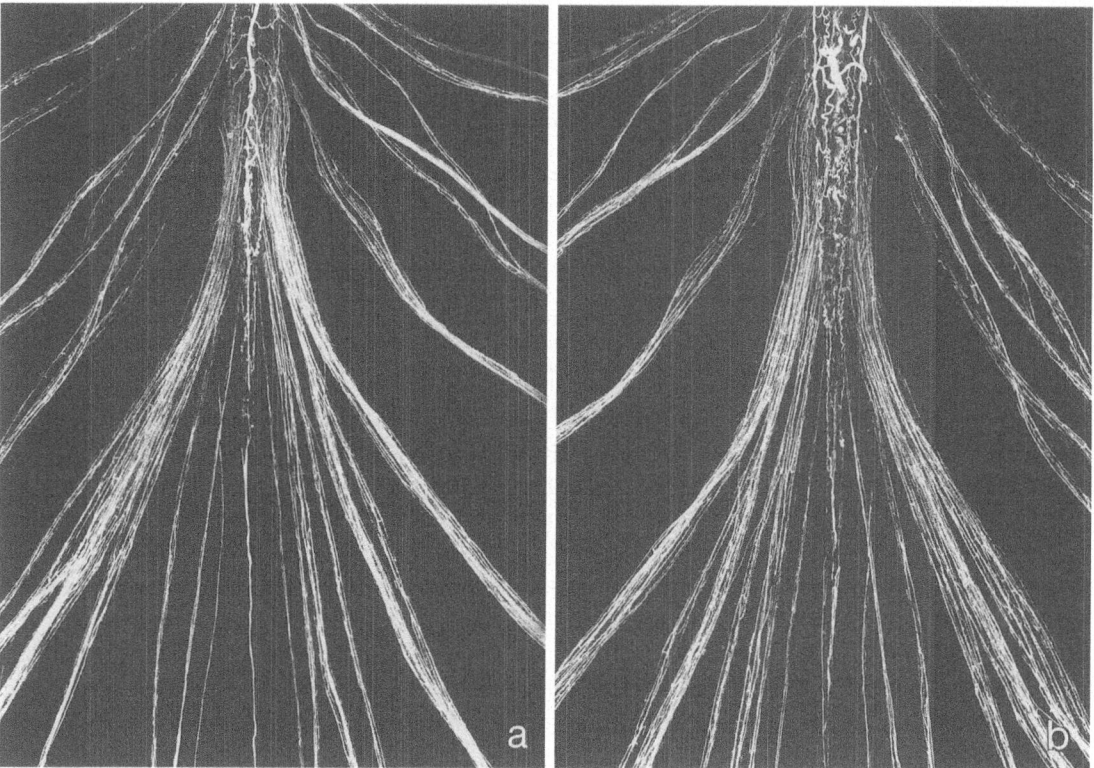

Figures 6.1 a, b. a A photograph of the anterior surface of the conus medullaris and cauda equina from a male aged 41 years, enlarged approximately one and a half times. In this specimen, the filaments of the cauda equina have been widely separated. *Their distal ends have been sectioned at the levels of their individual intervertebral foramina.* The arteries of the cauda equina and conus medullaris are clearly shown. Note the continuity of the vessels along the lengths of the filaments of the cauda equina, with the arteries on the surface of the spinal cord. Even at this magnification, the complexity of the arteries of the cauda equina can be appreciated. Note the numerous anastomoses, through ultra fine branches, between arteries coursing along adjacent nerve filaments. **b** A photograph of the dorsal aspect of the same specimen. The postero-lateral longitudinal arterial trunks, which in this specimen are rather fine, are clearly seen forming a loop distally at the tip of the conus, where they anastomose with the anterior median longitudinal arterial trunk of the spinal cord. The continuity of vessels extending along the course of the cauda equina to the arteries on the conus medullaris is shown. There is no suggestion of an area of hypo-vascularity in the region of the middle third of the cauda equina as previously described by Parke *et al.* (1981)

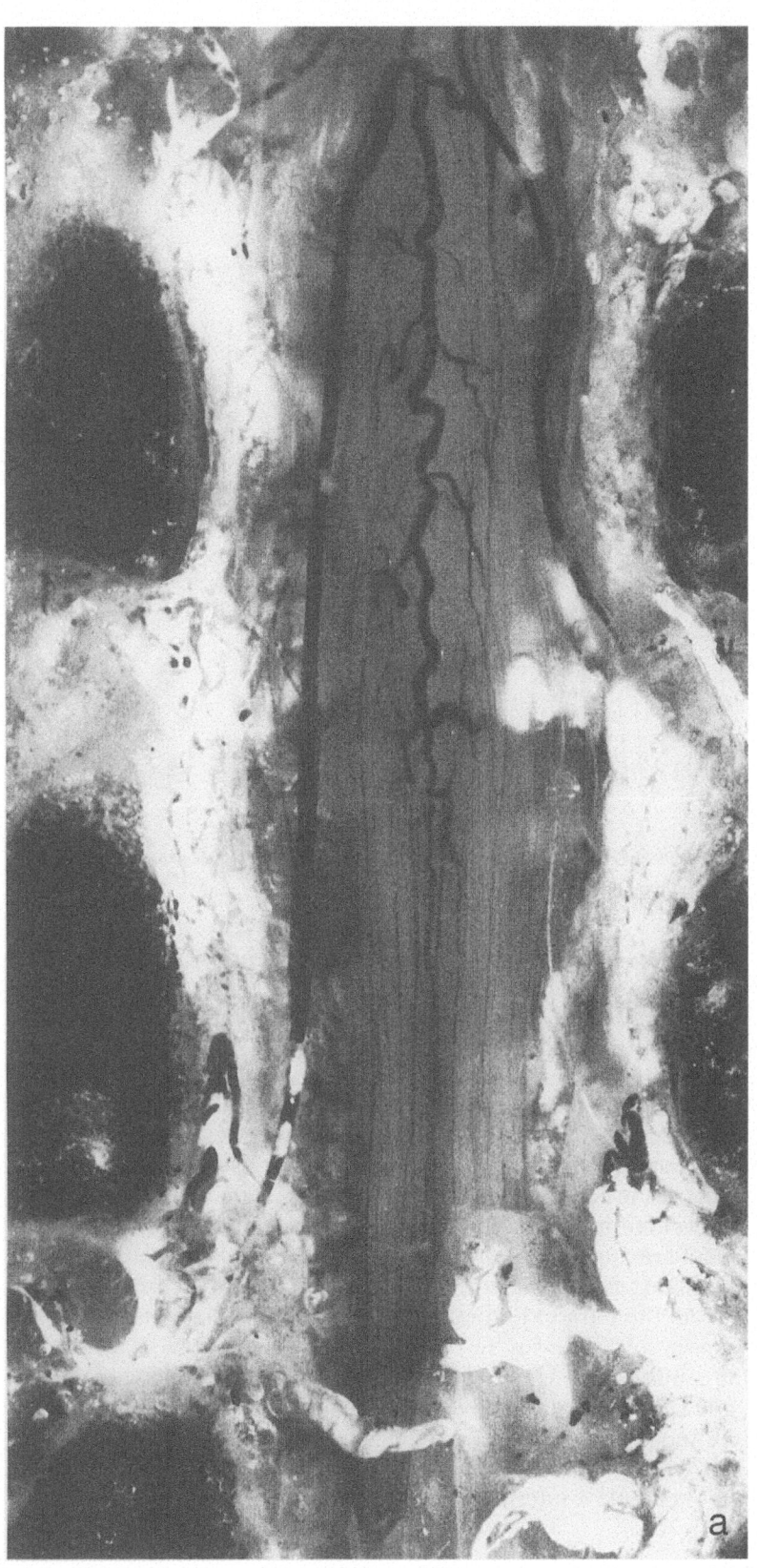

Figure 6.2a
(Legend see p. 190)

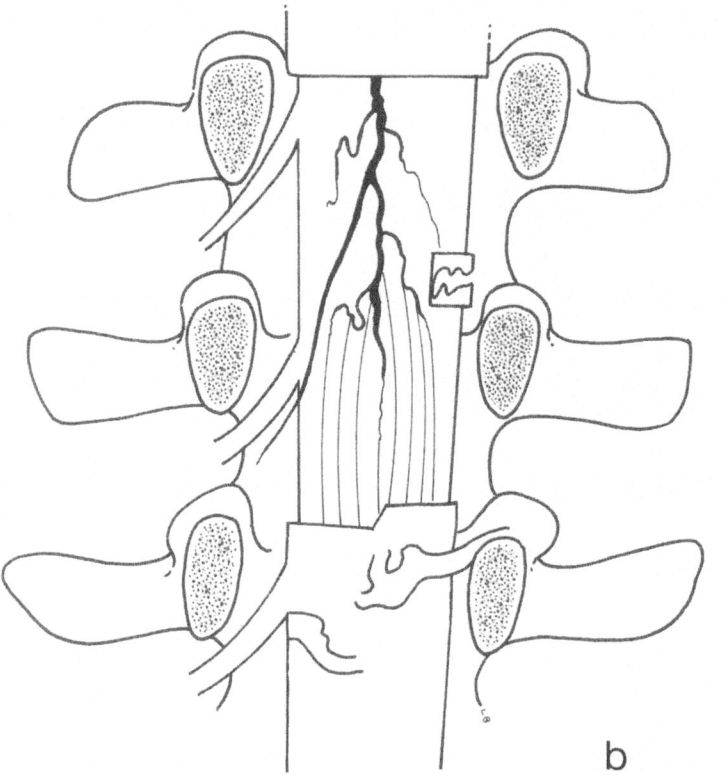

b   Figure 6.2 b

Figures 6.2 a, b. a A photograph of the posterior surface of the conus medullaris and lower part of the thoracic spinal cord from a male aged 65 years. The specimen is viewed from behind. The laminae of T 12/L1 and L2 have been removed. The pedicles of those vertebrae are seen on the left hand side. The dural sac is intact in the region of L2. Radicles of the *posterior internal vertebral venous* plexus (filled with white barium sulphate suspension) lie on its surface. They are in continuity with the anterior internal vertebral venous plexus on both sides. Above that level the dura, arachnoid membrane and pia mater have been removed. Note that the *anterior internal vertebral venous plexus* is completely filled with barium sulphate suspension. By contrast, the veins on the dorsal aspect of the conus are filled only with blood. On the left side of the specimen, a large dorsal radicular vein (dorsal vena radiculo-medullaris magna) is seen coursing downwards from the conus medullaris inside the dural sac. At the level of the pedicle of L1 vertebra two flecks of barium sulphate suspension lie within the clotted blood in this vein which tapers to a point as it emerges from the dura to join radicles of the anterior internal vertebral venous plexus in the epidural space. **b** A drawing to orientate the reader showing the conus medullaris and upper part of the cauda equina viewed from behind lying in the spinal canal from which the laminae of T12, L1 and L2 have been removed through their pedicles. The dural sac has been removed in part to show the veins on the surface of the conus medullaris and the course of the radicular vein on the left hand side extending from the surface of the spinal cord to penetrate the dural sac and join the anterior internal vertebral venous plexus

(Fig. 6.2 a see p. 189)

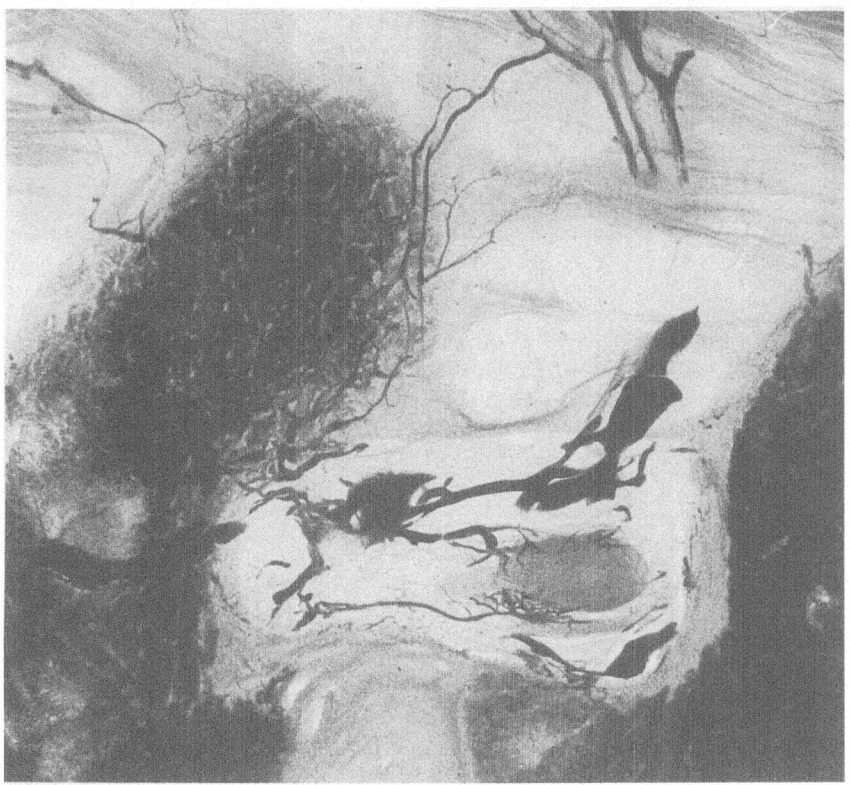

Figure 6.3. A photograph of a specimen from a male aged 68 years, cut in the sagittal plane through a lumbar intervertebral foramen. Details of the venous drainage of nerve roots in the foramen and their relationship to the anterior and posterior radicles of the internal vertebral venous plexus are shown. Note also the important relationship between veins in the pedicle and radicles of the internal vertebral venous plexus in the intervertebral foramen. [Reproduced with permission from "The Conus Medullaris and Cauda Equina in Man. An atlas of the arteries and veins", Crock *et al.*, Wien–New York: Springer, 1986]

the anterior and posterior surfaces of the spinal cord. There is no area of so-called hypo-vascularity in the cauda equina.

The venous drainage of the cauda equina rootlets is centrifugal, terminating after penetrating the dural sac in the region of the individual nerve root sleeves in the internal vertebral venous plexus. A valve-like mechanism between the intra-dural and extra-dural venous systems exists so that venous obstruction in the nerve root canals or intervertebral foramina will inevitably lead to engorgement of the intra-dural veins and nerve root oedema. The engorgement of these vessels has been beautifully demonstrated by Professor Ooi and co-workers (Figs. 6.4 a–c).

In the cervical and thoracic regions of the spine many of the pathological processes which lead to canal stenoses in these areas are related to the anterior surface of the spinal cord particularly in the mid-line. Compression of the arterial supply of the cord is probably the most important cause of the symptoms of myelopathy.

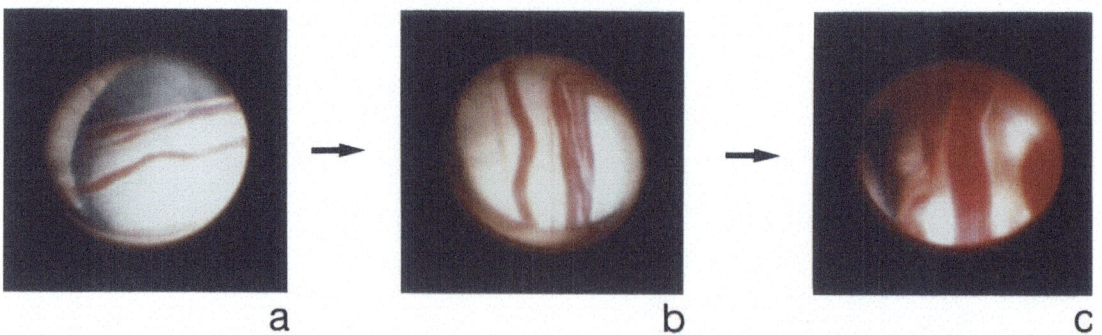

Figures 6.4 a–c. a Myeloscopic findings in a 48 year old man with multi-level lumbar canal stenosis during bed rest. **b** While standing. **c** While walking. Note the dilatation of the veins on the cauda equina. [Reproduced by kind permission of Professor Ooi and the editor of SPINE]

The causes of spinal stenosis may be classified as follows:

1. Congenital Causes
   a) Achondroplasia and other forms of dwarfism.
   b) Congenital small spinal canal, with short vertebral pedicles.
   c) Hemi-vertebrae with lumbar scoliosis.
   d) Congenital cysts arising from the dura or arachnoid, in an otherwise normal spinal canal.
2. Acquired Causes
   a) Degenerative spondylosis, including degenerative spondylolisthesis.
   b) Vertebral fractures, post-traumatic or pathological.
   c) Spinal infections.
   d) Paget's disease.
   e) Acromegaly.
   f) Following some spinal operations.

The experience of individual surgeons in treating cases of spinal stenosis due to different causes will vary, especially among those working in large cities where special units may be found dealing exclusively with spinal injuries, cancer patients and children (Figs. 6.5–14).

Spinal surgery has now emerged as a sub-specialty around the world and there are many surgeons devoted exclusively to its practice. It should no longer be regarded as exclusively in the realm of either orthopaedic surgery or neurosurgery so that the invidious comparisons between the skills of the two groups of surgeons should disappear.

Although Sarpenyer described congenital stricture of the spinal canal in 1945, Verbiest (1954) deserves much of the credit for focussing attention on the various clinical syndromes associated with stenosis of the spinal canal. Important contributions to the understanding of various aspects of spinal stenosis have been made by Kirkaldy-Willis, Paine, Cauchoix and McIvor (1974), Verbiest (1976), Weinstein, Ehni, and Wilson (1977). More recently, scholarly monographs on the subject have appeared, Postacchini (1989) and Nixon (1991).

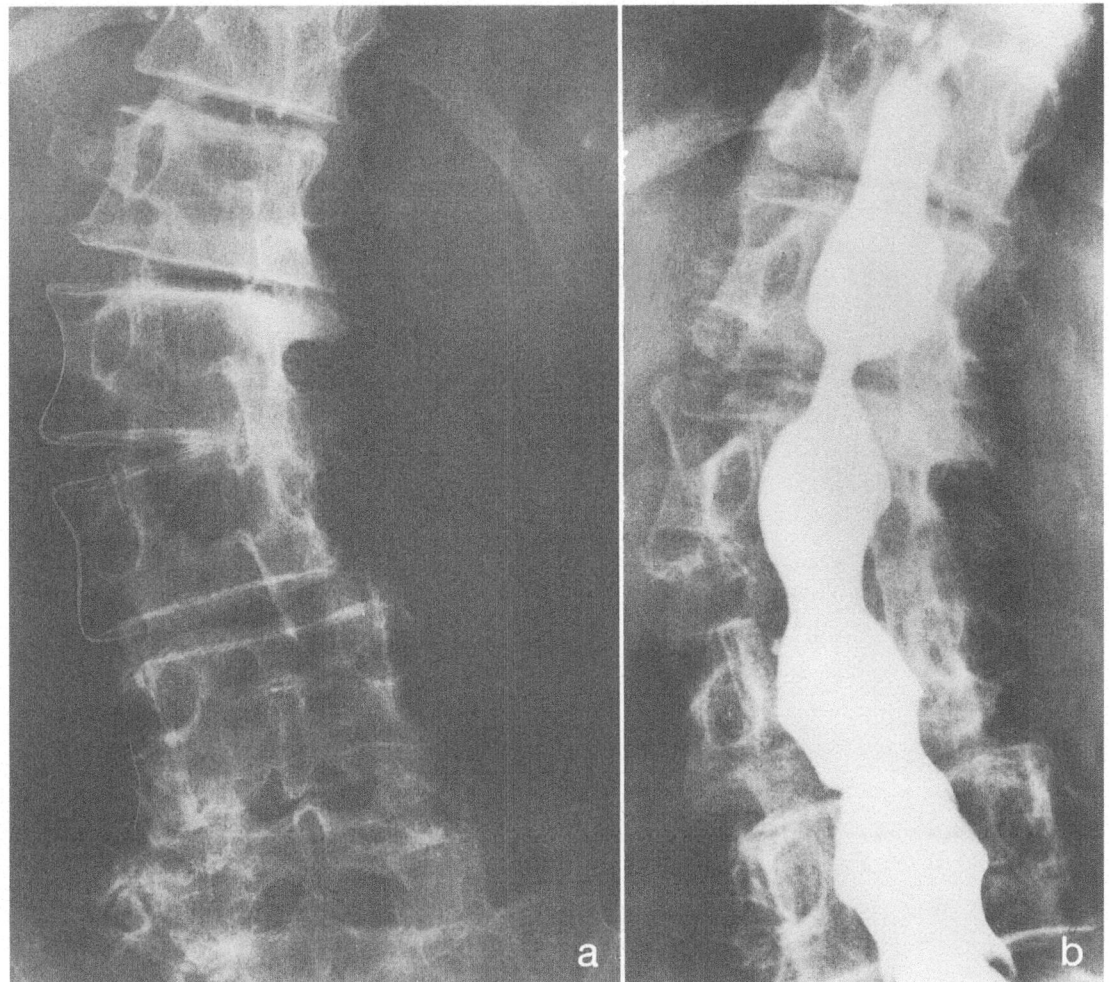

Figures 6.5 a, b. a An antero-posterior radiograph of the lumbar spine of a woman of 66 years showing congenital fusion of the vertebral bodies of L2 and L3 with resultant scoliosis, further aggravated by degenerative spondylosis at the disc between L1 and L2. This patient presented with a cauda equina claudication syndrome. **b** An antero-posterior radiograph of a myodil myelogram showing multi-level canal stenosis, most marked at the L1/2 and L2/3 regions. This patient's symptoms were greatly relieved following two level decompression of the spinal canal

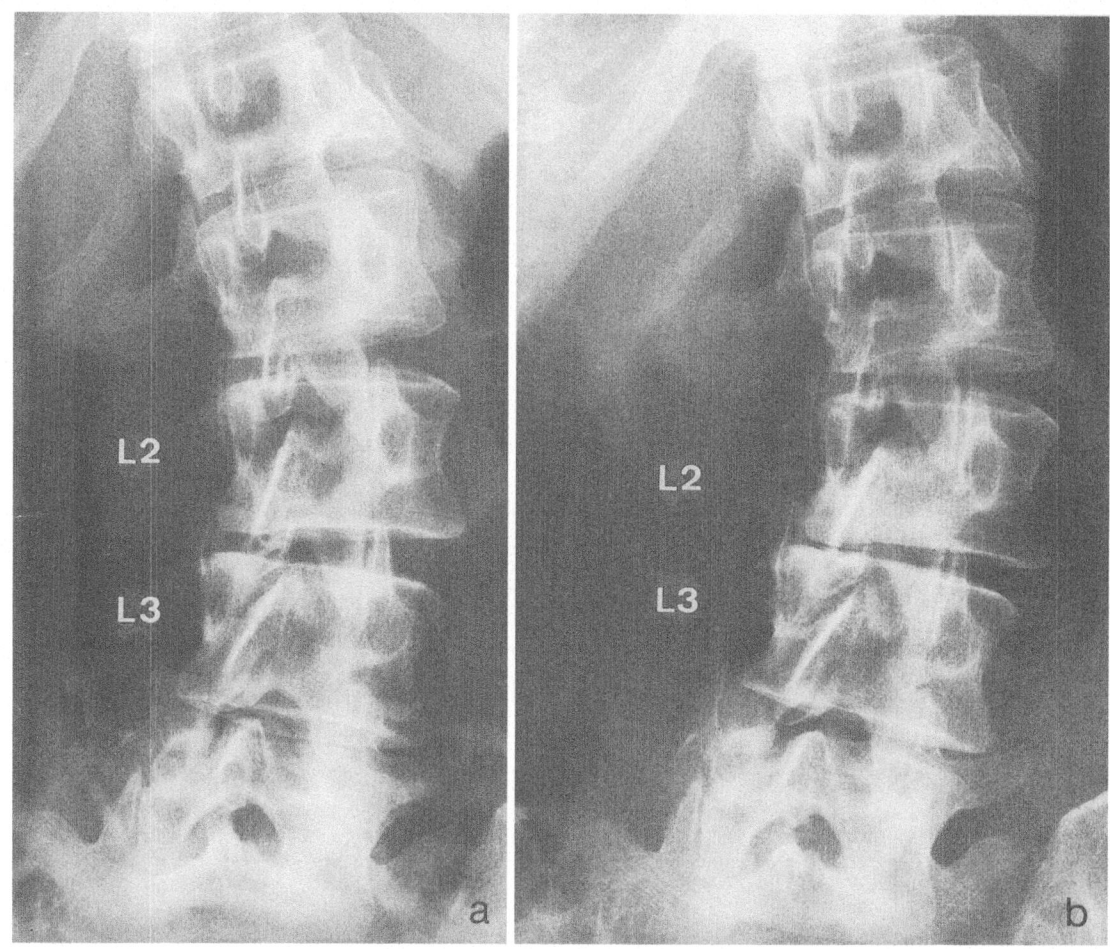

Figures 6.6 a, b

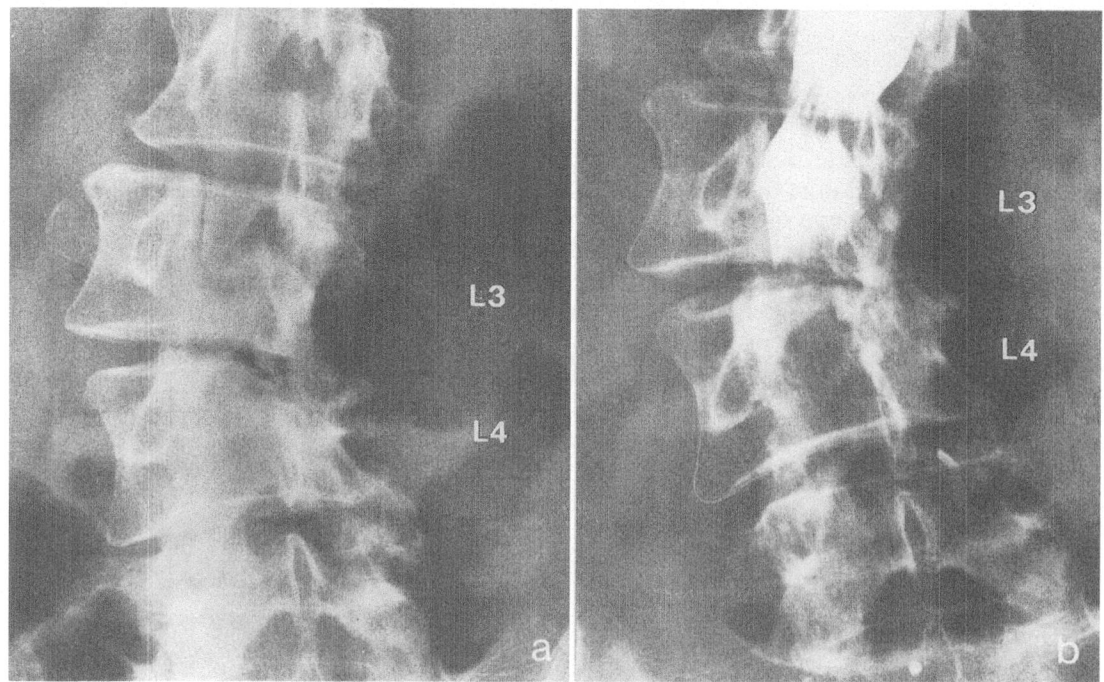

Figures 6.7 a, b

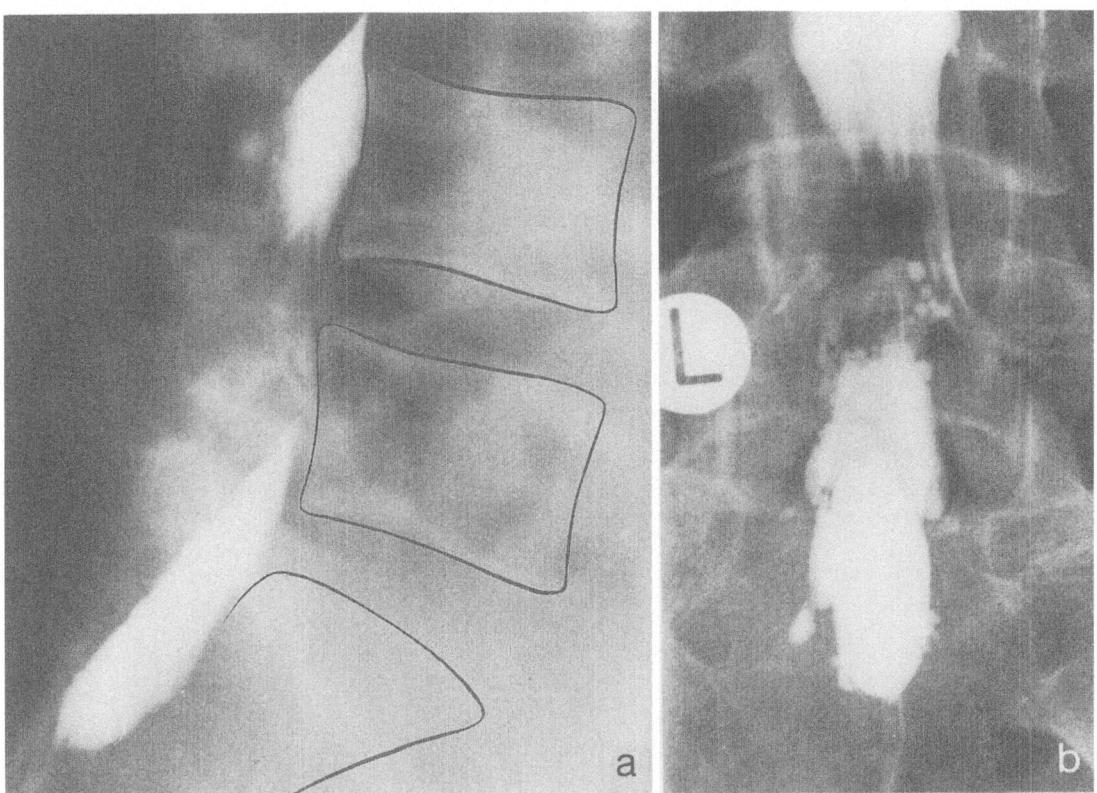

Figures 6.8 a, b. a A lateral radiograph of the lumbar spine of a man aged 47 years presenting with classical symptoms of cauda equina claudication. Note the myelographic defect and the normal disc height at L 4/5 and L 5/S 1. This is an example of incomplete obstruction and in such cases it is necessary to posture the patient at the time of myelography so that adequate studies of the flow of the dye can be obtained. What appears to be a complete obstruction may turn out to be incomplete if the patient is postured in the vertical or head down position. **b** An antero-posterior radiograph of the same spine showing the single level canal stenosis due to pathology in the roof of the spinal canal

---

Figures 6.6 a, b. a An antero-posterior radiograph showing early disc degeneration between the bodies of L 2 and L 3 causing scoliosis in a patient with four lumbar vertebrae. **b** The same spine three years later showing increased disc space narrowing with further increase in scoliosis. This form of degenerative lumbar scoliosis due to intrinsic disc disease is seen in middle-aged women, often with multiple discs involved. Many of these patients develop spinal stenosis

Figures 6.7 a, b. a An antero-posterior radiograph of the lumbar spine of a woman aged 55 years. Note the scoliosis with its apex at the L 3/4 level. This is one of the rare causes of degenerative scoliosis in middle-aged women due to acute vertebral end-plate necrosis. The deformities resulting from this lesion are often complex with both kyphotic and scoliotic components contributing to the overall deformity. **b** An antero-posterior radiograph of the myelogram in this case showing a complete block at the L 3/4 level with stenotic changes at L 2/3 above

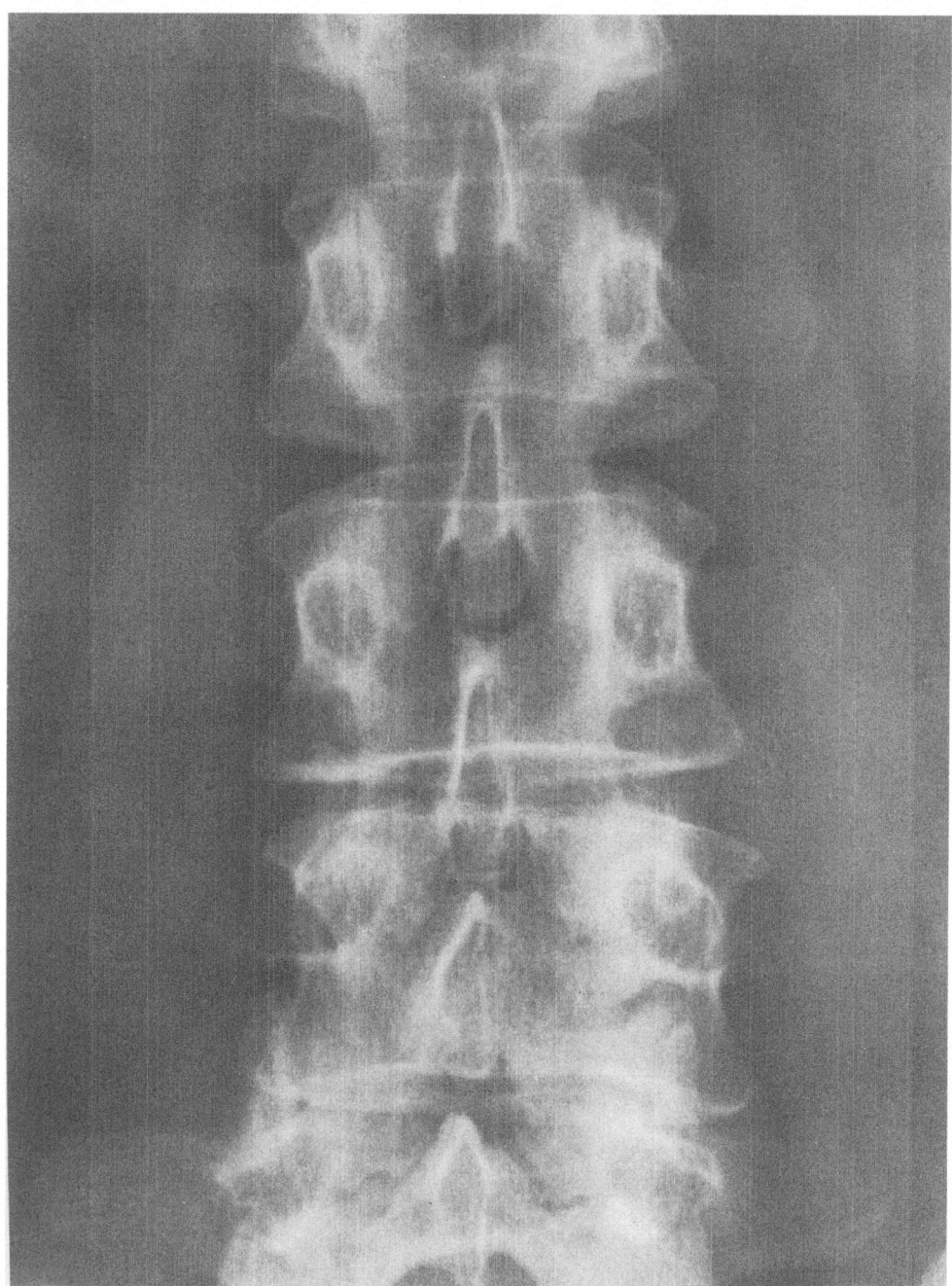

Figure 6.9. An antero-posterior radiograph of the lumbar spine in an adult in whom gross pathology is noted, particularly in the roof of the spinal canal. Although there is evidence of spondylosis at L3/4 with asymmetrical narrowing of the disc space, the major changes are in the laminal structures where facet hypertrophy, laminal thickening and spinous process interdigitation have reduced the interlaminar spaces at L2/3 and L3/4 to minute proportions

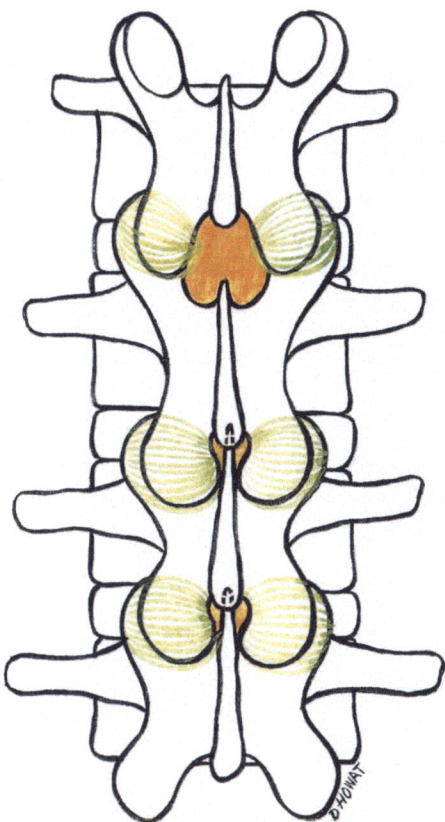

Figure 6.10. A drawing based on the X-ray shown in Fig. 6.9 to highlight the pathological changes which may occur in the roofing structures of the spinal canal leading to the development of multi-level canal stenosis. At the top of the drawing the ligamentum flavum is of normal proportions and there is wide separation between the medial margins of the capsules of the facet joints. In addition, the interspinous space is clearly defined. By contrast, at the lower two levels, note the interdigitation of the spinous processes, the hypertrophic changes in the facets and the almost complete occlusion from view of the ligamentum flavum at both of these levels

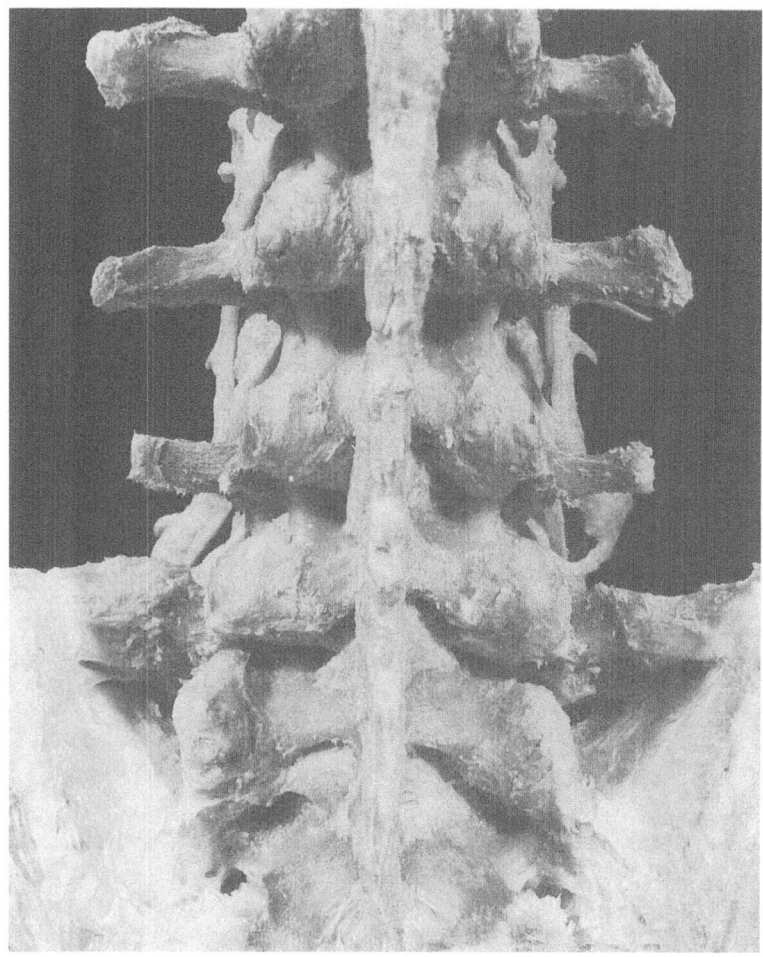

Figure 6. 11. A photograph of a dissection of a normal lumbar spine viewed from behind. Note the orientation of the facet joints at L3/4, L4/5, and L5/S1. These are separated widely from the mid-line, so that the ligamentum flavum can be seen clearly at each level. Shadows are cast on the ligamentum flavum by the lower margins of the laminae, highlighting the anatomical feature of the superior attachment of the ligamentum flavum to the anterior surface of the superior lamina at a particular interspace. (Dissected by Dr. M. C. Crock)

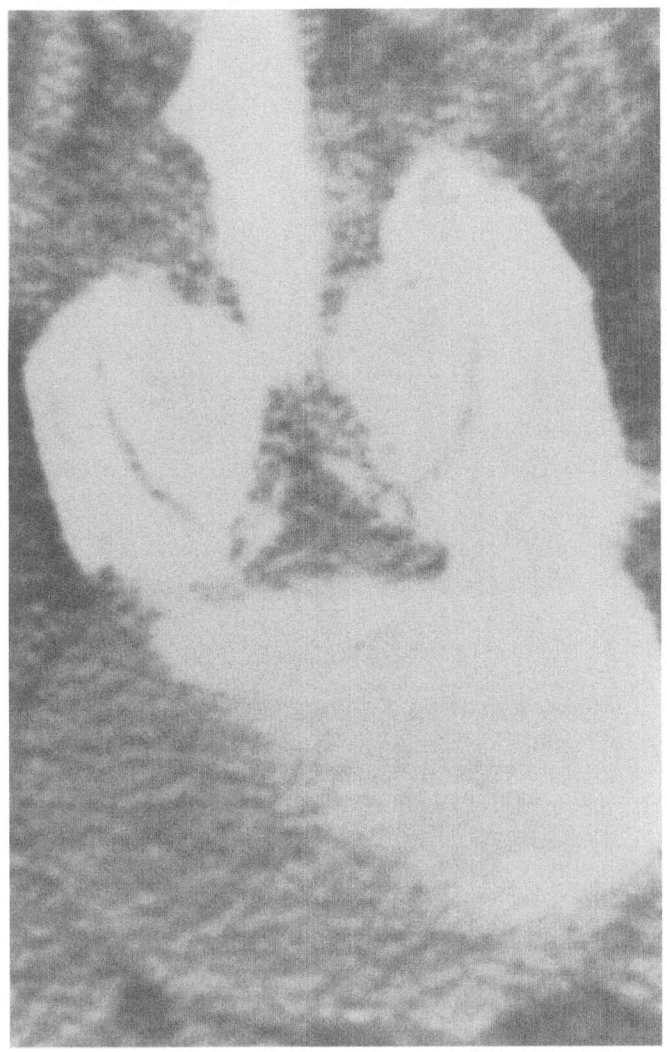

Figure 6.12. An axial CT image on the lumbar spine of an acromegalic patient aged 42 showing gross facet joint hypertrophy and osteoarthritis with ossification of the ligamentum flavum on both sides

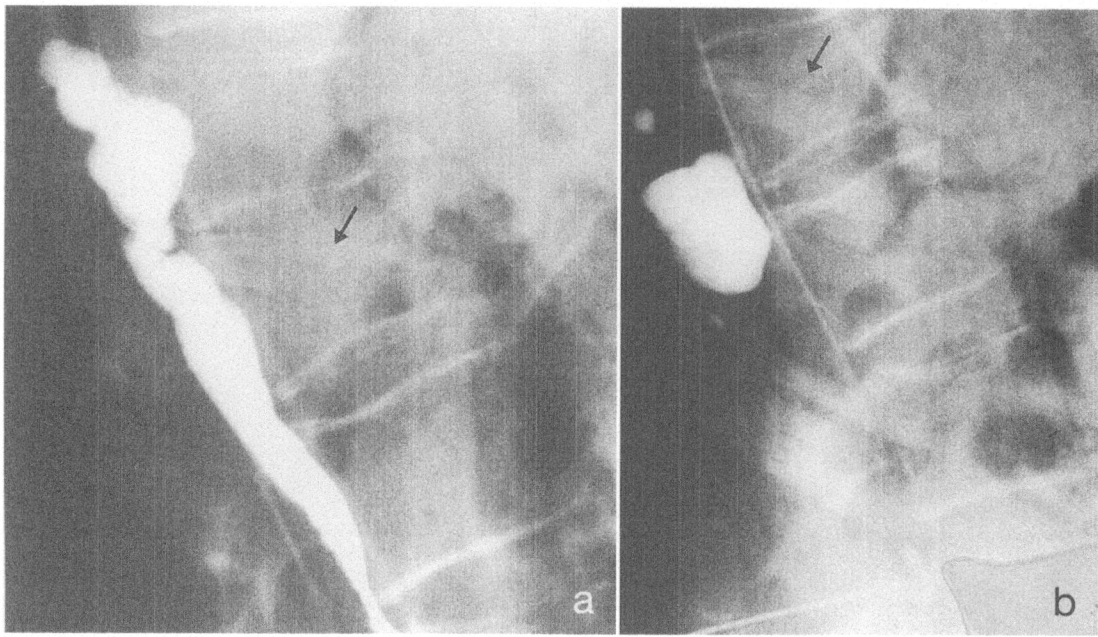

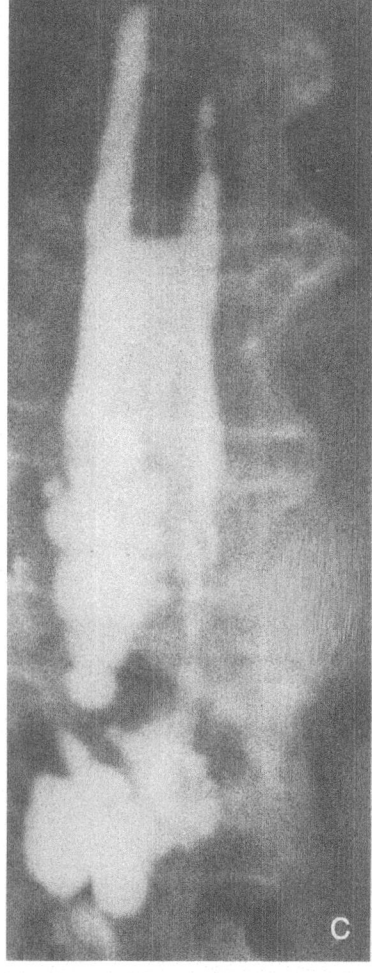

Figures 6.13a–c. a A lateral radiograph of the lumbar spine of a woman aged 68 years. The black arrow points to a crush-fracture of the vertebral body of L1, sustained following a fall from a bicycle. The myelogram was taken twelve months after this injury for the investigation of pain at the thoraco-lumbar junction with marked upper abdominal pain and gross abdominal distension. This patient had a post-traumatic arachnoid cyst which extended distally to the middle of the body of L2 and proximally to the level of T11. **b** A lateral radiograph of the same spine following removal of the myodil. Note the remnants of myodil trapped in the arachnoid cyst just below the vertebral fracture marked by the black arrow. **c** An antero-posterior radiograph to show the spatial distribution of the arachnoid cyst which produced a functional spinal stenosis responsible for the symptoms described. This patient had an extremely thin, transparent dural sac in the region of the thoraco-lumbar junction. The arachnoid cyst was easily identified at operation. Symptoms were relieved by multi-level decompression of the thoraco-lumbar canal. The arachnoid cyst was not ruptured and in view of the fact that the dural sac was abnormally thin, no attempt was made to find a rent in it – related to the fracture of the vertebral body – through which the cyst emerged. The patient's symptoms were relieved and the troublesome abdominal distension disappeared soon after operation

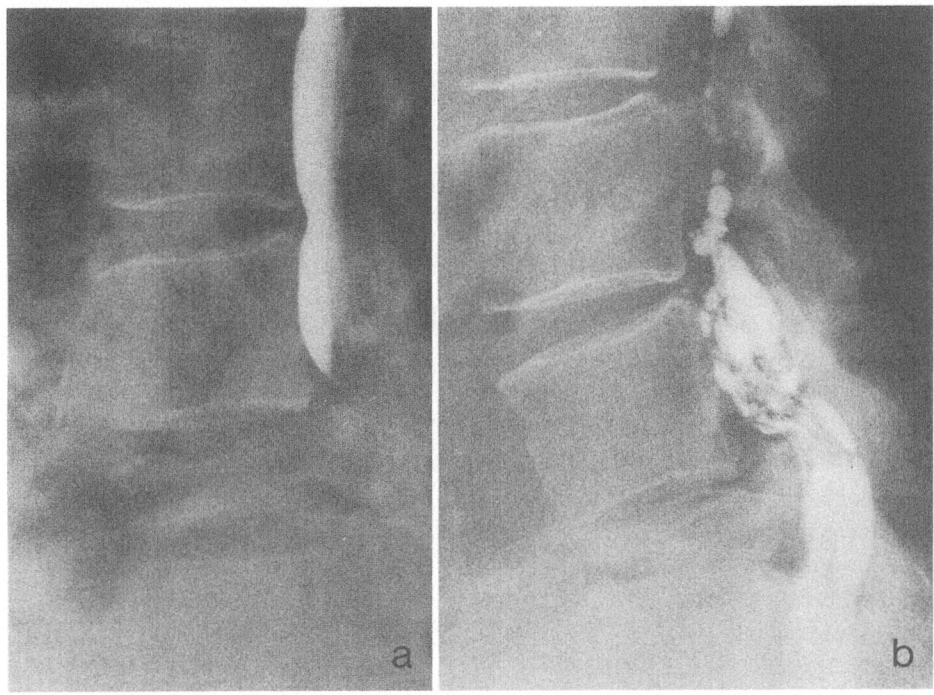

Figures 6.14a,b. **a** A lateral radiograph of the lower lumbar spine of a woman aged 59 years showing complete obstruction to the flow of myodil in a myelogram at the level of L4, the site of a pathological fracture of the vertebral body due to a primary tumour of bone. **b** Following decompression of the lumbar spinal canal, note the restoration of the flow of myodil. The patient's symptoms of referred leg pain were relieved and she lived for approximately nine months after this film was taken, dying with secondary pulmonary tumours. The primary lesion was sarcomatous

6.2. Clinical Features

a) Symptoms

Most patients describe a variety of symptoms which may include:

a) Back pain
   This is often aggravated by standing or walking. It may be the only symptom of which a patient complains in whom spinal stenosis can be demonstrated. Characteristically the back pain is relieved by bending forwards or by lying down.
b) Leg pain
   Of variable distribution, unilateral or bilateral, and often fluctuating.
c) Paraesthesiae
   Ranging from feelings of numbness and heaviness, sometimes with an associated burning pain, sometimes with a feeling of coldness in the limbs.
d) Weakness in the extremities
   Ranging from unilateral loss of power resulting in sudden falls, to paraparesis, related to walking and relieved by rest. In cases of cervical canal stenosis or of

thoracic canal stenosis, spasticity of gait may be a prominent feature. Upper extremity involvement with symptoms similar to those experienced in the lower limbs, in cases of lumbar canal stenosis, may be present in those with cervical myelopathy.

e) Restless legs

Uncontrolled leg movements experienced especially at night in bed.

f) Disturbances of bladder function

Ranging from frequency to incontinence after walking.

Despite wide-ranging descriptions of symptoms, all of these patients complain of claudication, related either to their pain, paraesthesiae, weakness or, occasionally, to all three symptoms together.

Intermittent claudication of vascular origin can usually be distinguished easily from cauda equina or nerve root claudication on clinical grounds. Pain in the legs of vascular origin is cramp-like and centres on the calf or buttock muscles. Impairment of arterial circulation is indicated by:

- loss of hair on the legs;
- absent peripheral pulses;
- the detection of audible bruits along the course of the main arteries in the lower abdomen or in the limbs themselves.

b) Physical Signs

There are no characteristic findings. Signs vary depending on the underlying pathological condition causing the spinal stenosis.

6.3. Radiological Investigations

a) Plain X-Rays

In congenital lumbar or cervical canal stenosis, certain findings can be important. For example, anomalies with block-vertebrae or hemi-vertebrae and scoliosis are frequently associated with stenosis. Narrowing of the spinal canal can be identified in lateral films when short pedicles and reduced inter-pedicular distances measured on AP films are found. Alterations in the pattern of orientation of facet joints at particular levels may also be important. In canal stenosis of degenerative origin, major changes are often found in the roof of the spinal canal, with gross hypertrophy of facet joints, shingling of laminae, and evidence of calcification or ossification of the ligamentum flavum. Gross lumbar scoliosis may occur due to asymmetrical narrowing of the disc spaces or to acute necrosis of the vertebral end-plates.

b) Computerized Axial Tomography

The use of this investigation has revolutionized the investigation of spinal stenosis in recent years, particularly in combination with radiculography. However, it has certainly not superseded the use of plain X-ray, radiculograms or MRI. Using bone windows and sagittal coronal and oblique reconstructions, when the technology is available, accurate estimates of the degree of stenosis at individual spinal levels can be made. Three-dimensional CT radiography shows promise of providing even more accurate depictions of stenoses in certain situations such as the occipito-cervical junction.

c) Radiculography

This investigation remains essential for planning surgical treatment wherever the sophisticated technology of CT scanning and MRI imaging is not available. Myelography provides information about the nature and severity of pathological changes at or below the site of obstruction, providing the movement of dye in the spinal canal is studied carefully. For example, by tilting the patient into head -down or erect vertical positions, the flow of dye can be observed with these changes in posture and distinctions drawn between complete and partial blockages, areas of arachnoiditis in the cauda equina can be identified and obstructions at multiple levels in the canal can be recognized (Figs. 6.5,6.7,6.8,6.13,6.14).

d) MRI

This is particularly valuable for identifying problems at the cranio-cervical junction, in the cervical spine or in the thoracic spine where it will provide the most accurate information about the changes induced in the dural sac or spinal cord. In the presence of cord involvement axial CT bone window studies should be used to identify the nature of the bony contributions to the stenotic lesions demonstrated in the MRI (see Chapter 7).

6.4. Conservative Treatment

Conservative measures must always be tried before surgery is recommended. Many patients with quite disabling symptoms will improve following physical therapy and the use of spinal supports. In very elderly people epidural injections of hydro-cortisone can be useful, though if the patient's symptoms are made worse, this may be taken as an indication that the stenosis is sufficiently severe to require spinal canal decompression.

6.5. Surgical Treatment

Traditionally many doctors have been reluctant to recommend surgical treatment for elderly patients with spinal stenosis, for those with post-traumatic stenoses, particularly if associated with neurological deficits and for cancer patients. Developments in anaesthesia and resuscitation and in spinal surgical techniques have now combined to improve the results of surgery so much as to render that reluctance obsolete. That is not to say that contra-indications to the use of surgery in any of these patients do not exist.

In elderly patients laminal bone is often osteoporotic and it bleeds readily. Conversely vertebral sclerosis may be found, the bone of the laminae being so dense that the use of chisels or diamond-tipped high speed burrs must be used to enter the spinal canal.

The normal ligamentum flavum is highly elastic, varying in thickness between 1.0 and 2.5 mm. Sometimes it is greatly thickened, retaining its elasticity. In other cases, while thicker than normal, it becomes inelastic and friable, containing visible patches of ectopic calcification. Complete ossification of the ligamentum flavum occurs in some cases following previous spinal surgery or spinal injury, in acromegaly and of course in ankylosing spondylitis. Occasionally it will be eroded by overlying osteophytes from the facet joints and its remnants may then be adherent to the dural sac.

Changes in the facet joints are common, with gangliform degeneration of joint capsules, hypertrophy of individual facets, osteophyte formation and intra-articular loose bodies.

Within the spinal canal, the epidural fat may be absent in the stenotic area though this is not an invariable finding. The dural sac and its contents also may show important changes; the dura may be thickened and opaque, or thin and extremely friable. In rare instances it may be absent due to erosion by osteophytes which have projected into the dorsal aspect of the spinal canal from the facet joints.

Arachnoiditis of the cauda equina may occur, identified on digital palpation of the dural sac at operation, by loss of the normal soft balloon-like consistency, the affected segment being firm and rubbery to touch, like a par-boiled sausage (Figs. 6.15–17).

Changes in the anterior wall of the spinal canal can be related to pathology of the intervertebral discs with herniation or sequestration of fragments. Osteophytes projecting backwards from the posterior margins of the vertebral body more frequently require to be removed in cases of cervical or thoracic canal stenoses. In the lumbar region, they may often be left undisturbed.

a) Selection of Levels for Decompression

Where multiple level defects have been demonstrated, it is usually advisable to perform decompressions of the nerve root canals and intervertebral foramina and of the central canal at each of these levels.

In patients with unilateral leg pain, pre-operative nerve root blocks have been used by Van Akerveeken and Hasue. These authors aim to produce anaesthesia in nerve roots related to individual intervertebral foramina and then restrict the decompression operation to that particular level. As a general rule, it is wiser to perform bilateral foraminal and nerve root canal decompressions rather than to restrict the procedure to one side of the spinal canal.

b) Technique

i) Exposure

Exposure of the affected vertebral segments is obtained using the techniques described on pp. 127–133. Identification of the affected level or levels should be

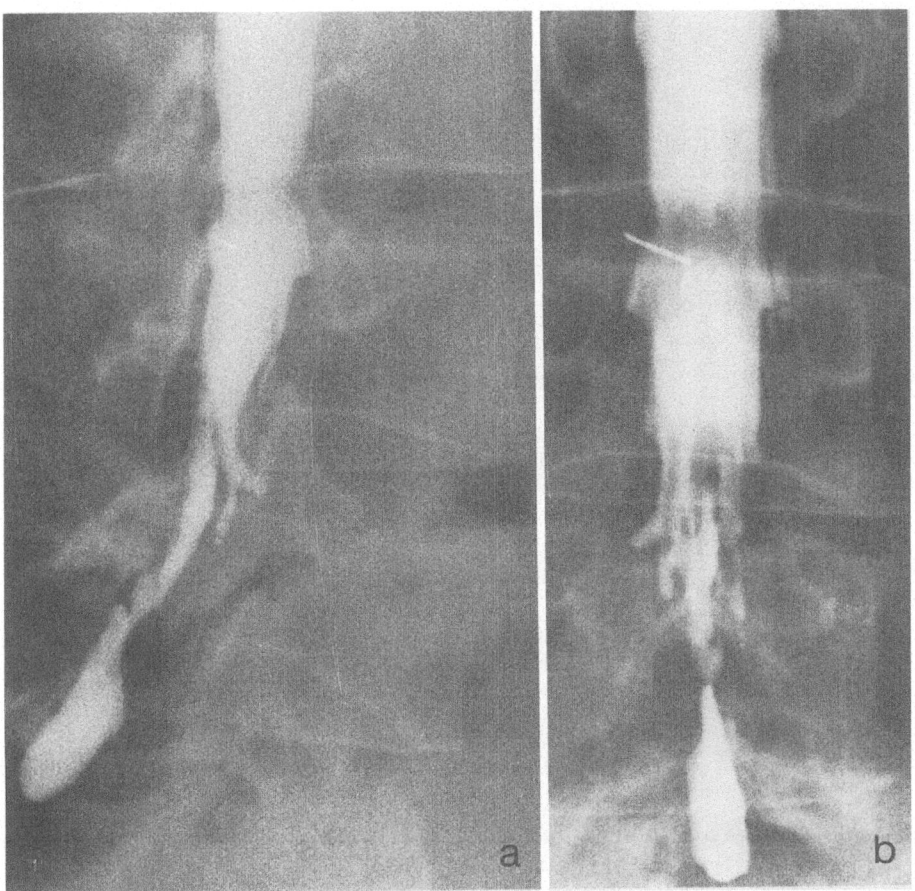

Figures 6.15 a, b. **a** An oblique radiograph of the lumbar spine of a man aged 47 years showing classical myelographic appearances of arachnoiditis of the cauda equina. **b** An antero-posterior radiograph of the same myelogram showing typical features of distortion of the column of dye due to arachnoiditis of the cauda equina (see Figs. 6.16 a–c)

confirmed by examining the patient's X-rays. X-ray control is not usually necessary, *providing the lumbo-sacral junction is identified visually as a routine, at least on one side of the S1 spinous process.* In patients with anomalous fused lumbo-sacral articulations, the first mobile segment of the lumbar spine should be identified.

At each level, after self-retaining retractors have been inserted, the laminal interspaces should be cleared of remnants of muscle fibres and fatty tissues. When the inter-laminar spaces are obstructed by hypertrophic facets, and the laminae override each other, it may be difficult to gain access to the spinal canal. The partes interarticulares of the laminae on both sides should be clearly exposed. Particular care should be taken in these cases to avoid damaging the arteries that supply the cauda equina. *The use of diathermy to coagulate bleeding vessels anterior to the pars interarticularis should be avoided.*

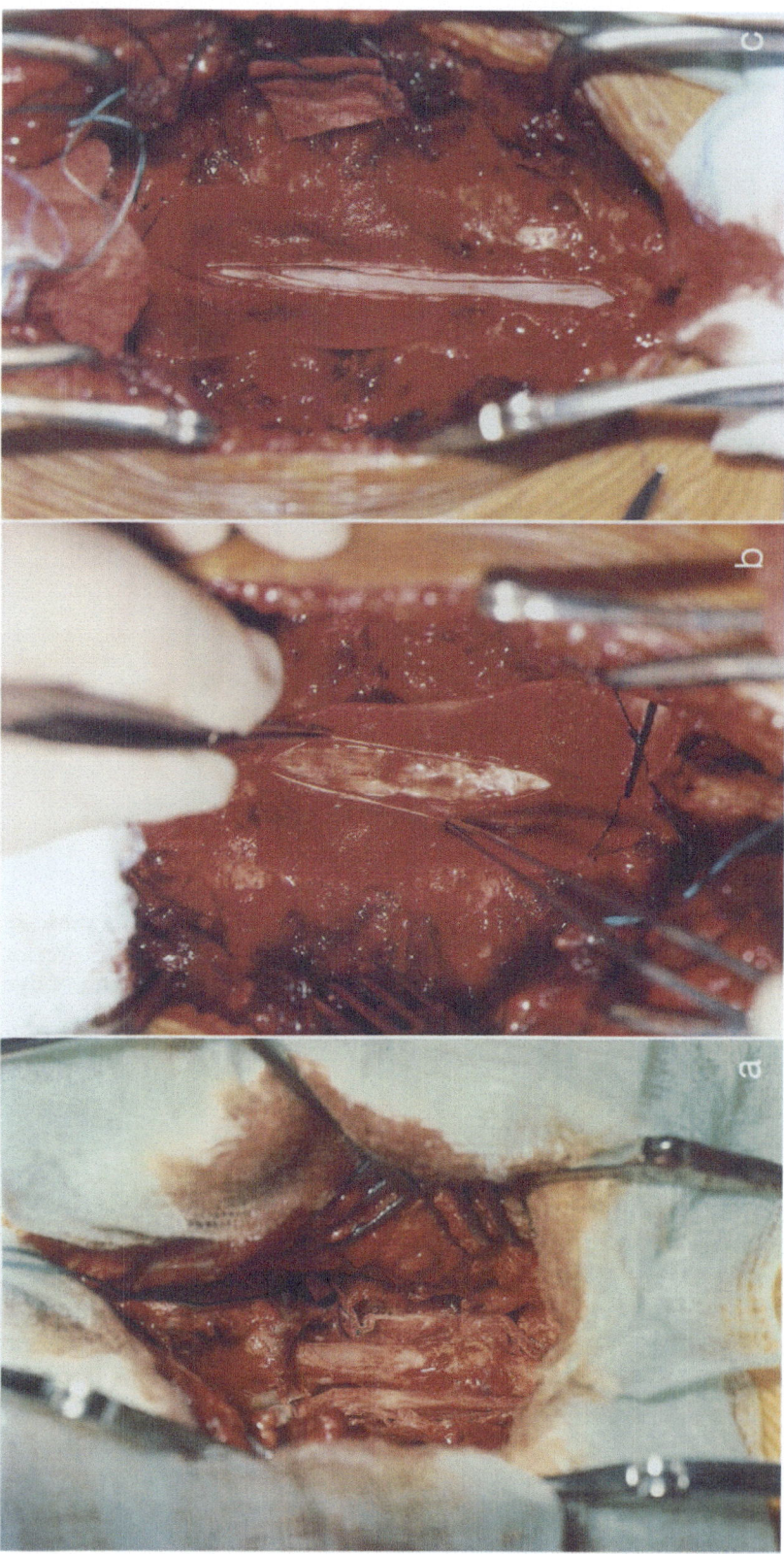

Figures 6.16a–c

ii) Enlargement of Bony Canal

The medial margins of the inferior facets at the level to be decompressed should be clearly defined. These are often very near the mid-line. Normal glistening silver fibres of the facet joint capsules are often obscured by masses of gangliform tissue projecting backwards from their inferior margins and covering their superficial fibres. This tissue should be incised and removed, paying particular attention to the lumbar vessels that may be adherent to it. The inferior capsular margin may be further obscured by an osteophytic outgrowth arising from the superior surface of the inferior lamina, the bar of bone projecting upwards to cover the capsular fibres of the adjacent joint. This bar of bone should be removed either with a high speed drill or with fine osteotomes. This will allow access to the hypertrophic medial margin of the facet joint which should then be excised, again, either with a high speed drill or with chisels, in such a way that the medial attachments of the facet joint capsule to the joint should not be disturbed, but sufficient bone and soft tissue should be removed to expose the underlying ligamentum flavum. These important stages in the procedure can be followed by examining in detail the dissection of the lumbar spine illustrated in Figs. 6.18–20.

The most effective technique for enlarging the laminal interspace, to expose the underlying ligamentum flavum, is to excise the medial aspects of these facets, using a fine osteotome, directed laterally and caudally. The cutting edge of the osteotome will emerge from the facet to strike the inferior lamina and the "non-articular" inner segment of the subjacent superior facet. If the laminae are osteoporotic, this manoeuvre can be carried out simply with a straight, short pituitary rongeur.

When the ligamentum flavum has been widely exposed, it may be thinned with a rongeur and then removed in the usual manner to expose the spinal canal.

Using a Watson-Cheyne probe, the pedicles should be palpated above and below, separating the dura carefully from the walls of the spinal canal. Having identified the medial margin of the inferior pedicle at the interspace, the medial edge

---

Figures 6.16a–c. a A photograph taken during operation to show the appearance of the dural sac in the lower lumbar spine in the patient whose myelogram is illustrated in Figs. 6.15a,b. The dura is totally opaque and on digital palpation, in contrast to the normal sensation of feeling a soft balloon, the consistency of the contents can be likened to that of a par-boiled sausage. **b** A photograph taken following opening of the dural sac. Note the markedly thickened glistening arachnoid. It is impossible to identify individual filaments of the cauda equina. **c** A photograph of the cauda equina extending from L2 to the upper border of L4 in a woman aged 52 years who presented with a complete block on a myelogram at the level of the lower border of L2. Clinically, this patient had severe paraparesis and at operation, classical features of multi-level lumbar canal stenosis were found along with severe arachnoiditis of the cauda equina. In this photograph, at the top of the picture, it is possible to identify individual filaments of the cauda equina with some blood vessels on the surfaces inside the arachnoid membrane which is normal at this level. In the lower half of the picture, note the thickening of the filaments of the cauda equina and the opacity of the arachnoid. In this remarkable case, when the dura was opened throughout the whole course of the lumbar spine, the cerebrospinal fluid leaked gradually downwards within the exposed arachnoid sheath, until it reached the level of the L3 vertebral body at its lower border. This patient's paraplegia recovered rapidly following operation for decompression of the canal, the dural sac being left widely open following operation

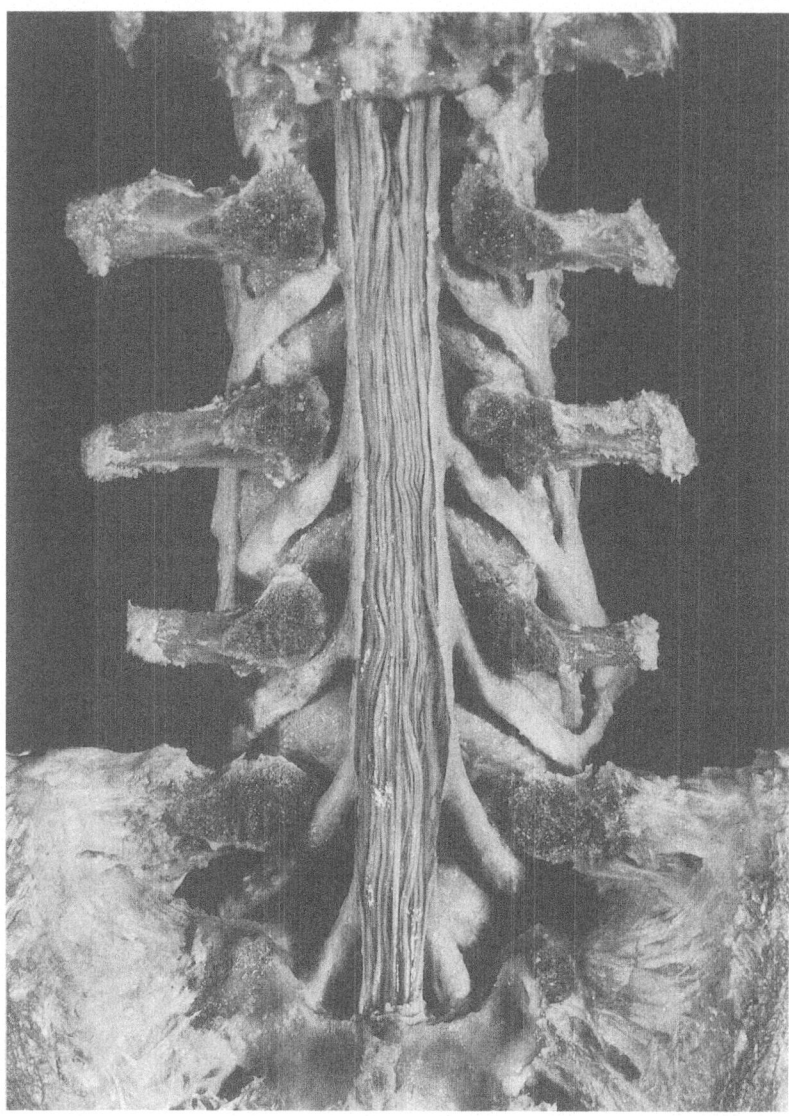

Figure 6.17. A photograph of a dissection of the lumbar spine from a woman aged 46 years. The posterior part of the dural sac has been removed to show the cauda equina which is still ensheathed in transparent arachnoid membrane. During explorations of the lower lumbar spine the dural sac is usually transparent and filaments of the cauda equina can be seen floating in the cerebrospinal fluid. (Dissected by Dr M. C. Crock)

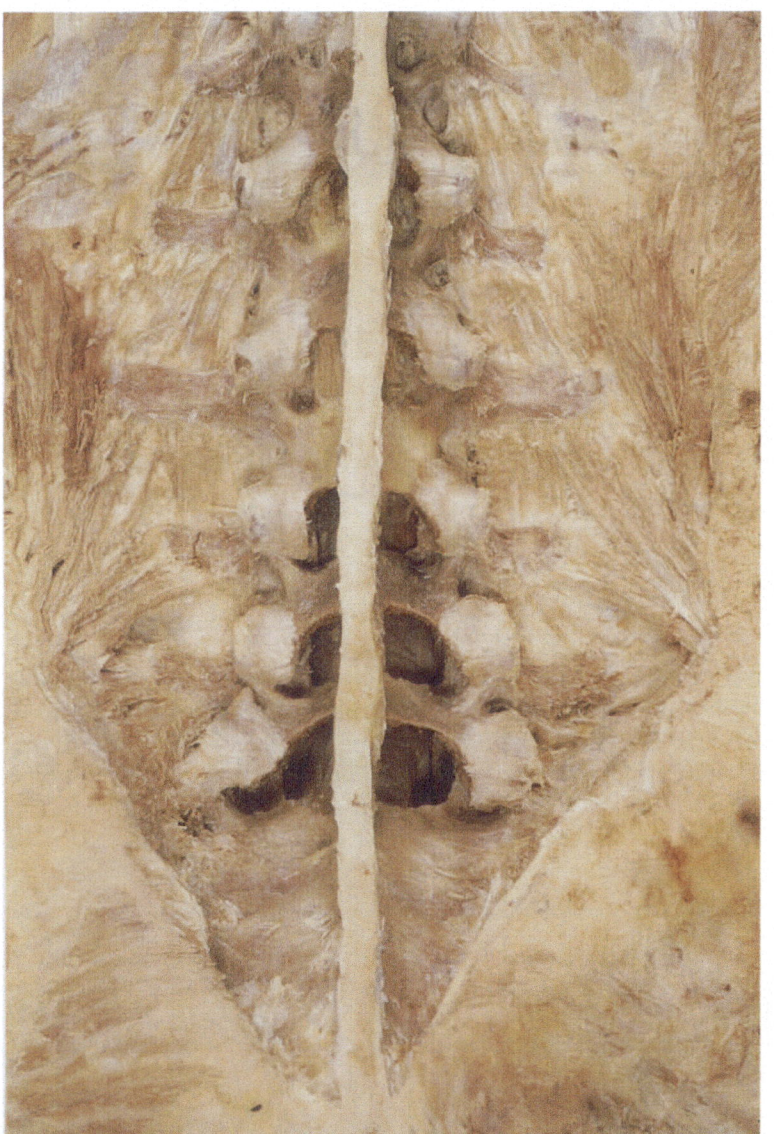

Figure 6.18. The photograph of a dissection of the lumbar spine to illustrate aspects of the technique of multi-level lumbar canal, bilateral foraminal and nerve root canal decompressions preserving the mid-line bony structures and interspinous and supraspinous ligaments. Towards the top of the picture at the L2/3 level the preliminary procedure which involved removal of the medial portion of the inferior facet of L2 along with the capsular extension on to the ligamentum flavum and including a few millimetres of the inferior laminal margin of L2 has been performed on both sides exposing the fibres of the ligamentum flavum. Note the striking difference in colour between the capsular fibres and the bright yellow of the ligamentum flavum itself. *The importance of stressing the appreciation of the normal anatomical colour of specific spinal structures cannot be overstressed. It is a valuable guide to the surgeon at every stage of spinal surgery but most valuable when difficult re-explorations of the spinal canal are undertaken.* At the L3/4, L4/5 and L5/S1 interspaces the decompression is complete. The dural sac and nerve roots can be seen and on the right side of the picture the outline of the internal vertebral venous plexus can be made out running parallel to the slightly glistening S1 nerve root sheath. (Dissected by H. V. Crock and reproduced by kind permission of Professor S. Sinatamby and the President and Council of the Royal College of Surgeons of England)

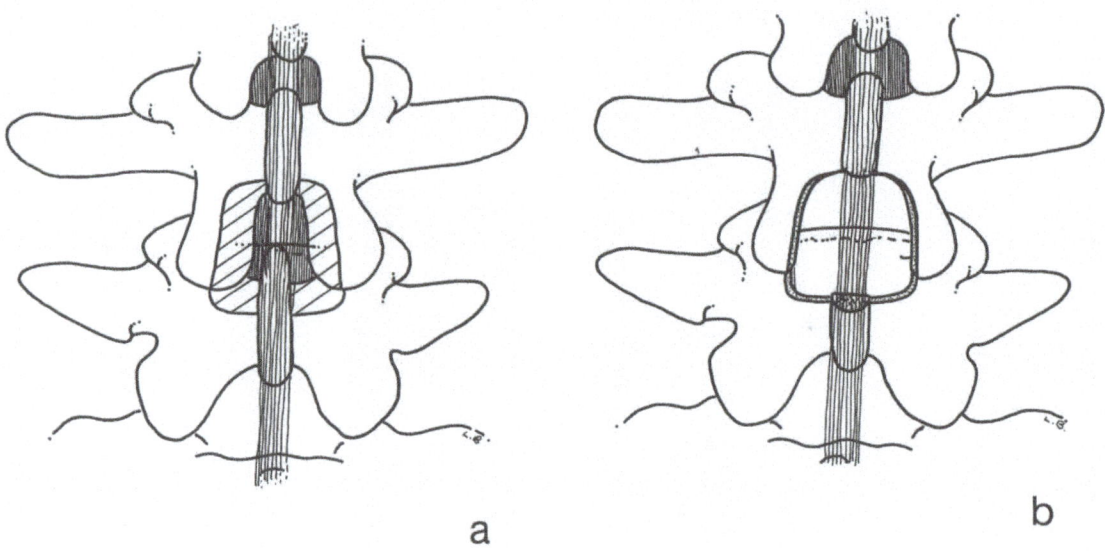

a   b

Figures 6.19 a, b. a A schematic drawing depicting typical pathological changes of facet hypertrophy at the L4/5 level. The hatched area outlines the extent of the dissection usually required to decompress the canal. **b** A schematic drawing showing the decompression completed with the interspinous ligaments and supraspinous ligaments still intact. The lateral extent of the bony dissection is in line with the medial borders of the pedicles of L5

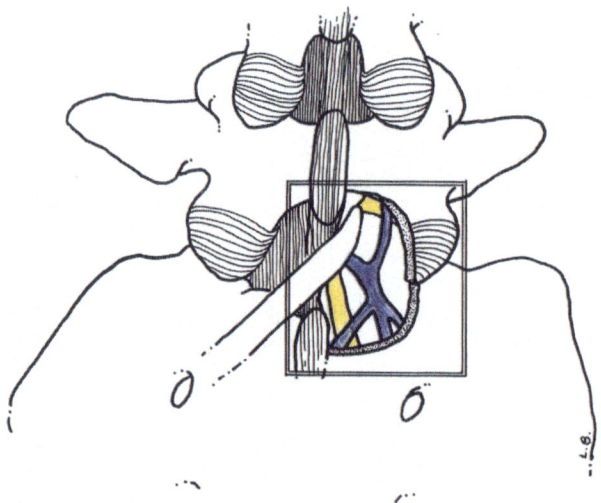

Figure 6.20. A schematic detailed drawing to show the typical appearances following successful nerve root canal and foraminal decompressions at L5/S1 on the right hand side. The probe is retracting the lateral margin of the dural sac and at its tip, the outline of the L5 nerve root can be seen. Refilling of the internal vertebral venous plexus and lumbar vein tributaries is prominent. Note that these vessels are often as large as the nerve roots which they surround and accompany

of the superior facet related to this pedicle should be excised flush with the inner margin of that pedicle. The line of this cut in the facet, where it emerges from the lamina, should mark the lateral extent of removal of bone.

In almost every case, even in those with degenerative lumbar scoliosis, it is possible to produce satisfactory decompressions of the spinal canal without disturbing the integrity of the supra-spinous and inter-spinous ligaments and the spinous processes to which they are attached, Tsuji (1991). Further details of the technique have already been described in Chapter 3 (Figs. 6.21 a, b).

Where it becomes necessary to remove the spinous processes and central segments of the laminae, the partes interarticulares should be preserved at each vertebral level on both sides of the canal. Removal of the facets in toto should be avoided, as this will lead to serious vertebral instability in some patients (Fig. 6.22).

Bleeding from the cut surfaces of the laminae should be controlled by the application of bone wax regularly as the decompression is proceeding. This will help to reduce blood loss significantly in elderly patients with osteoporosis.

Once the canal has been exposed on both sides, the dural sac should be inspected carefully and palpated.

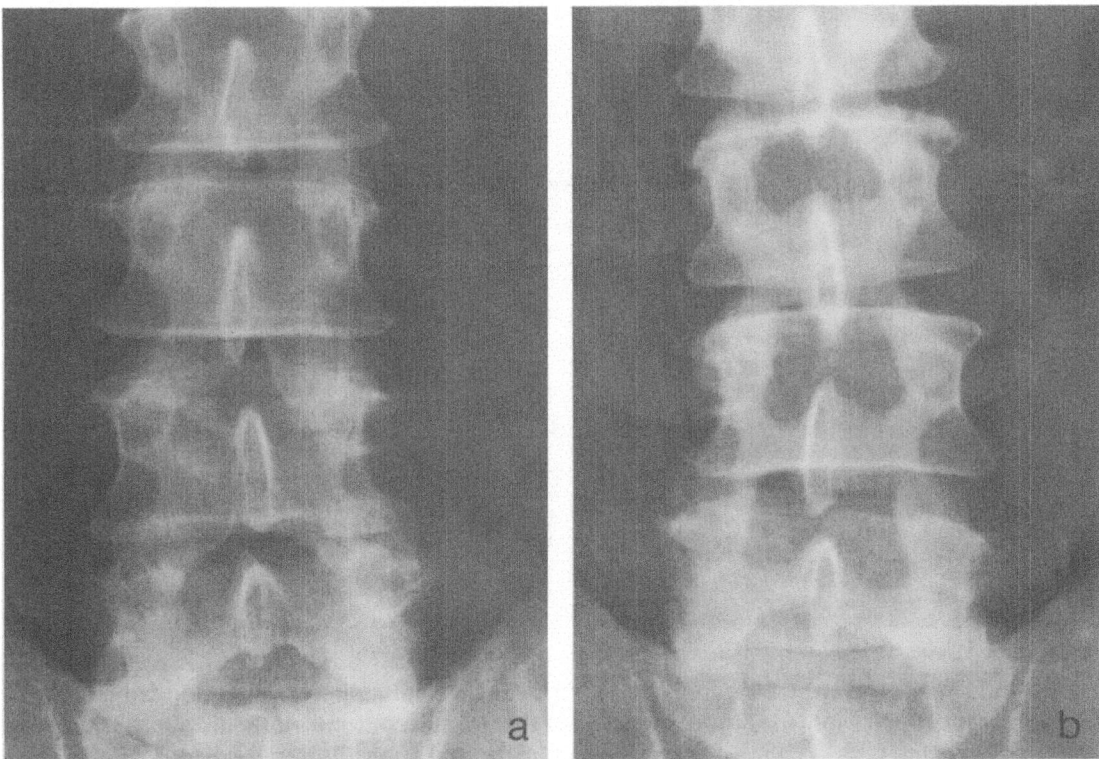

Figures 6.21 a, b. a Antero-posterior photograph of the lumbar spine in a middle aged male patient with multi-level lumbar canal stenosis confirmed by radiculography. **b** The post-operative appearance following nerve root canal and foraminal decompressions at L2/3, L3/4 and L4/5 with preservation of the spinous processes and interspinous ligaments, followed by reattachment of the lumbo dorsal fascia at the end of the procedure

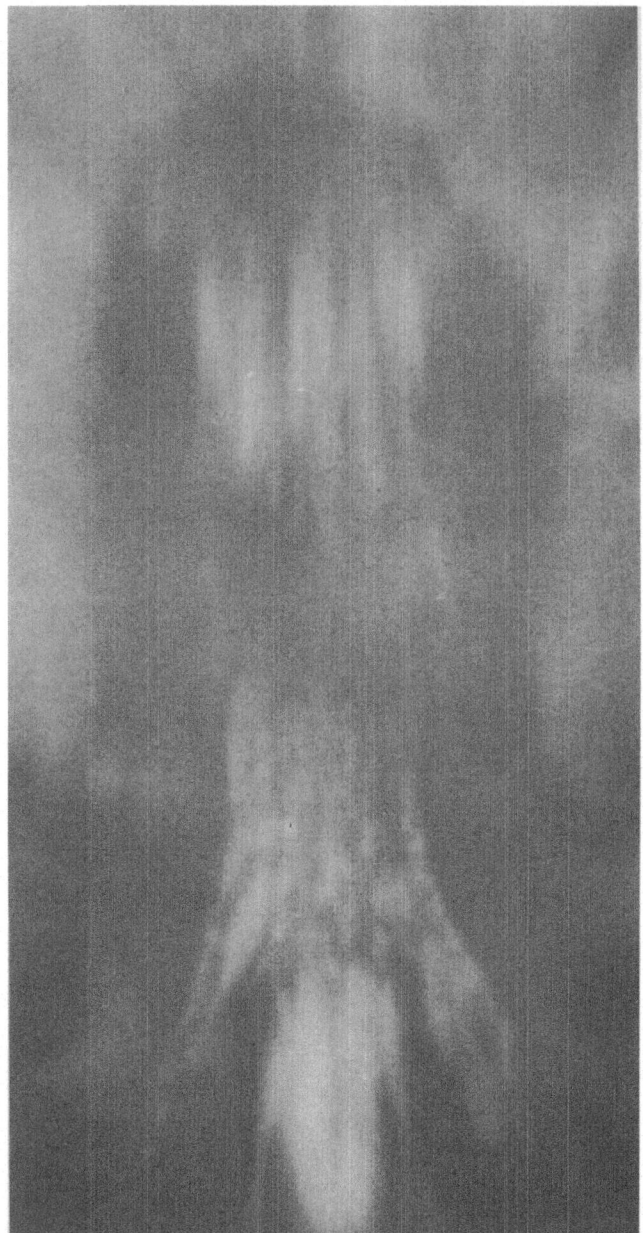

Figure 6.22. An antero-posterior tomogram of the lower lumbar spine taken following decompression of the spinal canal to show restoration of the normal contours of the dural sac following treatment for single level canal stenosis at L4/5. Note the smooth margins to the laminae on both sides of the vertebral column. The technique of spinal canal decompression should be such that the post-operative films have this appearance, with preservation of the partes interarticulares and greater portions of the facet joints on both sides. The lateral extent of laminal dissections should not proceed beyond the medial margins of the pedicles at each level. Multi-level decompressions of the lumbar canal may be carried out in this manner without fear of causing vertebral instability

iii) Haemostasis

Haemorrhage from the internal vertebral venous plexus on either side of the dural sac should be controlled by packing strips of a suitable haemostatic agent, such as gelfoam, along the antero-lateral margins of the spinal canal. The gelfoam should be covered with moistened linteen strips until the posterior surface of the dura is outlined on either side by these strips and the field should, by then, be bloodless.

iv)　Dural Opening

Arachnoiditis of the cauda equina should be suspected if the dura is opaque and non-pulsatile. Digital palpation will confirm the suspicion when the firm texture, described above, is felt. If this condition is diagnosed, the surgeon should first complete the decompression over the planned length of the spine. The dural sac should then be opened carefully in the mid-line over a segment firm to the touch of the surgeon's finger. The dura will be quite thick, but its edges will be distinct from the underlying greyish-pink thick arachnoid. The filaments of the cauda equina will not be visible, as they are ensheathed by the inflamed arachnoid membrane.

The aim in exposing the inflamed arachnoid membrane is to leave the dural sac widely open and sutured to the laminal margins, thereby helping to relieve the venous obstruction between the intra-dural and extra-dural venous channels. Dissection should continue proximally either to the level where the dural sac pulsates or to a point where cerebrospinal fluid can be seen contained by the transparent arachnoid membrane.

The margins of the opened dura should be fixed with a few interrupted sutures to the muscles along the lateral edge of the bony margins of the spinal canal over the area of the decompression.

Assuming that no other lesions, such as prolapsed disc fragments, have been found during the operation, the wound may now be closed, without drainage. Particular care should be taken to ensure that the lumbo-dorsal fascia layer is tightly sealed.

6.6.　Results of Surgical Treatment for Arachnoiditis

Although this is a rare complication of severe lumbar canal stenosis, more than twenty cases have been treated by this method. Managed post-operatively by early mobilization, the patients have been given daily doses of Aspirin 100 mg with multivitamin tablets for three months. The rationale of this therapy has been that the fine circulation in the vessels supplying the cauda equina should be thereby enhanced. Two of these patients had been paraparetic before surgery. Many had complained of intractable severe bilateral leg pain, and a number were addicted to narcotics as a result of prolonged usage for pain control.

Both paraparetic patients recovered full motor power in their lower extremities. At least four patients returned to work. Among those apparently addicted to narcotics, only two continued to require non-narcotic analgesics for pain control.

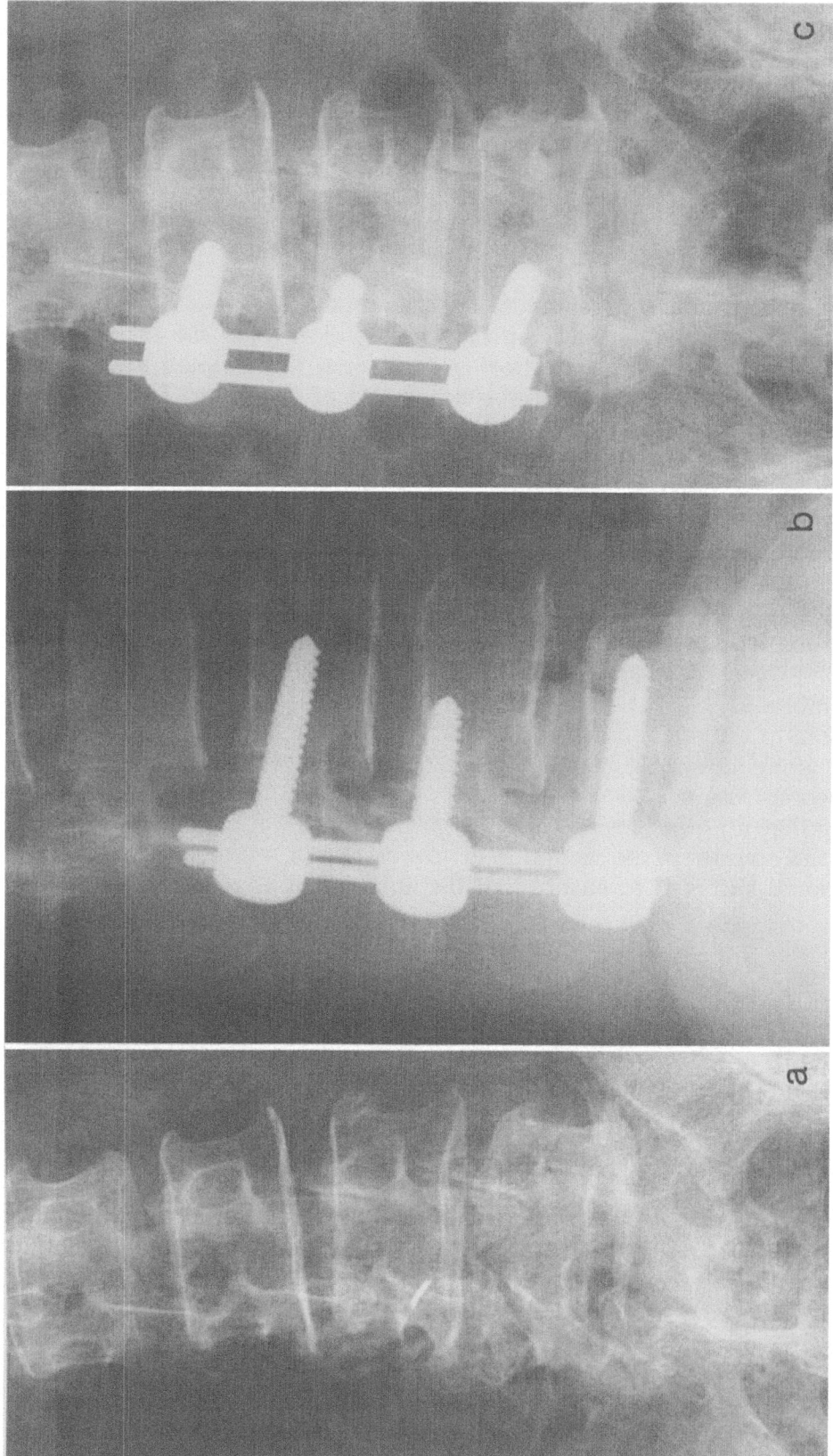

Figures 6.23a–c. **a** An antero-posterior photograph of the lumbar spine of a 57 year old Japanese lady with degenerative spondylolisthesis of L4/5 with symptoms of back pain and intermittent left sided sciatica related to effort. **b** A lateral radiograph following insertion of three pedicular screws with the Crock Pericic spinal fixation system. **c** An antero-posterior view of the same patient's spine following facet fusion. This patient remained symptom free three years after operation

6.7. Recognition and Treatment of Associated Pathological Conditions

In the course of decompression operations in the lumbar spinal canal, particularly in patients with degenerative scoliosis, care should be exercised to ensure that other lesions are recognized and treated, for example, disc prolapses and nerve root canal stenosis.

Vertebral instability may occur following removal of a large volume of intervertebral disc tissue, or in rare cases of acute vertebral end-plate necrosis with massive disc sequestration leading to kypho-scoliosis. In some of these cases, inter-pedicular pedicle screw fixation devices may be used with spinal fusion, either in the form of inter-transverse fusions, facet fusions or posterior interbody fusions (Fig. 6.23 a–c).

The introduction of the pedicle screw system for vertebral fixation has certainly provided an excellent method for spinal stabilization in selected cases. Complications resulting from the use of these devices have tended to run at an unacceptably high level, Esses *et al.* (1991).

These authors presented a careful review of 617 surgical cases in which various designs of implants had been used. They recorded the following complications:

Unrecognized screw misplacement	5.0%
Post-operative deep infection	4.2%
Pedicle fracture and CSF leakage	4.0%
Aortic perforation and death occurred in one case.	
Transient neuropraxia	2.4%
Permanent nerve root injury	2.3%
Screw breakage	2.9%
Overall they reported *a complication rate of*	*27.4%*

6.8. Wound Closure

Using the conservative method of bilateral foraminal and nerve root canal decompression combined with enlargement of the central portion of the spinal canal where indicated by removing the upper attachments of the ligamentum flavum at each level, and thinning the laminal bone on its deep surface, followed by reattachment of the lumbo-dorsal fascia on both sides to the mid-line supra-spinous and inter-spinous ligaments, the post-operative results have been superior to the older method of extensive lumbar canal decompression involving excision of the spinous processes and central portions of the laminae. In the first instance, reconstitution of the normal anatomical relationships between the spinous processes and related ligaments and lumbo-dorsal fascia has obviated the necessity for wound drainage even after multi-level decompressions. The paraspinal muscles no longer bow-string across the decompressed segment of the vertebral column. Spinal stability appears to be enhanced and the necessity for using internal fixation devices with spinal fusion has been greatly restricted.

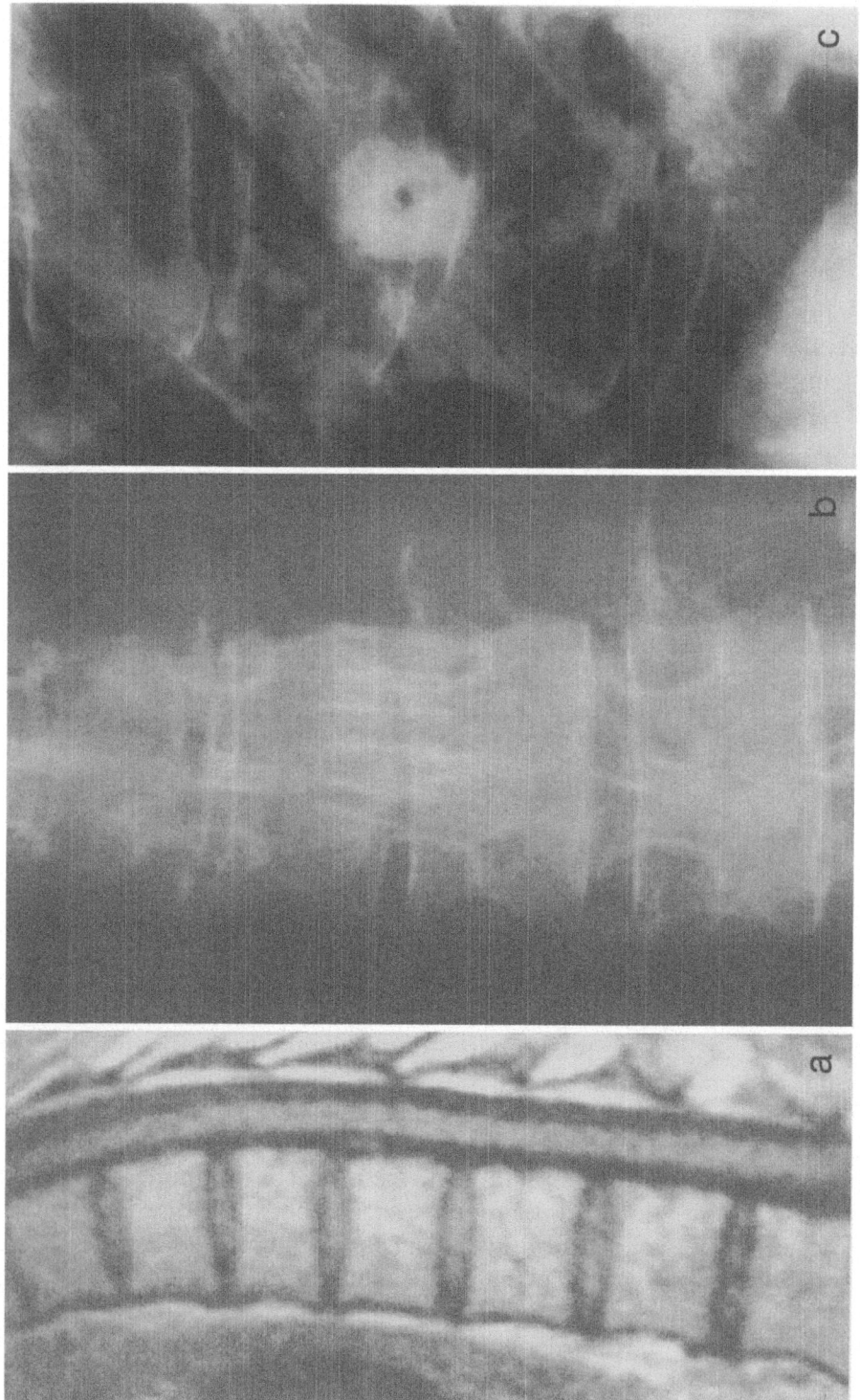

Figures 6.24a–c. a A mid-sagittal MR T2 weighted image of the thoracic spine of a female aged 56 showing a sequestrated disc fragment at the T 8/9 level. **b** An antero-posterior photograph of this patient's spine taken six months after interbody fusion. Note the separate discs of bone cut from the rib removed at the time of thoracotomy. **c** A lateral view of the same spine showing the proximity of the grafts to the spinal canal. Before inserting the grafts the disc prolapse was easily removed

6.9. *Thoracic Canal Decompression*

Stenotic lesions producing spinal cord compression are rare. Ossification of the posterior longitudinal ligament is sometimes associated with ossification of the ligamentum flavum. Ossification of this ligament may also occur following trauma. Intra-dural lesions, other than tumours, which may compress the cord, such as post-traumatic arachnoid cysts (Fig. 6.13 a–c) or localized ossific arachnoiditis may all respond to simple thoracic laminectomy.

The major lesions which cause thoracic canal stenosis and impairment of cord function are usually found in the anterior wall of its canal. Thoracic disc prolapse, ossification of the posterior longitudinal ligament, and calcific disc prolapses are all dealt with most safely by a trans-thoracic approach to the thoracic spine. Localization of these lesions is often difficult and very careful radiological and MRI studies are needed for that purpose. Depending on the siting of the lesion, the chest may be opened either from the right or left side excising portion of the rib proximal to the vertebral level of the lesion. Sometimes these approaches can be accomplished by an extra-pleural approach though often in healthy people the parietal pleura is very thin and easily ruptured, so that the operation is performed transpleurally and post-operative chest drainage is then necessary.

Providing appropriately long instruments are available, many of these lesions can be dealt with through quite limited approaches following removal of the middle third of a rib, retracting the anterior margin of the latissimus dorsi muscle without dividing it.

Once the chest has been opened, the parietal pleura should be incised along the mid-lateral line of the vertebrae. Most of the pathological processes that require surgical treatment involve only one or occasionally two intervertebral discs. These can be dealt with without dividing the overlying sympathetic nerve fibres and without division of any of the regional intercostal vessels. However, if extensive exposure is required when dealing with inflammatory lesions of the spine or with neoplastic lesions, then several intercostal arteries may need to be divided. This can be safely done without damage to the spinal cord circulation providing the vessels are divided at about the mid-point between their aortic origins medially and the intervertebral foramina laterally.

Thoracic disc prolapse can usually be satisfactorily removed by incising the peripheral annular fibres and removing the disc in toto with long fine straight pituitary rongeurs.

For the removal of large sequestrated fragments or calcified nuclear material, it is wiser to construct a dowel cavity from one side of the vertebral column to within a few millimetres of the other. Ellipses of bone and intervening disc are then removed and through this large cavity the remaining disc tissues posterior to the dowel can be removed from the front of the spinal canal itself.

To determine the actual level of the posterior vertebral margins, it is often necessary to excise the head and neck of the rib and to work across the floor of the canal with the aid either of a high speed drill or fine angled curettes until the anterior surface of the dural sac has been completely decompressed.

With this method, using a cutter one size larger than that used to prepare the dowel cavity, a series of discs can be cut from the excised rib fragment and these are then impacted into the dowel cavity from one side of the vertebral bodies to the other (Figs. 6.24, 25).

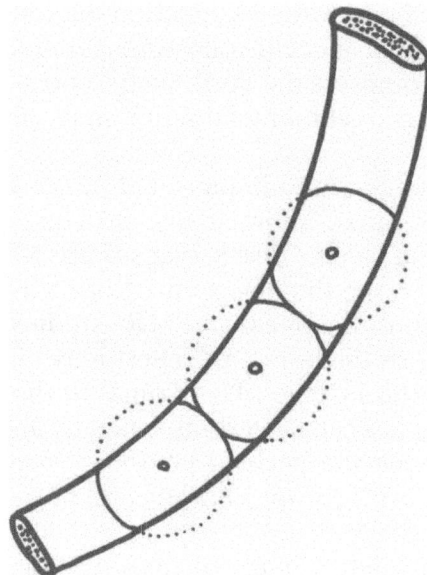

Figure 6.25. A schematic drawing showing the methods of preparation of rib grafts for inter-body fusion when the dowel technique is used

7

Surgery of the Cervical Spine

7.1. Introduction

The surgical management of lesions of the cervical spine is now dominated by the operation of anterior interbody fusion. This procedure was introduced for use in the neck in 1955 by Robinson and Smith. Their technique was modified when Cloward introduced special instruments for dowel grafting in 1958.

In the course of performing anterior cervical interbody fusion operations a wide range of pathological lesions can be dealt with safely and effectively. For example, some of the space-occupying lesions which project into the anterior wall of the cervical canal can be removed before the grafts are inserted, lesions such as central disc prolapses, sequestrated disc fragments, or osteophytic bars of bone. The incidence of severe neurological deficits, including quadriplegia, was formerly so high following the use of "laminectomies" for posterior approaches to these lesions that surgery in general, in the cervical spine, had a very poor reputation.

The operation of cervical laminectomy still retains an important place for use as follows:

1. For decompression of the spinal canal in cases of multi-level stenosis.
2. For the relief of persistent stenosis of the canal after anterior interbody fusion operations, rarely.
3. For drainage of epidural abscesses.
4. For the treatment of spinal cord tumours.

However, its use to gain access to lesions which lie anterior to the spinal cord has been abandoned.

Posterior cervical spinal fusion between the arch of C1 and the lamina and spinous process of C2, for the treatment of un-united fractures of the odontoid process, remains the treatment of choice for this problem. Apart from this indication, and that of internal fixation following open reduction of some fracture-dislocations in the neck, this operation has been superseded by that of anterior cervical interbody fusion (Figs. 7.2 a, b).

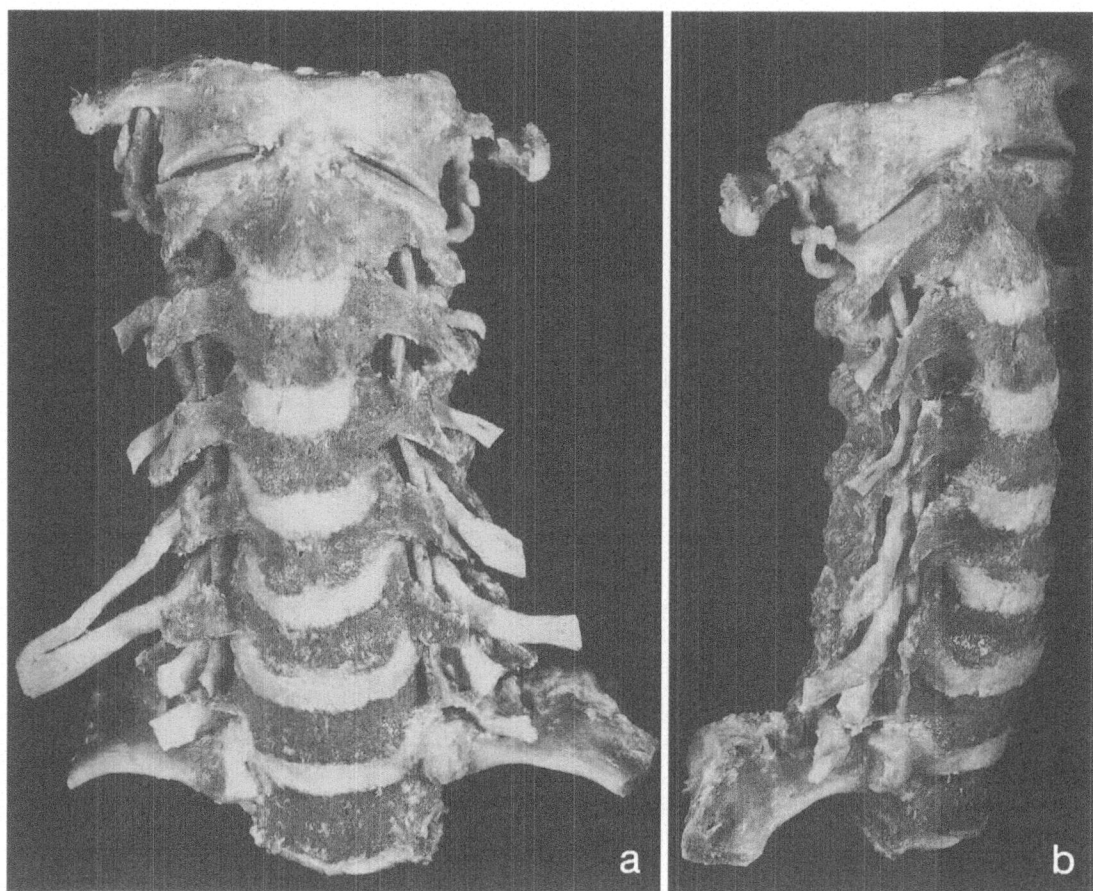

Figures 7.1a,b. a A photograph of a dissection of the cervical spine and the cervico-thoracic junction viewed from in front. All the soft tissues have been removed with the exception of the intervertebral discs and the vertebral arteries on both sides. The emerging nerve roots are also shown. Note the proximity of the vertebral arteries to the lateral margins of the intervertebral discs in the region of the unco-vertebral joints. Note also the dimensions of the intervertebral discs particularly in the transverse plane. They increase gradually in size from above downwards (dissected by Dr. M. C. Crock). **b** A photograph of the same specimen viewed obliquely from the right side showing the relationships of the vertebral artery and the emerging cervical nerve roots

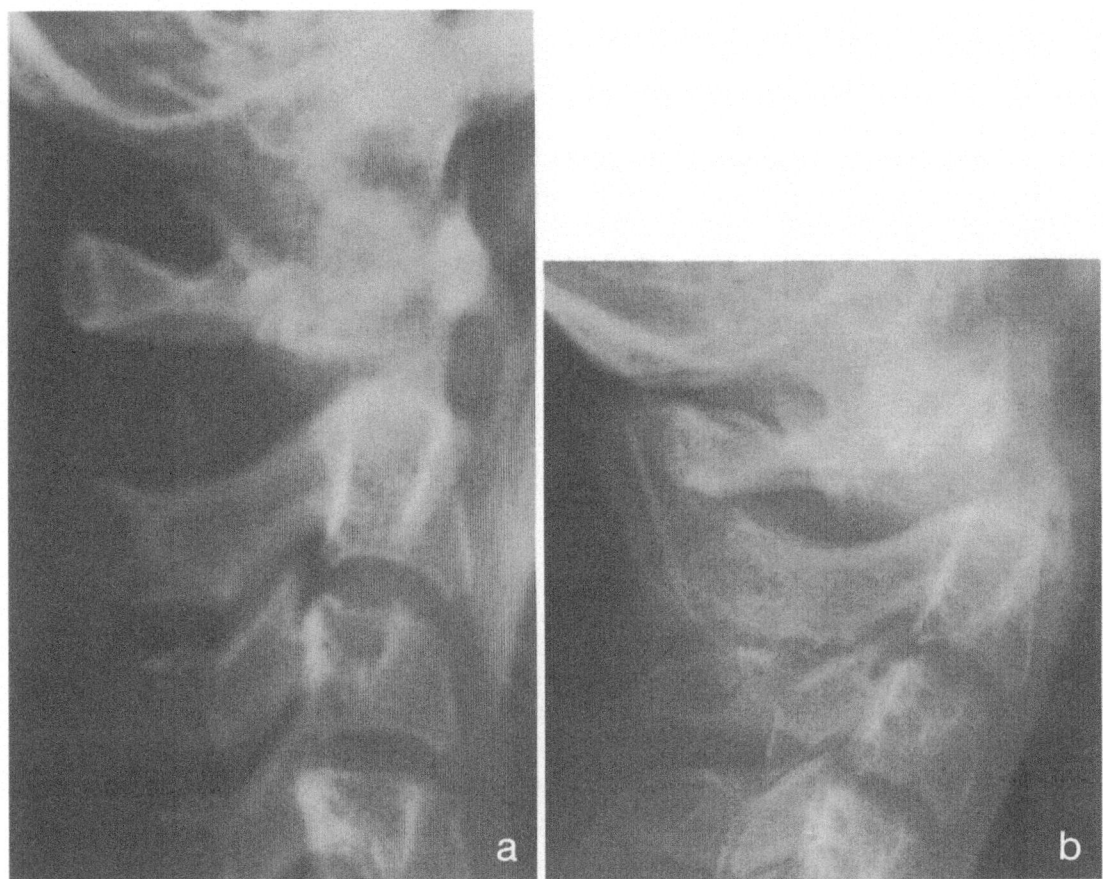

Figures 7.2 a, b. a A lateral radiograph of the upper cervical spine of the patient aged 22 years, showing an un-united fracture of the odontoid following a neck injury sustained in a motor vehicle accident. **b** A lateral radiograph of the upper cervical spine of a man aged 22 years who sustained a severe head injury following a motor vehicle accident in which the odontoid peg was fractured. C1/2 fusion is solid, though the reduction of the odontoid fracture is incomplete. The patient had no neurological signs or symptoms following union of the graft. At operation the grafts were held in place with heavy braided nylon which does not appear on the X-ray film

7.2. Indications for Surgery

a) Cervical Spondylosis

In the preface to their book "Cervical Spondylosis and Other Disorders of the Cervical Spine", Brain and Wilkinson (1967) wrote: "Cervical spondylosis was hardly recognised twenty years ago". Now, twenty-five years later, the most widely accepted indications for surgical treatment in the cervical spine would be for problems complicating that condition. Occurring as a disorder localized to one intervertebral segment or in a more generalized form, it gives rise to a variety of syndromes which can be related largely to the variable pathology resulting from the disc-space narrowing and osteophyte formation which characterize the condition (Figs. 7.3–5).

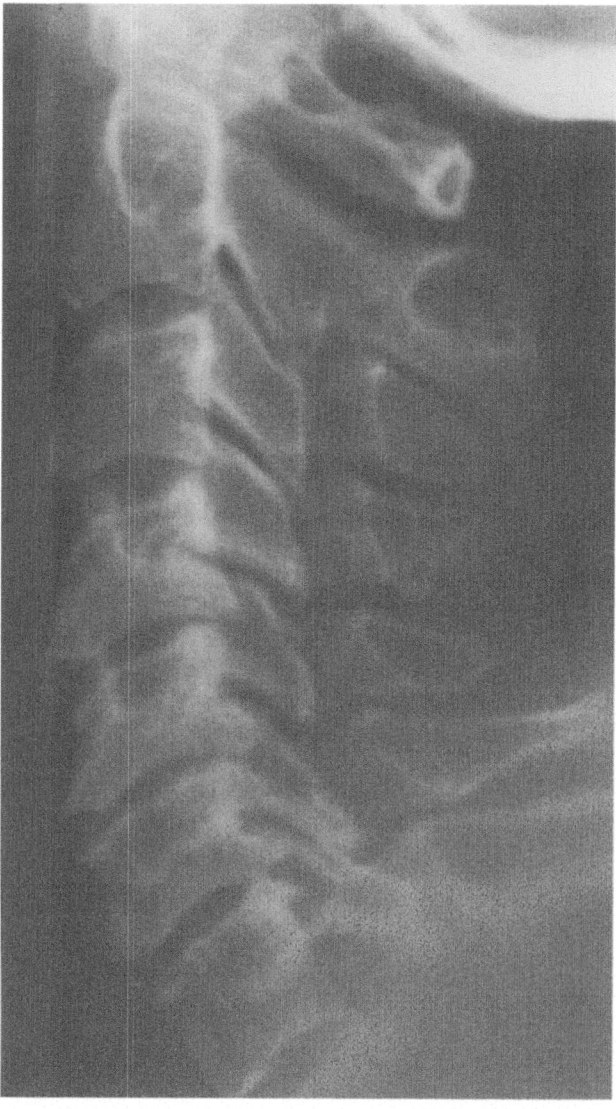

Figure 7.3

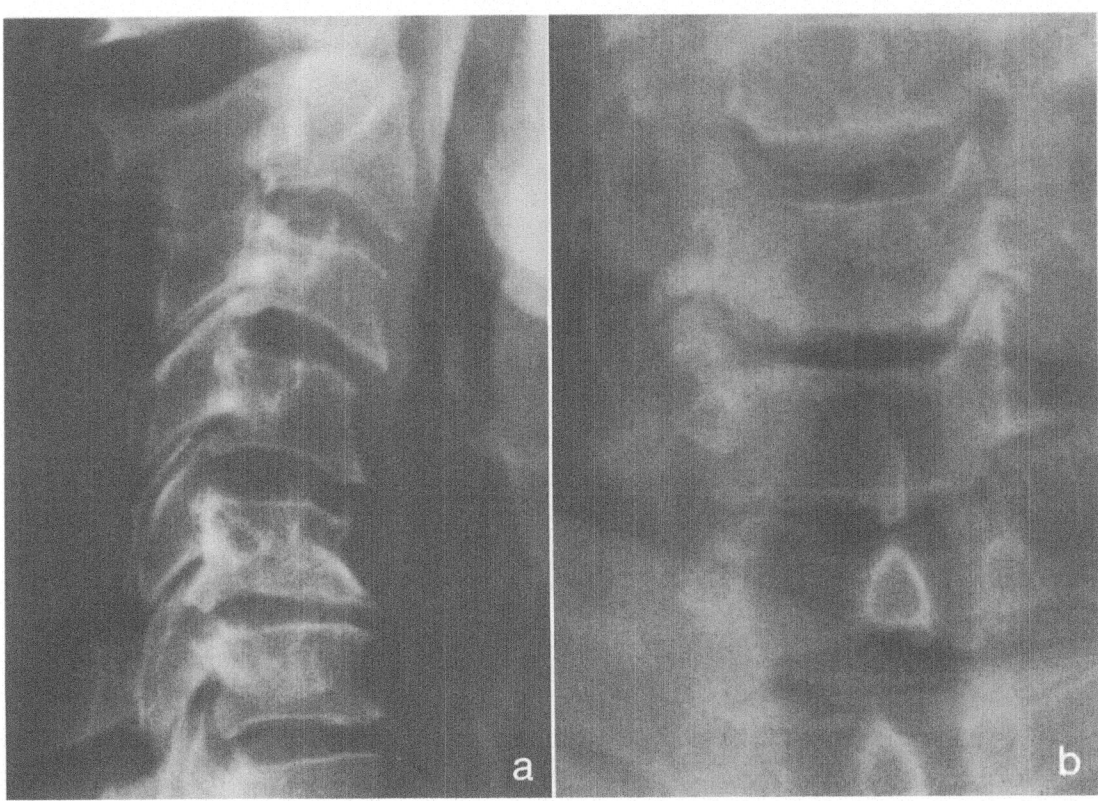

Figures 7.4 a, b. a A lateral radiograph of the cervical spine of a patient aged 55 years showing localized advanced cervical spondylosis at C5/6 with marked disc space narrowing and large osteophytes projecting backwards into the cervical spinal canal. **b** An antero-posterior radiograph of the spine of the same patient showing the advanced degenerative changes which affect the unco-vertebral joint regions, with osteophytes projecting laterally into the spaces through which the vertebral arteries pass on both sides

Figure 7.3. A lateral radiograph of the cervical spine of a woman aged 45 years showing advanced cervical spondylosis affecting the discs between the vertebral bodies of C4/5, C5/6 and C6/7. Large osteophytes project backwards into the spinal canal. This is an example of post-traumatic disc degeneration and post-traumatic cervical spondylosis, the patient having fallen from the height of 40 feet at the age of 8 years, injuring her neck. [Reproduced by kind permission of the Editors from: Handbook of Clinical Neurology, Vol. 25, Fig. 1, p. 483, Amsterdam–Oxford: North-Holland, 1976]

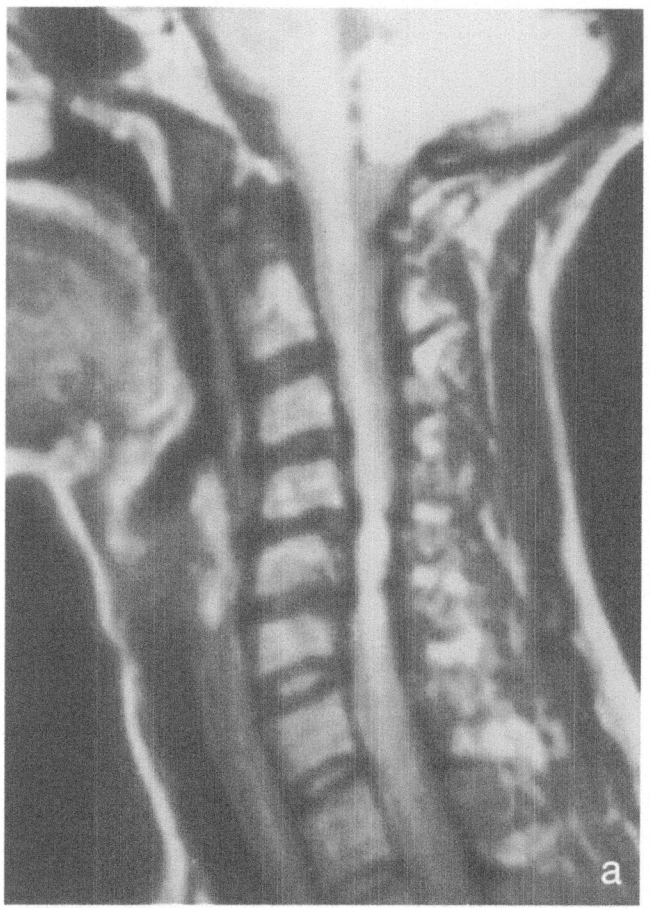

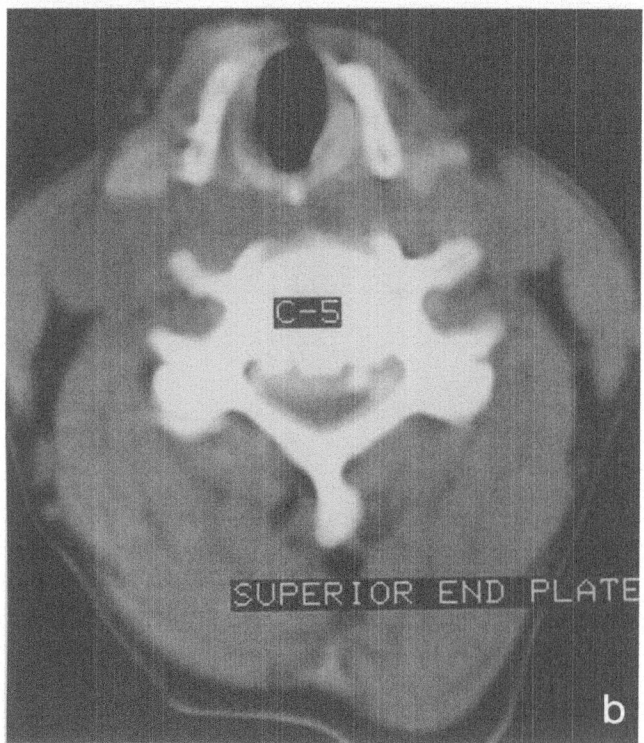

Figures 7.5 a, b. a A central sagittal view of the cervical spine in a female patient aged 41 years, T2 weighted sequence MRI. Note the hour-glass shaped deformations of the spinal cord commencing at the C3/4 disc level and increasing in degree at C4/5 and C5/6 levels. The bony components of the tissues indenting the anterior surface of the dural sac are not defined in this MRI sequence **b** An axial image from the CT radiculogram in the same patient. The dense irregular osteophytes that form a bar projecting backwards into the spinal canal can be clearly seen. This patient presented with increasing weakness of her arms and legs, with severe neck pain and occipital headache. Symptoms had commenced insidiously two years previously

Surgical treatment may be indicated in the management of cervical spondylosis as follows:

a) For the relief of persistent neck pain, neck stiffness and occipital headache, in the absence of abnormal neurological signs.
b) For the relief of neck pain and brachial neuralgia, with or without abnormal neurological signs.
c) For the relief of symptoms or signs resulting from cervical myelopathy, complicating stenosis of the cervical spinal canal due to the projection of spondylitic osteophytes into the anterior wall of the canal.
d) For the relief of dysphagia. This is a rare complication which may follow the development of a massive osteophyte projecting forwards and compressing the oesophagus. Simple excision of the osteophyte may suffice to relieve the dysphagia.
e) For the relief of stenosis of the vertebral artery or arteries due to mural pressure by osteophytic outgrowths from the regions of the unco-vertebral joints. The results of surgery for this problem are unpredictable and often unrewarding.

b) Cervical Disc Lesions

i) *Cervical disc prolapses* are uncommon. Sequestration of relatively large volumes of disc material into the cervical spinal canal may follow manipulation of the spine, performed in the course of conservative treatment for the relief of neck and arm pain. Surgical treatment may be indicated for the management of these lesions and again, there would be general agreement among surgeons on the specific indications for operation. These are in common with those outlined in Chapter 3, p. 120, for the management of lumbar and thoracic disc prolapses (Fig. 7.6).

ii) *Post traumatic internal disc disruption.* The incidence of neck injuries following motor vehicle accidents has increased dramatically in the past twenty years. In particular, the number of rear-end collisions, which occur when a moving vehicle strikes the rear-end of a stationary one, has increased enormously in most cities with large numbers of motor vehicles.

The much vaunted "whiplash injury of the neck" is usually sustained by the occupants of stationary cars in accidents of this type. There is no consensus of opinion among surgeons about indications for the use of surgical treatment in such patients.

Biomechanical studies have shown that enormous forces are transmitted through the head and cervical spine following this mechanism of injury.

Acting on the results of many of these investigations, car manufacturers have modified seat designs, incorporating head supports and restraining straps for the trunk. Such measures have been quite effective in reducing the morbidity arising from head and neck injuries in many of these accidents.

Despite the improvements in car design and the growing awareness of the hazards of neck injuries that may follow rear-end collisions, many patients still sustain these injuries which often cause protracted disability. Opinions among doctors vary widely, not only on the question of the causes of persisting symptoms in these patients, but also on the methods of treatment which should be used to treat them.

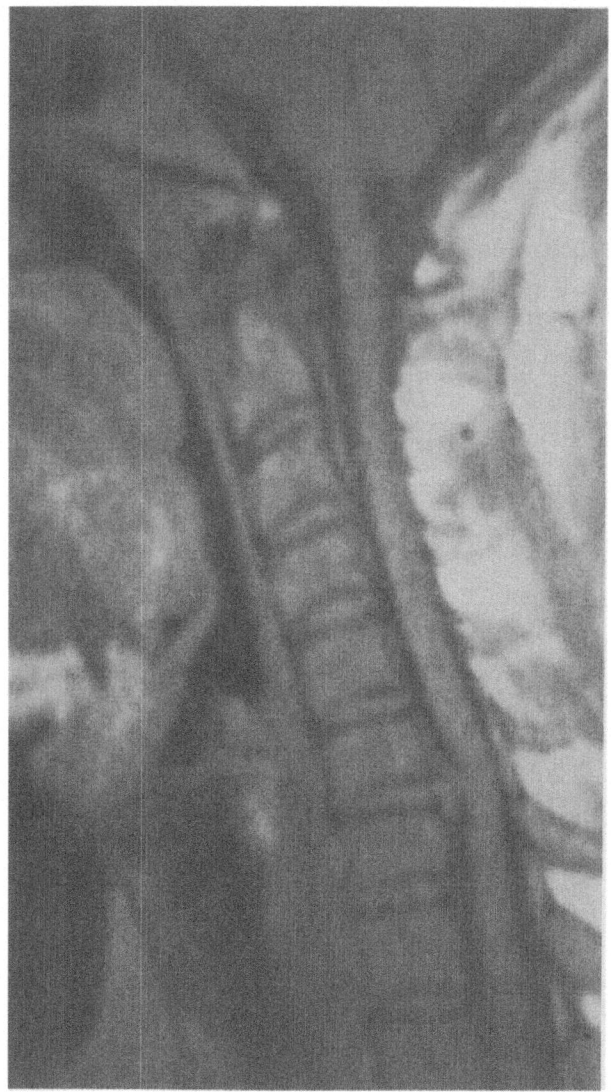

Figure 7.6. A sagittal MRI of the cervical spine of a female patient aged 36 years, showing a large disc lesion at C6/7 indenting the spinal cord

The range of symptoms described may include the following:

- Severe neck pain, neck stiffness.
- Occipito-frontal headaches, often with orbital pain.
- Earache and intolerance for loud noise.
- Mental depression.
- Defective memory after the accident.
- Giddiness.
- Varying patterns of arm pain with paraesthesia.
- Feelings of heaviness or weakness of the arms.
- Exacerbation of pain following physical activity or after physical exercise in the course of physiotherapy treatment.

Clinical examination is usually unremarkable. Apart from minor degrees of restriction of neck motion, there may be no objective abnormal physical signs, with particular reference to neurological examination. The only striking findings may be that the patients appear to be in severe pain, looking pale and downcast.

Having cared for many hundreds of victims of whiplash injuries of the neck in the past twenty-five years, a number of facts have impressed me:

1. The adverse effects of injuries are likely to be greater and disability more protracted following high speed impacts when the "victims" have been seated in vehicles without head rests on their seats.

2. These patients often seek treatment from many different doctors, each of whom may order new X-rays of the spine.

3. Many patients attend specialists only to be discouraged from further attendance if they fail to improve over the course of a few months.

4. The patients are often confused by conflicting advice about the diagnosis of their problems and by diametrically opposed views about treatment as they move from one doctor to another in their search for relief.

5. Despite the fact that abnormal neurological findings are rarely found on clinical examination, many of these patients will be subjected to cervical myelography, which is almost invariably normal. That information is often used, then, to re-enforce the advice that there is no surgical treatment indicated in their case.

6. These patients do not "get better with the passage of time" or after settlement of their court action.

7. Insurance payments to which they are legally entitled may be summarily reduced or stopped on the advice of a doctor acting for the insurance company on the basis of:
   a) Negative physical findings, except for the fact that the patient looks ill and pain-ridden.
   b) Normal spinal radiographs.
   c) Normal myelogram.

8. The most useful diagnostic test, indicated after failure of carefully supervised conservative treatment, in a patient with a history of significant mechanism of injury, is cervical discography, to identify the level, or levels, of cervical disc disruption.

9. Many of the patients can be cured after cervical disc excision and interbody fusion.

   Neglect of the use of cervical discography has been disastrous for those unfortunate patients suffering from post-traumatic internal disc disruption after injuries to the cervical spine.

   Unquestionably, soft tissue injuries of the neck may occur in cases following "whiplash injury". Disability from muscle tears, haematomas and ligament "strains" cannot be the cause of protracted disability of the order of magnitude described by many patients. When conservative measures of treatment have been tried for four to six months after injuries of this type, and have proven ineffective, then it is time to think of the possibility of a non-prolapsing disc injury, post-traumatic internal disc disruption, as the underlying cause of the continuing symptoms. It is time then to order cervical discograms (Figs. 7.8 a, b).

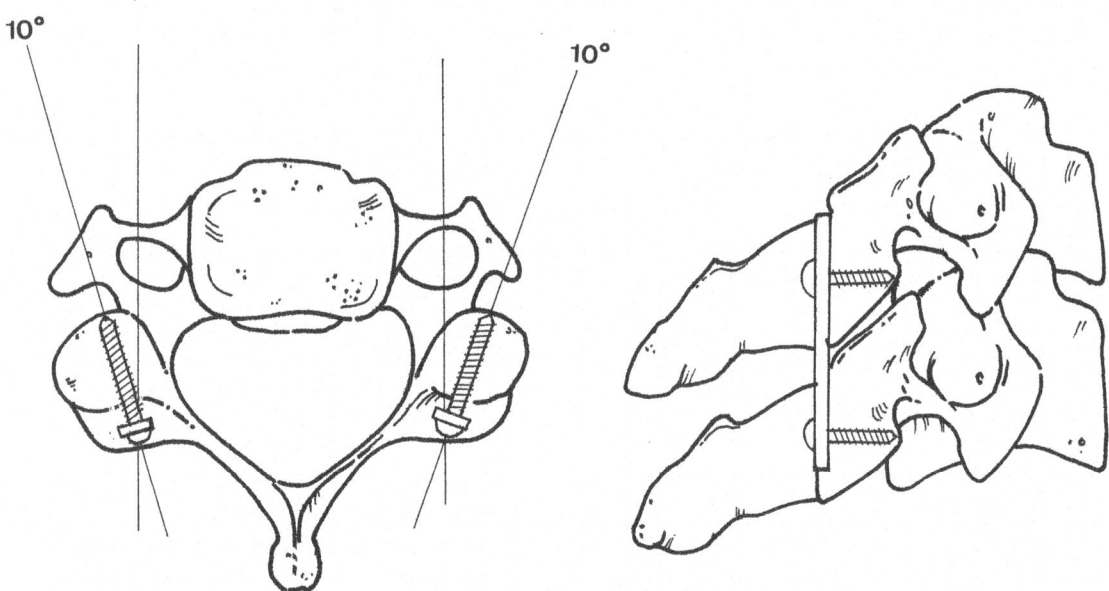

Figure 7.7. Drawings to illustrate the orientation of screws and a plate for cervical vertebral fixation

Figures 7.8 a, b. a A lateral radiograph of the cervical spine in a girl aged 20 years showing discograms between the vertebral bodies of C4/5, C5/6 and C6/7. Extra-thecal leakage of dye has occurred in both of the upper discs while the C6/7 discogram is of normal appearance. **b** An antero-posterior radiograph of the spine of the same patient, showing a normal discogram at C6/7, with marked disruptive changes at C4/5 and C5/6 discs, in both of which dye leaks transversely across the vertebral interspace towards the unco-vertebral joint regions. This patient was suffering from post-traumatic internal disc disruption following a whiplash-mechanism of neck injury. Symptoms of intractable neck pain and occipital headache were relieved by anterior interbody fusions between C4/5 and C5/6. Reviewed 16 years later, she remained symptom-free without radiological evidence of disc degeneration above or below the sites of the fusions

c) Spinal Injuries

Indications for surgery following cervical fractures and dislocations have been expanded considerably in the past ten years. European surgeons (Magerl, Grob, Roy-Camille and Böhler) have introduced innovative fixation techniques and devices which can be applied to the cranio-cervical junction and to lower regions of the neck for the treatment of many of these lesions, shortening hospital stay and speeding rehabilitation (Fig. 7.7). The use of screw fixation for odontoid fractures, either introduced from in front, as recommended by Böhler, or from behind, using trans-articular screws and C1-C2 grafts as described by Magerl and reported by Grob *et al.* (1991), has revolutionised the care of this injury (Figs. 7.9 a, b).

The management of burst fractures and fracture dislocations with cord involvement, formerly treated with rigid conservatism, has also changed. Emphasis in many centres now focuses on urgent anterior decompression of the cervical canal with interbody fusion and if necessary plate and screw fixation.

Following spinal injuries, without associated neurological damage, spinal fusion may be required occasionally, as follows:

a) For the treatment of persisting vertebral instability after dislocations or subluxations (Fig. 7.10).
b) For the treatment of non-union of fractures of the odontoid.
c) For post-surgical deformity of the cervical spine, a difficult problem which often follows extensive laminectomies for spinal cord tumours (Fig. 7.11).

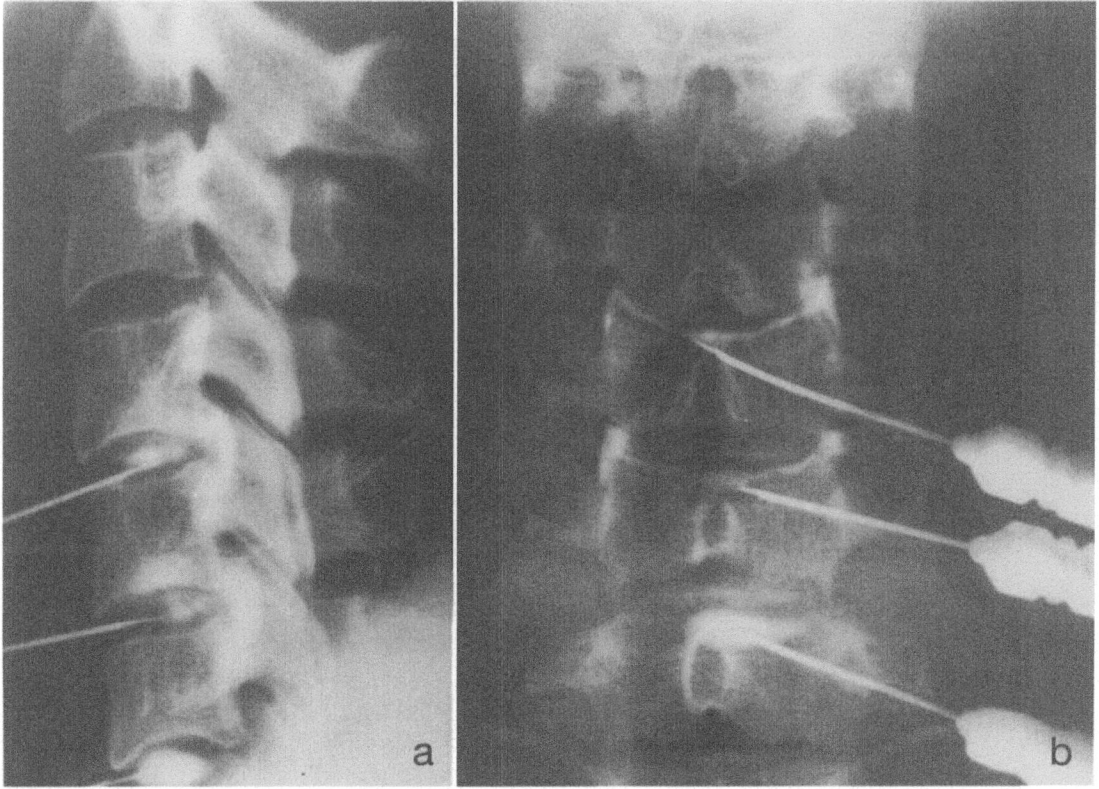

Figures 7.8 a, b

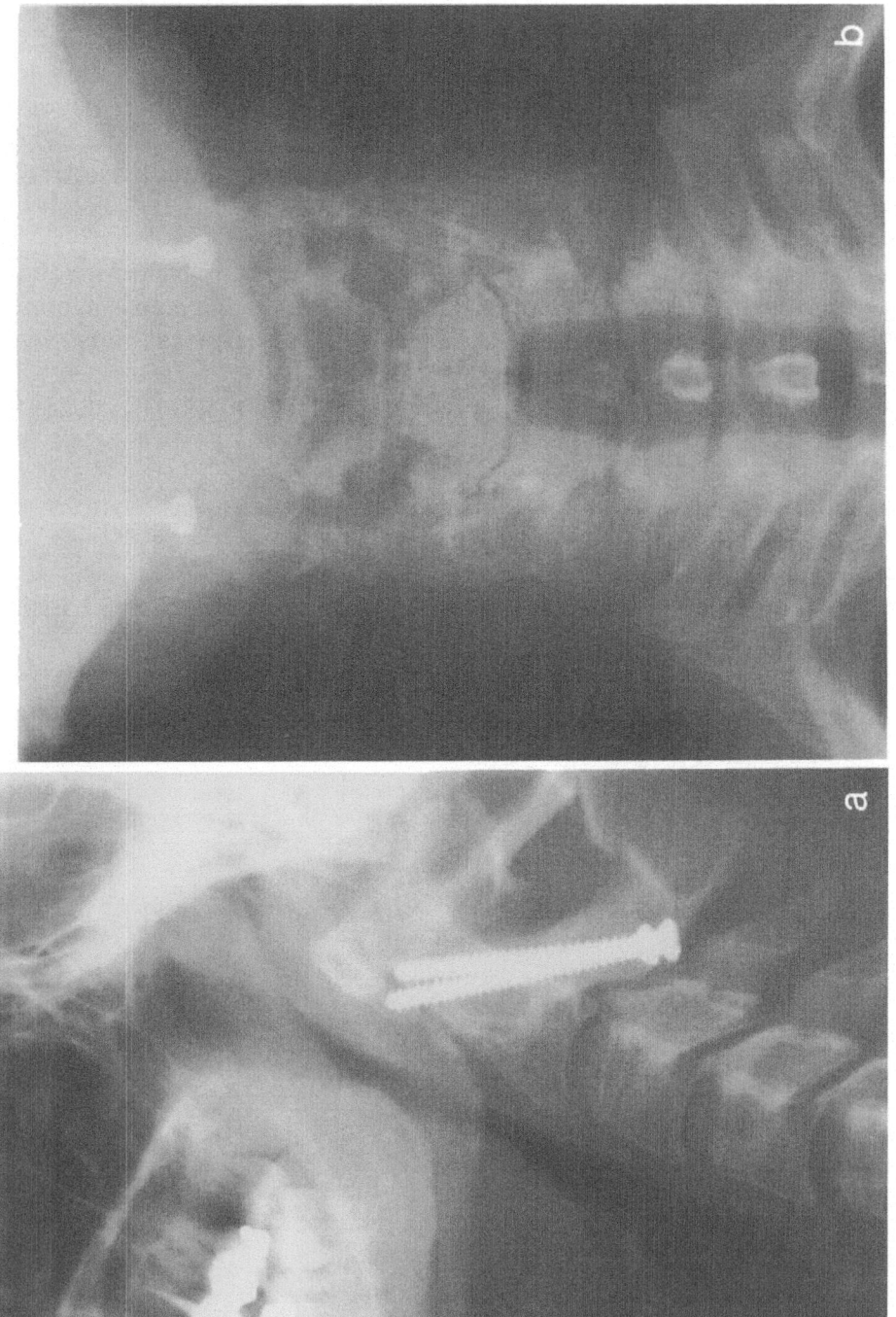

Figures 7.9 a,b. a A lateral radiograph of the upper cervical spine in a male patient showing the Magerl, Grob method of trans-articular screw fixation of C1/C2 vertebrae with an inter-laminar graft between C1 and C2. **b** An antero-posterior view of the same spine. This operation was kindly performed on this patient in London by Dr. Dieter Grob, orthopaedic surgeon, Schulthess Clinic, Zurich, Switzerland, for post traumatic rotatory subluxation of C1 on C2

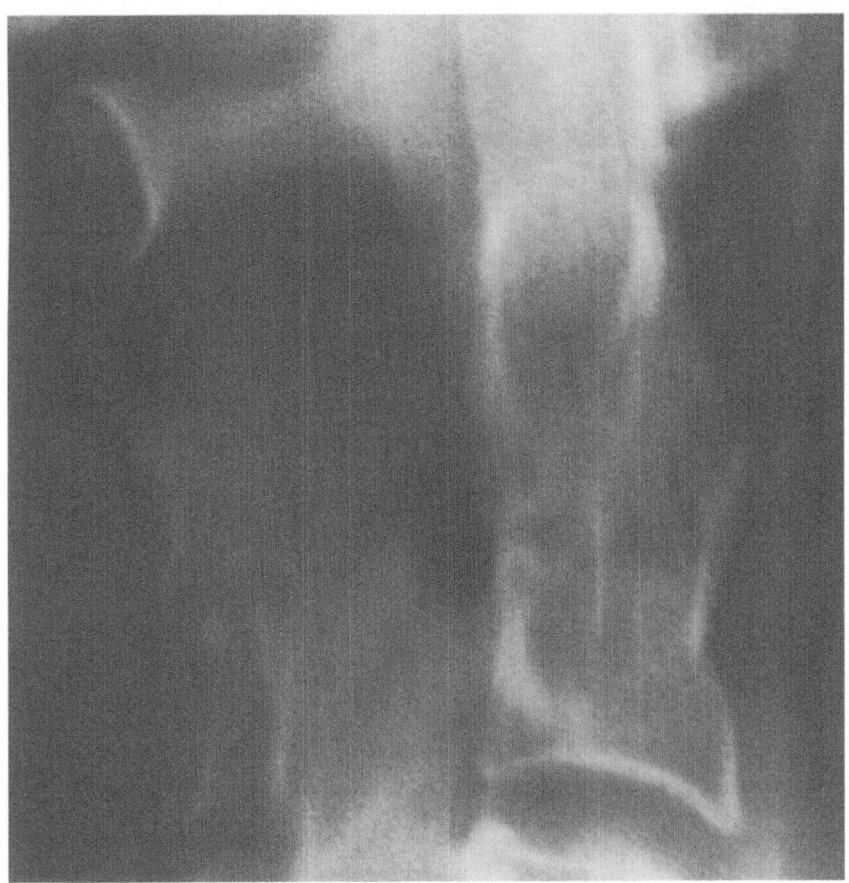

Figure 7.10. A lateral tomogram of the upper cervical spine in a man aged 24 years showing an anterior interbody fusion at the C2/3 level six months after operation. The indication for treatment was for persisting subluxation of C2 on C3 following a neck injury sustained in a motor vehicle accident when his car overturned

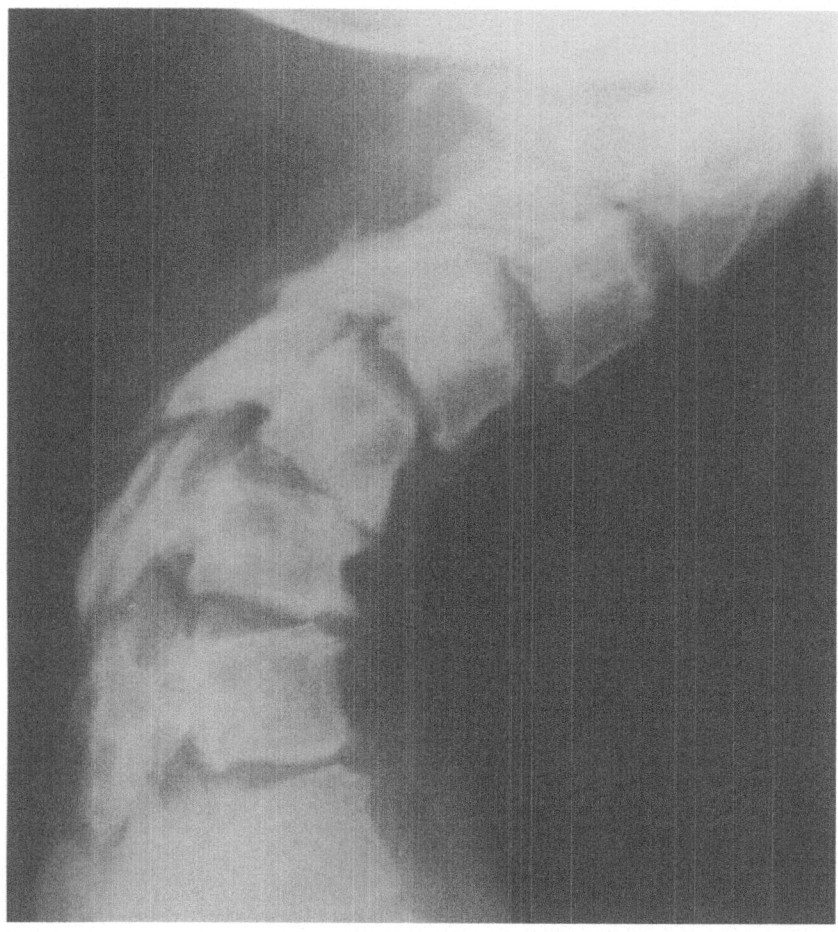

Figure 7.11. A lateral radiograph of the cervical spine of a patient showing gross kyphotic deformity with localized degenerative changes between the vertebral bodies of C5/6 and C6/7 – following an extensive laminectomy for the treatment of syringomyelia

d) Inflammatory Disorders

Rheumatoid arthritis involving the upper cervical spine may result in instability between the first and second cervical vertebrae. Complications resulting from this disease at the base of the skull sometimes pose most challenging problems in surgical management (Von Torklus and Gehle, 1972). These patients are usually frail with delicate skin, making it difficult to fit supporting braces (Figs. 7.12 a–c). Roy-Camille (1980) has designed plates for the fixation of the occiput and upper cervical spine, fixed with screws, passing into the inner table of the occiput and into the lateral masses of the cervical vertebrae. Posterior cervical fusion is not always applicable because of the severe osteoporosis of the laminae and erosion of the posterior arch of C1. Cervical myelopathy often complicates rheumatoid disease at the C1, C2 junction where large soft tissue masses may compress the spinal cord or brain stem. Trans-oral decompression combined with posterior spinal stabilisation has emerged as the treatment of choice. This sophisticated surgery is best carried out in specialised units, Crockard (1988).

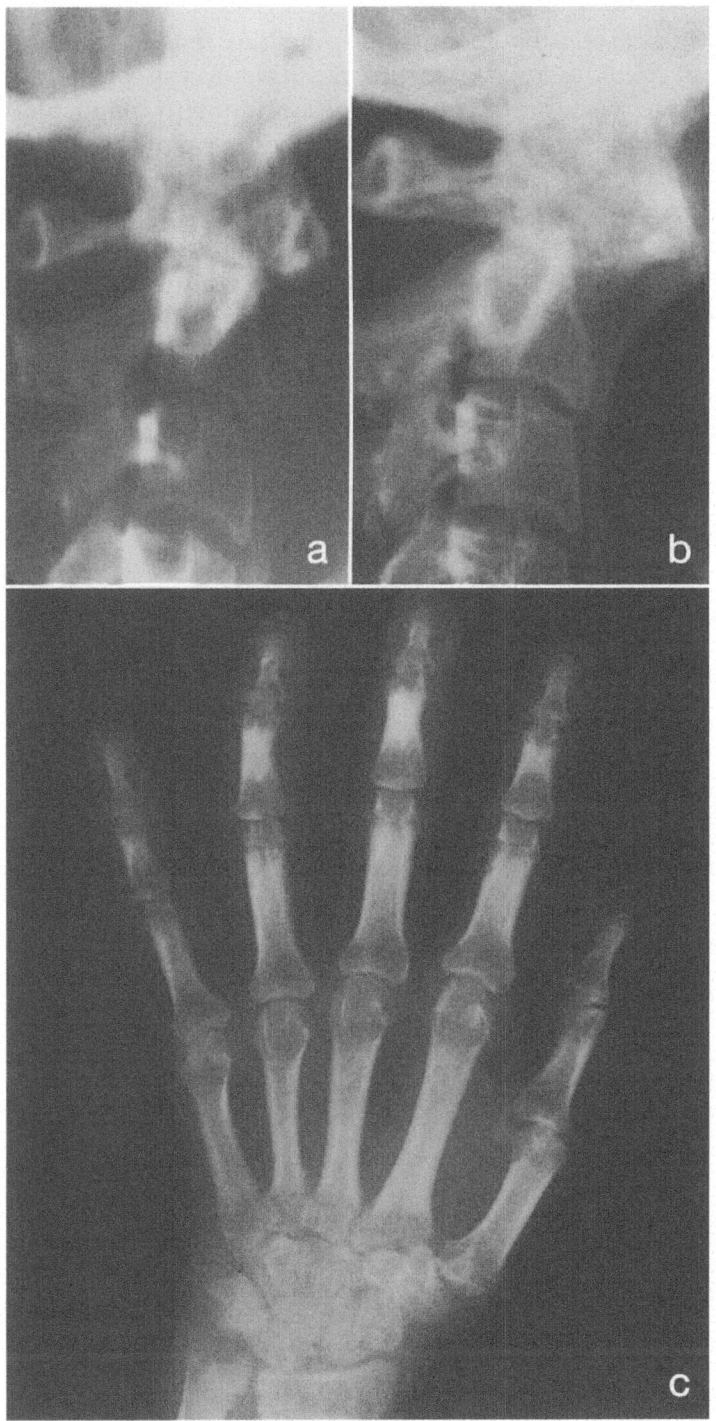

Figures 7.12 a–c. a A lateral radiograph of the upper cervical spine in a woman aged 30 years, showing erosive changes in the region of the odontoid peg due to rheumatoid disease. **b** A radiograph of the same area of the spine in flexion, showing instability between C1 and C2 due to rheumatoid joint disease at that level. **c** A radiograph of the bones of the wrist and hand of the same patient showing the changes of juxta-articular osteoporosis in all the digital joints due to rheumatoid arthritis

e) Infective Lesions

Acute haematogenous osteomyelitis affecting the cervical spine may lead to acute or chronic compression of the spinal cord due to associated epidural abscess formation or to pathological subluxation of the vertebrae. Patients presenting with quadriplegia need urgent investigation, appropriate surgical treatment being planned on the results of myelography or MRI. In the case illustrated in Chapter 8 (Figs. 8.4 a–c), it was on the basis of the myelographic findings that the decision was taken to perform a decompression laminectomy to drain the epidural abscess. Subsequently, the associated spinal deformity was treated conservatively, using skull traction in extension. Spontaneous interbody fusion followed, union occurring without significant residual spinal deformity.

f) Tuberculous Infection

This may cause gross deformity in the neck. Trans-oral fusion of C1/2 involving the facet joints on both sides of the odontoid may be required (Fig. 7.13).

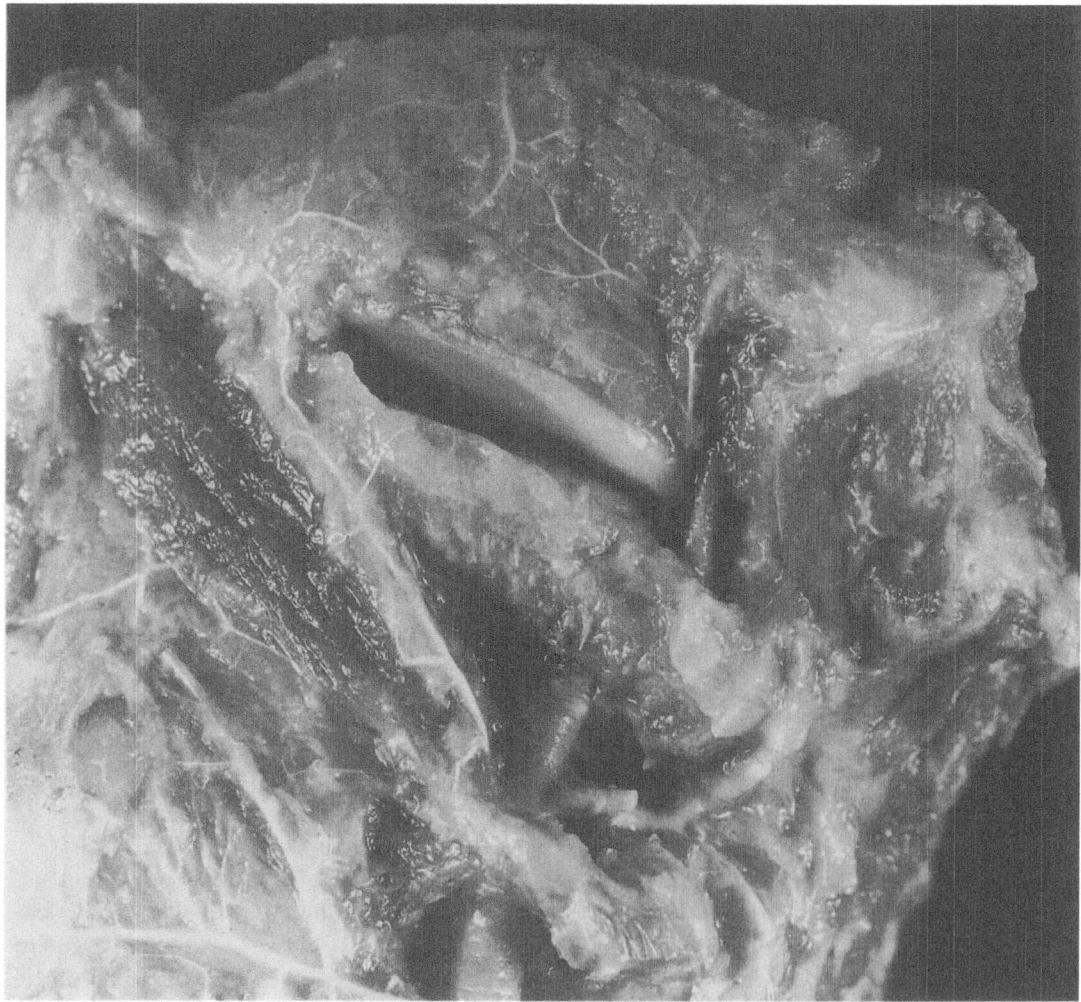

Figure 7.13

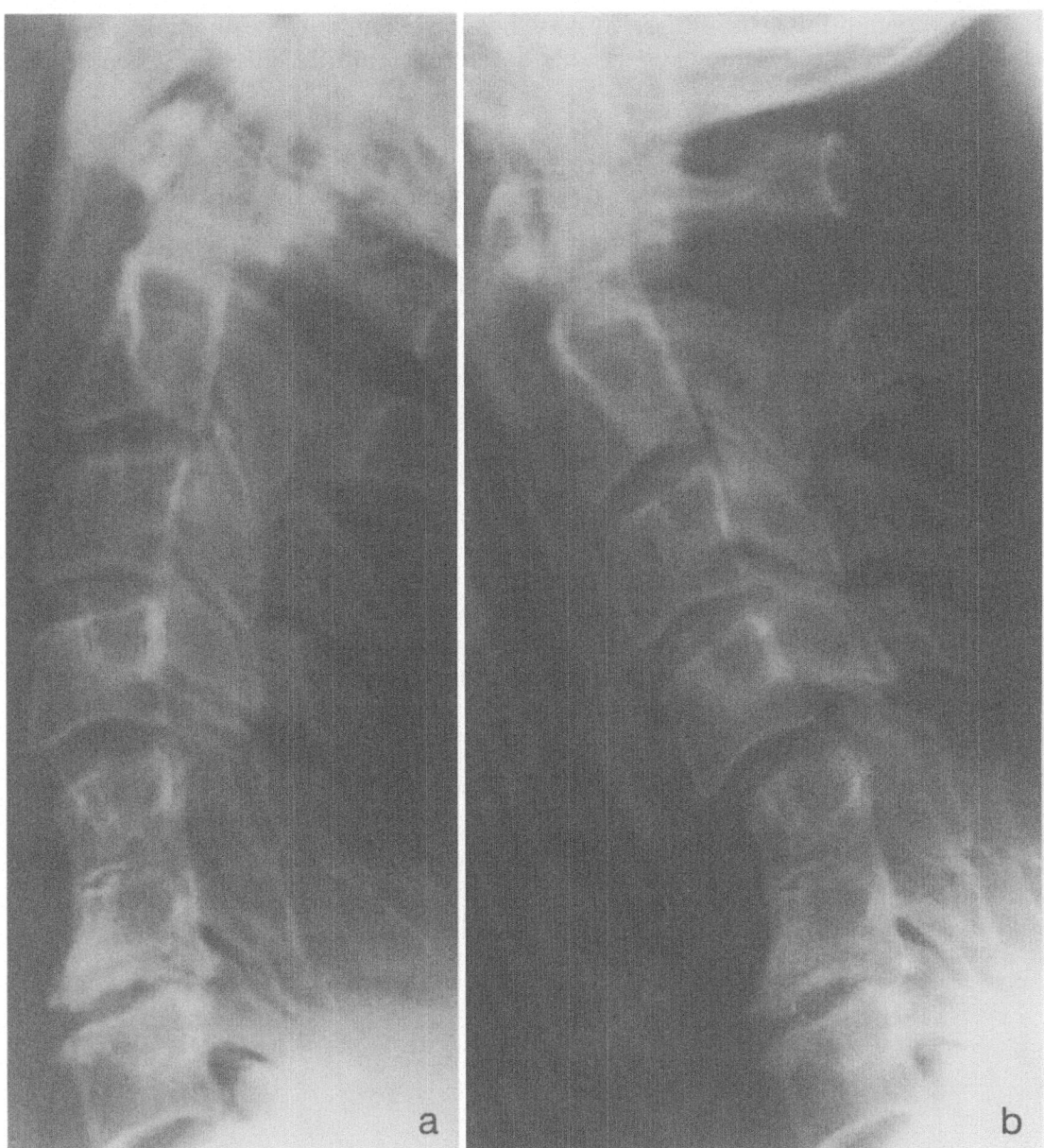

Figures 7.14 a, b. **a** A lateral radiograph of the cervical spine of a patient aged 40 years. Note the congenital fusions between the bodies of C5 and C6. Advanced degenerative changes have occurred at the disc between C6 and C7 with large osteophytes projecting posteriorly into the spinal canal. The disc between C4 and C5 appears normal in this view. **b** A lateral radiograph of the same spine in flexion showing instability at the C4/5 level

Figure 7.13. A detailed view of the facet joint between C1 and C2 on the left side of the specimen illustrated in Fig. 7.1. Note the relationships of the vertebral artery to this joint from which the bulk of the capsule has been excised. In the operation of trans-oral fusion of C1 and C2, grafts are inserted into this joint space after removal of the articular cartilage and sub-chondral bone plates. The lateral capsule of the joint should be carefully preserved to avoid damaging the vertebral artery on the lateral aspect of the joint

More commonly, the disease affects lower cervical vertebrae where it is best treated by local debridement of carious tissue and anterior interbody fusion, see Chapter 8 (Figs. 8.12 a, b).

g) *Congenital Abnormalities*

Congenital fusion of cervical vertebral bodies is relatively common. Severe degenerative spondylosis is usually found in the adjacent vertebral segment below the fusion early in adult life. Occasionally vertebral instability will be found in the segment above or below the congenital fusion. Anterior cervical interbody fusions may be required for the treatment of either or both of these lesions (Figs. 7.14a,b).

7.3. *Cervical Discography*

The test is performed on the conscious patient with light sedation. The needles used for this investigation are smaller in calibre than those used in the lumbar spine (Fig. 7.15). They are usually inserted through the right side of the neck, anteriorly, by pushing the mid-line structures of the neck across to the left side with the

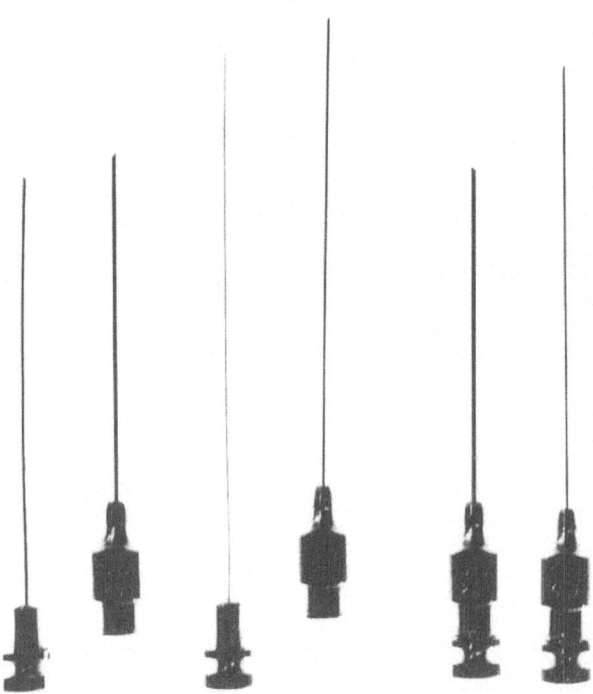

Figure 7.15. A photograph showing a gauge 25 "discogram needle" on the right of the picture with a gauge 22 "guide needle" alongside. On the left of the picture the stilettes are shown alongside their respective needles

operator's index finger. Control X-rays are taken in antero-posterior and lateral planes to ensure accurate placement of the tip of each "discogram needle" in the centre of the nuclear zones of the discs before dye is injected (see Chapter 2, pp. 66–69).

Spread of dye beyond the zone of the nucleus pulposus may occur into the unco-vertebral joint areas on both sides, while leakage backwards into the spinal canal (extra-thecal) may indicate a posterior disc disruption. Spread of dye results from incompetence of annular fibres and is not necessarily an indication of disc prolapse.

The pain response provoked by injection of dye into the disc is not related to the volume injected or to the resultant increase in intra-discal pressure; rather, it is due to irritation, by the dye, of the sensitized pain fibres within the disrupted disc itself. Hence, the pattern of pain distribution is not strictly segmental and it does not follow the dermatomes in the upper limbs, as has been suggested by some writers. Use of cervical discography should be reserved for the investigation and demonstration of non-prolapsing disc disorders. By contrast, neither myelography nor C.T. scanning will help to identify the level of a disc with internal disruption. Those investigations find their proper application in the investigation of cases with disc pathology producing space-occupying lesions in the vertebral canal.

MRI, particularly with gadolinium enhancement, though useful, has not yet been found superior to discography in helping to confirm the diagnosis of post-traumatic internal disc disruption.

7.4. Technique of Anterior Cervical Interbody Fusions

a) Instruments

Dowel cutting instruments permit these operations to be performed accurately at each attempt. Their use in most cases is preferred to the use of chisels or osteotomes for this reason and for the added safety afforded, during the operation, by the safety devices built into the design of Crock cutters. Photographs of essential instruments are found in Figs. 7.16–20 with descriptive legends outlining details of their assembly and use.

b) Positioning

Patients are placed supine on the operating table. A small wedge-shaped pillow should be placed under the shoulders, with a rolled towel supporting the hollow of the neck, the occiput resting in a rubber ring. The patient's eyes should be protected and the anaesthetic tubes securely fixed to the patient's forehead (Fig. 7.21).

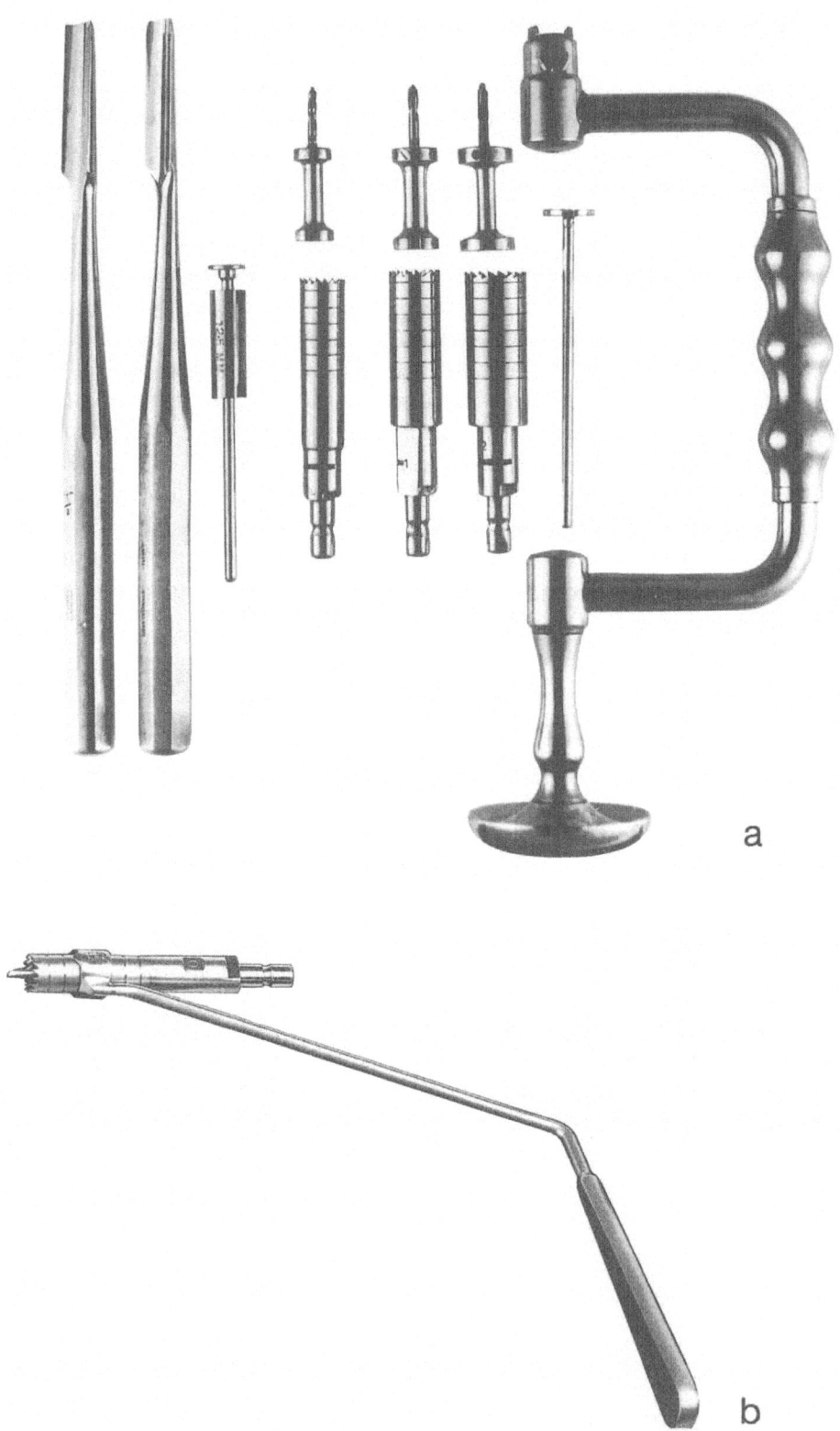

Figures 7.16 a, b

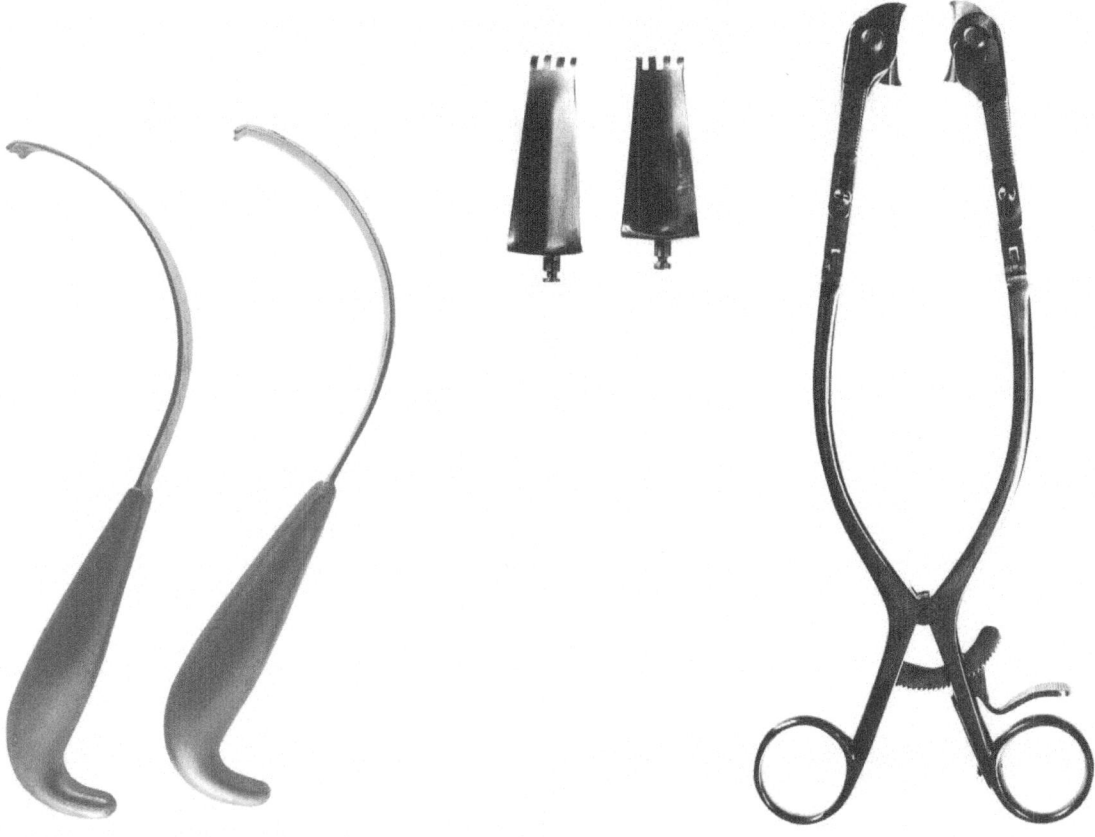

Figure 7.17   **Figure 7.18**

Figure 7.17. A photograph of two cervical retractors with smooth excavated ends designed to be held transversely across the anterior surfaces of the cervical intervertebral discs

Figure 7.18. A photograph of the self-retaining retractor designed by Cloward for use in anterior cervical fusions

---

Figures 7.16 a, b. a A photograph showing the Crock instruments used for dowel cutting in the operation of anterior cervical interbody fusion. On the right of the picture is a Hudson brace. Cutters of three sizes are shown. The starter centre pieces have been removed from each of these. On the right of the cutters is a pusher, which fits inside the cutters and can be used to eject the starter centre pieces or graft bone. On the left of the cutters a pusher is shown with a tubular segment of metal measuring 12.5 mm in depth. When this "dummy" is slotted into the cutter it acts as a guard, preventing the cutter from penetrating deeper than 12.5 mm into the cervical vertebral bodies. Dummies are provided in three sizes, 10 mm, 12.5 mm and 15 mm, for use according to the vertebral dimensions in individual cases. On the left of the photograph, two tooled gouges are shown, which will fit into the cuts made into adjacent vertebral bodies. Their use is illustrated in Figs. 7.28 a–c. Note that the cutters have circular rings marking their outer surfaces, at intervals of 5 mm. Instruments manufactured exclusively by Thomson and Shelton Instrumentation Company, 6119 Danbury Lane, Dallas, TX 75214, U.S.A. **b** A photograph of guide sleeve with two prongs which penetrate the disc – allowing the cutter to be inserted without snagging surrounding soft tissues

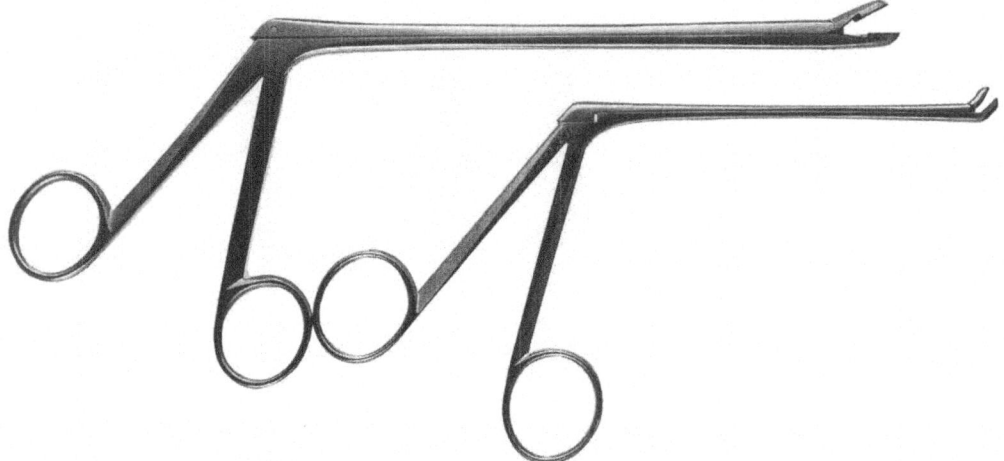

Figure 7.19. A photograph showing fine, straight and forward-angled pituitary rongeurs suitable for use during anterior cervical interbody fusion operations, for removing remnants of vertebral end-plates and disc tissue following curettage of the disc space

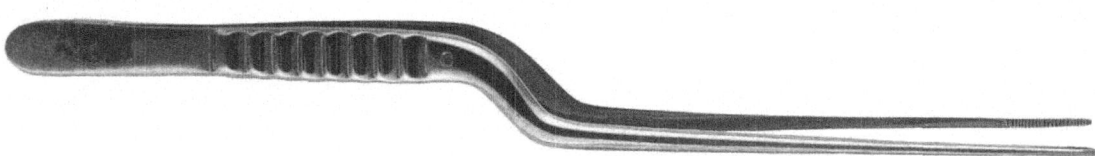

Figure 7.20. A photograph of a Bayonet forceps with a fine tip, essential for use in cervical spine operations

c) Incisions

A right-sided hemi-collar incision can be used for approaches to any of the cervical discs, from that between C2 and C3 vertebrae to the lowest in the cervical spine. The use of longitudinal incisions may result in unsightly scars, though they may be necessary in special cases requiring multi-level spinal fusions.

The platysma muscle is exposed by separating subcutaneous fat from its superficial surface before the muscle is split in the line of its fibres. The encircling layer of deep cervical fascia is then incised along the anterior border of the sterno-mastoid muscle, allowing access to the space between the carotid sheath laterally and the mid-line structures of the neck medially. Inserting the index finger into the space now created, the surgeon can palpate the front of the vertebral column. By moving the finger deliberately and carefully along the antero-lateral margin of the vertebrae, a plane of cleavage can usually be opened easily in the loose fascia between the carotid sheath and the mid-line structures of the neck over a distance sufficient to allow exposure of one, two or three of the cervical intervertebral discs.

Most cervical fusions are performed at the levels of C4/5, C5/6 or C6/7. Having cleared the space as indicated, retractors may then be inserted, orientated trans-

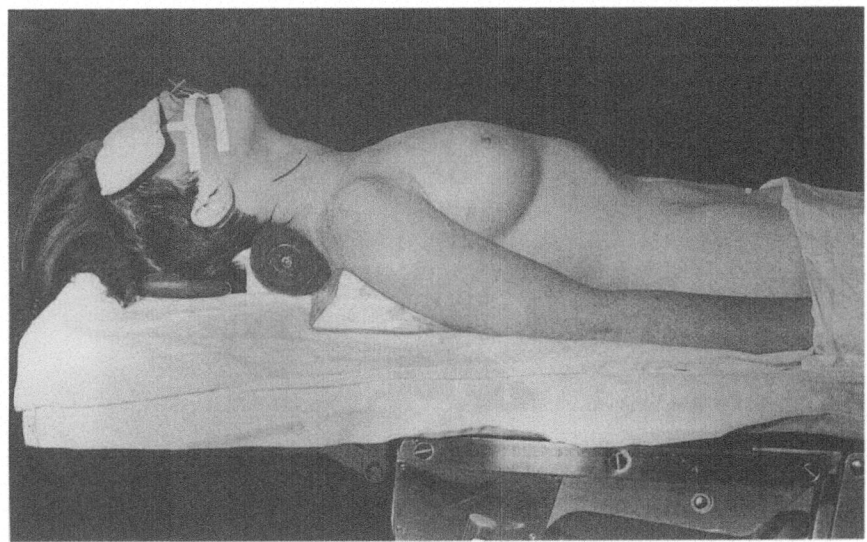

Figure 7.21. A photograph of a patient postured on the operating table for anterior cervical interbody fusion. Note the triangular-shaped pillow underneath the shoulders, the rolled towel (in black) under the neck, and the rubber ring on which the occiput rests. The endo-tracheal tube and the reinforced rubber airway adjacent to it are strapped to the patient's face. Note the pad covering the eyes, to prevent pressure on the orbits during surgery. Assistants have been known to press on the eyes during the operation. Irreparable ocular damage has been reported from this cause. Note also the outline of the hemi-collar incision extending from the anterior border of the sterno-mastoid muscle to just behind the mid-line. Through this incision two or three cervical discs can be exposed. For exposure of the disc between C2 and C3 vertebral bodies, the incision needs to be placed in the sub-mandibular region, care being taken to avoid damaging the mandibular branch of the facial nerve. Note that both arms are by the patient's side, to allow traction on the hands for lowering the shoulders while control X-rays are being taken during the operation

versely and applied to the anterior aspect of one of the intervertebral discs. Up to this point the only major anatomical structures encountered will have been those already mentioned. Only occasionally will it be found necessary to ligate and divide an anterior cervical vein or some un-named venous tributary of the internal jugular vein. The superior thyroid vessels may be seen, but it is rarely necessary to ligate and divide them.

The pre-vertebral fascia, that thin, filmy, opalescent membrane which sheaths the pre-vertebral muscles and the cervical column itself, is split longitudinally in the mid-line and the retractors re-positioned to give a clear view of the intervertebral discs and anterior aspects of the vertebral bodies. The medial edges of the right and left-sided longus colli muscles can be seen clearly and, using a fine bayonet forceps, the vessels related to the muscles at their attachments along the antero-lateral aspects of the vertebral bodies are coagulated with diathermy (Fig. 7.22). These muscular attachments are then separated from the vertebrae and discs, so that the cervical retractors may be replaced beneath their freed medial margins to expose the disc or discs to be removed. The risk of obstructing the carotid vessels during operation is thereby reduced, either with the use of the hand held retractors (Fig. 7.17) or with self retaining types (Fig. 7.18).

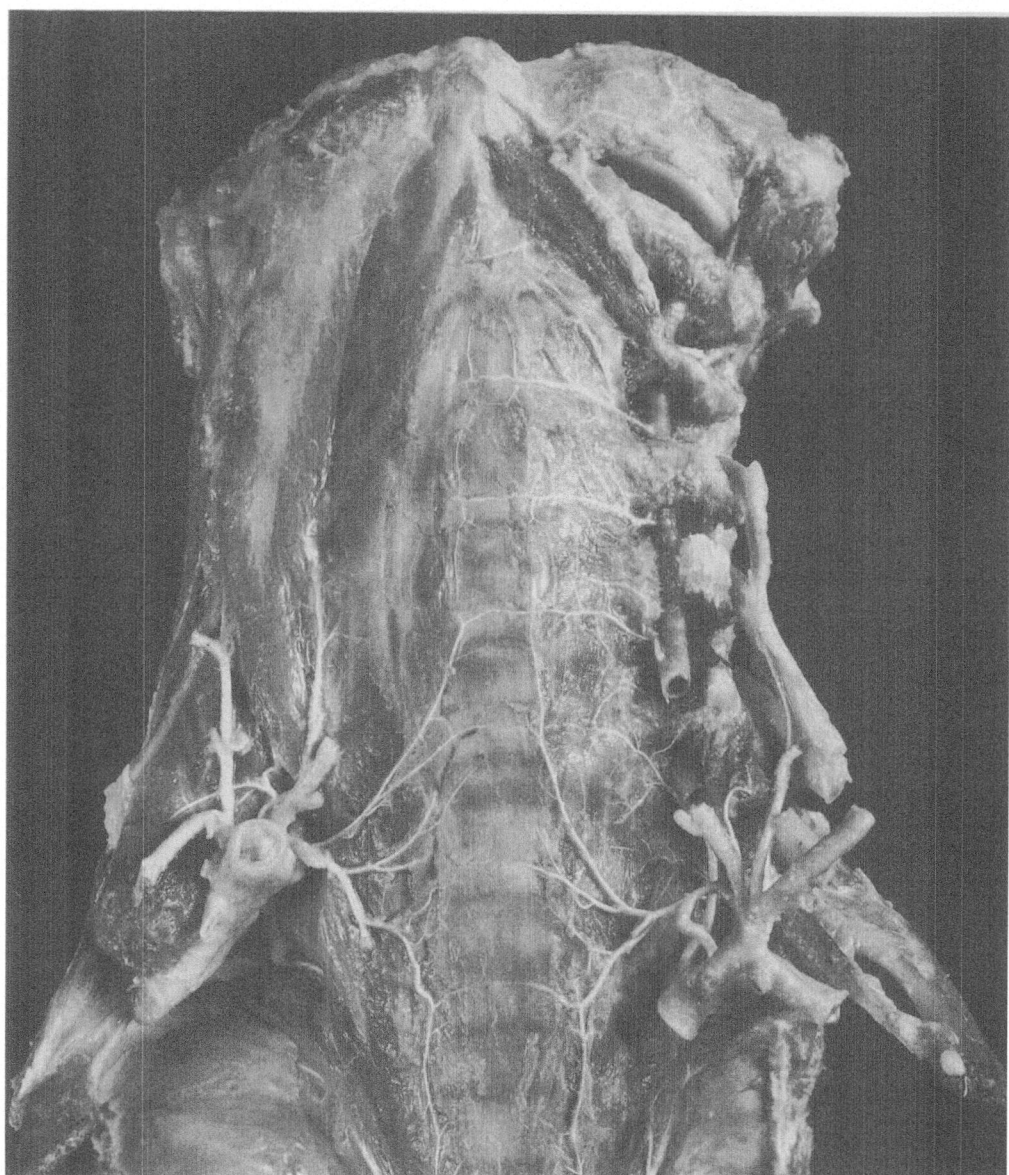

Figure 7.22. A photograph of a dissection of the anterior aspect of the cervical and upper thoracic spine of a female child aged 3 1/2 years, showing the origins and courses of arteries supplying the antero-lateral aspects of the vertebral bodies. The longus colli muscles have been removed from the left side of the specimen. The pre-vertebral fascia has also been removed but the anterior margin of the longus colli at its attachment to the antero-lateral aspects of the vertebral bodies on the right side is intact. Note the vertical chain of arterial anastomoses running along the margin of this muscular attachment, forming a parallel vascular channel with corresponding vessels on the left side of the vertebral column. (Dissected by Dr. H. Yoshizawa) [Reproduced from: Crock, H. V., Yoshizawa, H.: The Blood Supply of the Vertebral Column and Spinal Cord in Man. Wien–New York: Springer, 1977]

d) *The Thyroid Gland*

Before planning cervical discography and anterior cervical spine surgery in any patient, the surgeon should examine the patient's thyroid gland. On three occasions in twenty-five years of practice, I have had patients in whom thyroidectomy has been required before satisfactory access to the anterior aspect of the cervical vertebral column was possible.

e) *Control X-Rays to Identify Individual Intervertebral Discs*

The use of a disposable needle with a Z bend in it, inserted into the disc, is recommended before lateral X-rays are taken. The needle serves the dual purpose of identifying the disc level and allowing the precise measurement of its antero-posterior width. (Fig. 7.23 a–c). *Never remove the needle before the control X-ray has been exhibited in the operating room confirming the level of the disc to be removed.*

f) *Preparation of the Dowel Cavity*

The relevant anatomy of the spine and the steps in this critical phase of the operation are illustrated in detail in Figs. 7.22–28. Once cutting instruments have been applied to the vertebral bodies the potential hazards of injuring the vertebral arteries or the neural structures in the spinal canal must be borne in mind (Figs. 7.1 a, b).

Having made the preliminary cut across the disc space, the starter centre piece is removed from the cutter. The surgeon then selects the "safety dummy" of predetermined size, by re-checking the antero-posterior measurements of the disc space and then personally assembles the cutter ready for use by inserting the "dummy", which is held in place by the "pusher device". Both the assistant surgeon and theatre sister should check the preparation of the cutter with the "dummy" and cross-check the disc space measurements before the surgeon re-inserts the cutter, after stage one, to commence the final preparation of the dowel cavity.

Errors made at this stage could lead to catastrophic accidents during the operation. The equipment illustrated in this chapter has been used by the author since 1962 without any instance of spinal cord or cervical nerve root injury occurring up to the present time (1991).

Having re-fitted the cutter into the preliminary circular slot cut during stage one (Fig. 7.25 a–c), it should be oscillated clockwise and counter-clockwise, avoiding any wobbling motion as the Hudson brace is being rotated. No force is to be exerted on the proximal end of the brace, other than that required to steady it with one hand, while the surgeon's other hand holds the off-set control bar through which the oscillating motion is transmitted to the cutter.

As the cutter advances slowly into the vertebral bodies and intervening disc tissue, the operator becomes aware of a grating sensation at its cutting end, from which an audible grating sound is emitted. The "dummy" inside the cutting cylinder will abut against the anterior surface of the disc and adjacent vertebral margins when the cutter has reached the depth that is determined by the length of the "dummy" (Fig. 7.26 a, b). Further penetration of the cutter into the vertebral bodies is thereby prevented. At this stage, the grating sensation ceases and the cutter spins smoothly

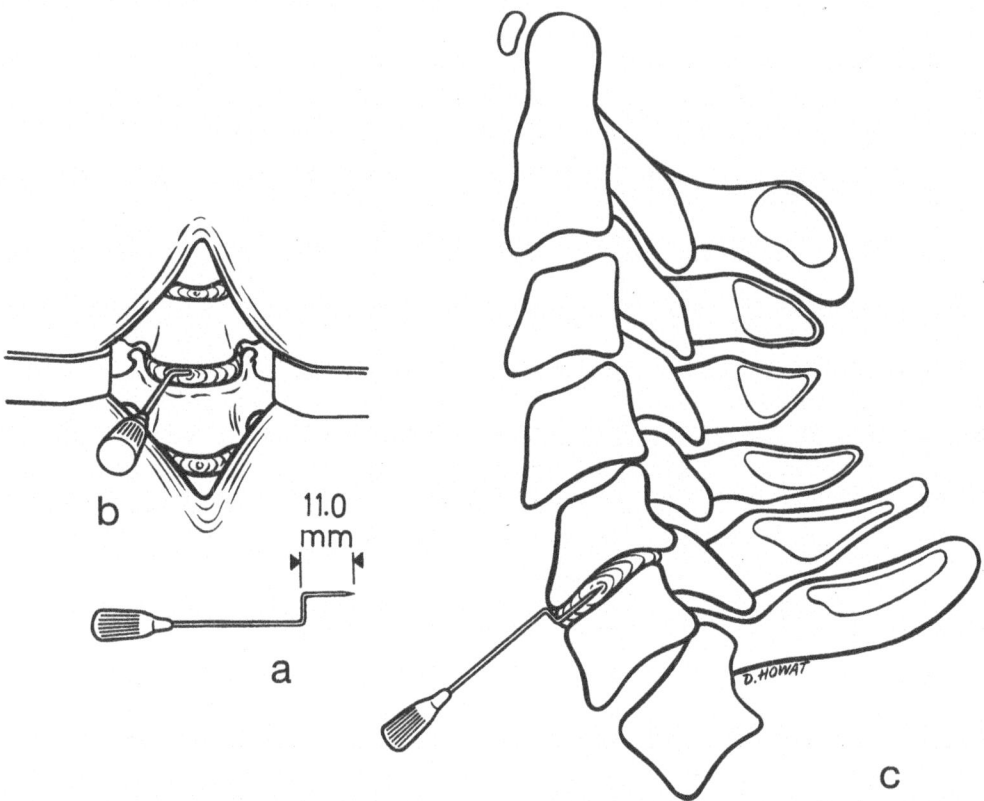

Figures 7.23 a–c. **a** A drawing to illustrate the use of a bent needle recommended by the author for use during control X-rays in the neck. A disposable 19 gauge needle is prepared by bending it in the jaws of an artery forceps. A right-angle bend is made near the tip and the measurement between the tip and the first right-angle bend taken. Usually 11.0–12.5 mm is satisfactory, depending on the size of the patient. **b** A drawing to depict the front of a cervical intervertebral disc with the needle in place for control X-ray during operation. **c** A drawing of the cervical spine shown from the side depicting the use of the bent needle for control X-ray. The right angle bend prevents penetration of the needle into the cervical canal, a potential risk if a straight needle is inserted. It has the added advantage of allowing precise measurement of the intervertebral disc space on the control X-ray

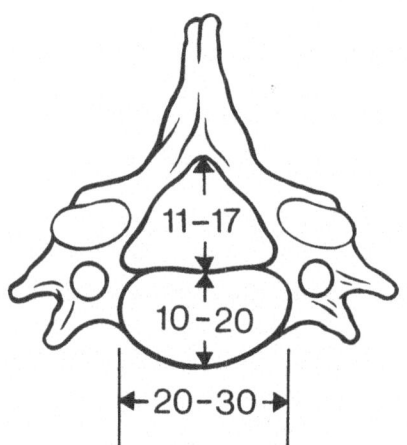

Figure 7.24. A drawing of a typical cervical vertebra with the ranges of measurements in millimetres of the transverse and antero-posterior diameters of the vertebral body and the antero-posterior diameter of the cervical canal

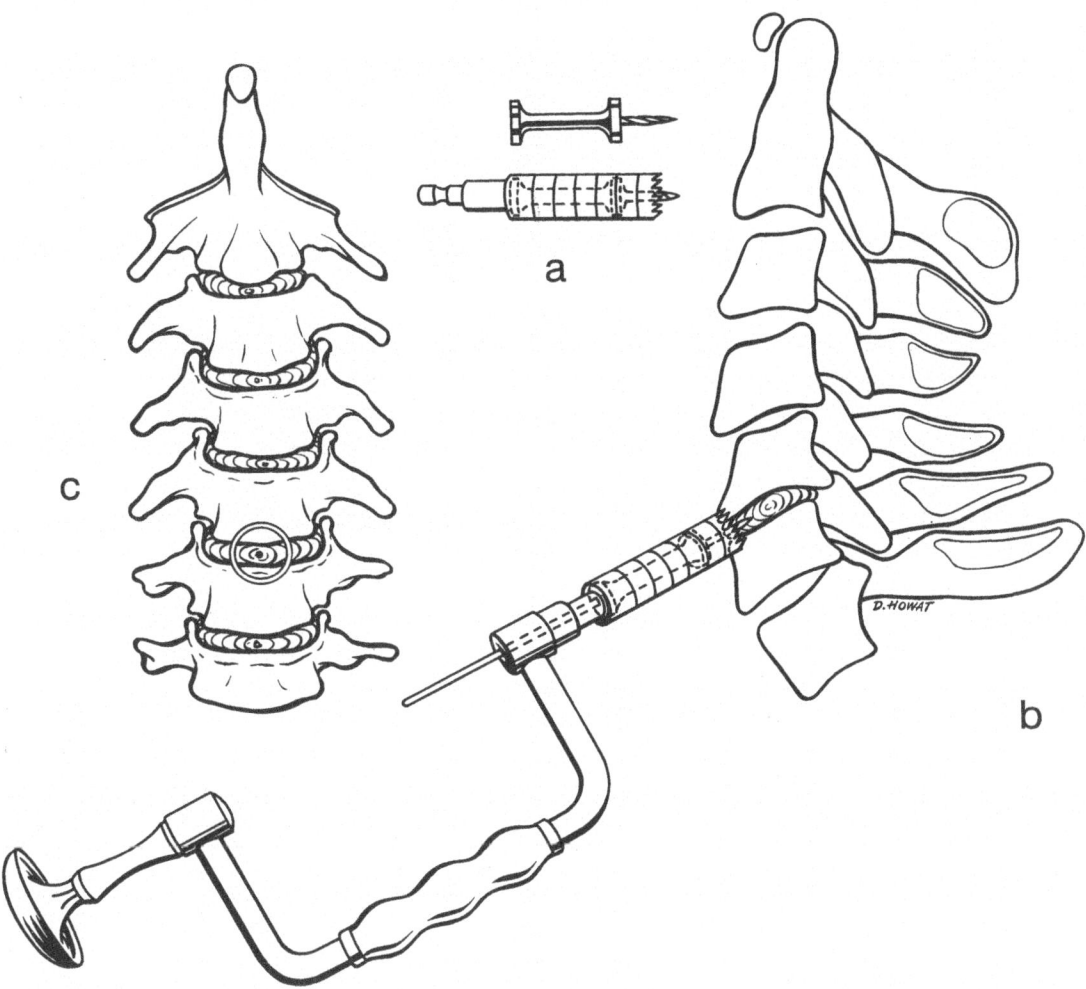

Figures 7.25 a–c. a A drawing showing a starter centre piece at the top. Below it, the starter centre piece is shown in outline, assembled in the zero-size cutter. Note the circumferential markings on the cutter, each separated from the other by 5 mm. **b** A drawing of the cervical spine, viewed from the side, showing the cutter assembled on a Hudson brace with the starter centre piece in position and the pusher within the tube. The drawing depicts the method of commencing the preparation of a dowel cavity between the vertebrae of C5 and C6. **c** A drawing of the cervical spine viewed from in front, showing the outline of the cut in the mid-line between the vertebral bodies of C5 and C6, at the first stage of preparation of the dowel cavity

and silently. For added safety, while the cutter is being oscillated, the surgeon may check the measurement of its advancement by counting the rings on its outer surface.

In the third stage of the preparation of the cervical dowel cavity a special tooled gouge is used to displace the fragments of vertebral bodies and intervertebral disc from the spine (Fig. 7.28 a). This has been manufactured specifically to fit accurately into the dowel cavity between the cut margins of the vertebral bodies, so that the central plug of disc attached to elliptical segments of the adjacent vertebrae can be levered out and removed. This instrument must be handled with caution, introduced without undue force as it is directed into the depth of the cut, so that it fits snugly into the vertebral body before a simple levering force is applied to snap off the ellipse of vertebral body, first on one side of the disc, then on the other. *The gouge should not be rotated so that it lies transversely across the disc space.* It will not then be effective in fracturing the ellipses of vertebral bone to which the disc is attached. *It is designed specifically for use as described.* It is usually possible to remove the plug of bone and intervening disc tissue in one piece.

In cases of advanced spondylosis, where the opposing vertebral end-plates are sclerotic, being separated by thin unyielding remnants of disc tissue, it may be necessary to curette the remnants of the disc tissue from between the arcuate segments of vertebral bodies in order to create a gap in the intervertebral space into which these bony fragments can be displaced with the gouge. If the vertebral bone is extremely dense, one of the segments may need to be removed with a high speed drill, the other being removed then in the manner set out above.

When the base of the dowel cavity has been exposed, brisk haemorrhage may occur from arteries and veins in the vertebral bodies. This is controlled easily by applying small quantities of bone wax to the cut surface of the vertebral bodies, only at the site of bleeding.

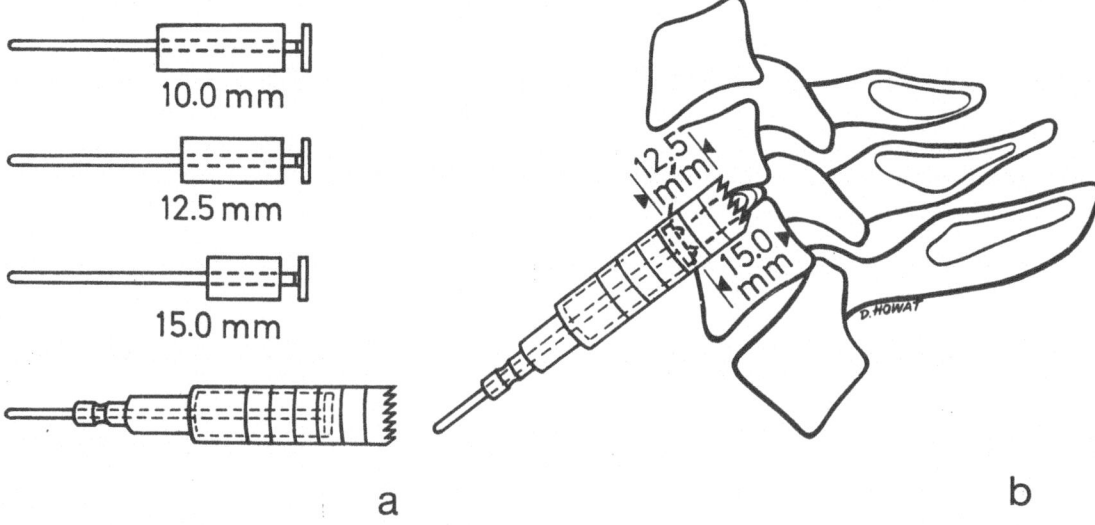

a   b

Figures 7.26 a, b

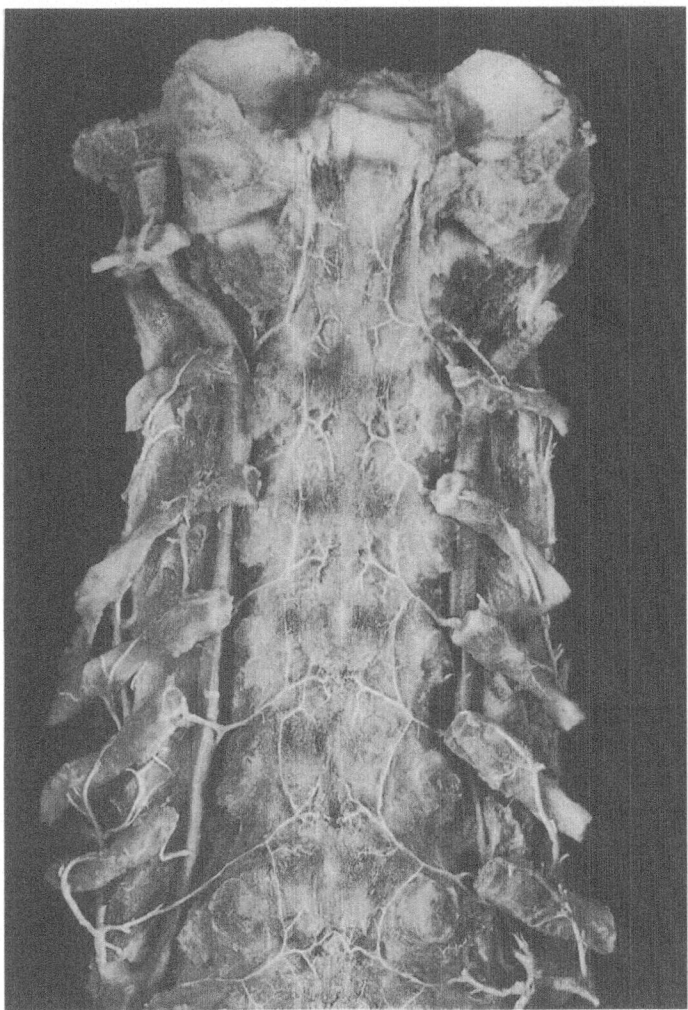

Figure 7.27. A photograph of a dissection of the posterior aspect of the cervical and upper thoracic spine of a male aged 34 years. The posterior aspects of the vertebral bodies have been exposed and portions of the posterior longitudinal ligament have been removed from a number of vertebral bodies in the lower part of the specimen. In the upper part of the specimen on both sides, the origins of the anterior spinal canal branches of the vertebral arteries can be seen. In the neck, these vessels form the familiar arcuate arterial pattern on the anterior surface of the spinal canal which is found along its length. The vessels contribute to the intra-osseous arterial supply of the vertebral bodies, anastomosing with branches from the vascular chains demonstrated in Fig. 7.22 on the anterior aspect of the vertebral column. In the operation of anterior cervical interbody fusion the blood supply of the vertebral body remains largely intact, ensuring rapid vascularization of grafts

---

Figures 7.26 a, b. a A drawing to show the range of metal dummies available for insertion into the zero-size cutter, allowing the preparation of dowel cavities of pre-determined depth, depending on the depth of the disc space in individual patients. The depth of the space is checked at operation by control X-ray with the use of the bent needle as indicated in Figs. 7.23 a,b,c. At the bottom of the drawing, note the dummy assembled inside the cutters. **b** A drawing to depict the cutter in use, demonstrating the mechanism of safety protection provided by the 12.5 mm dummy which has been inserted after removal of the starter centre piece. Note also that the surgeon is able to count the rings on the outer side of the cutter, providing a double safety factor. (See pp 243 for a detailed description of the technique for cutting the dowel cavity)

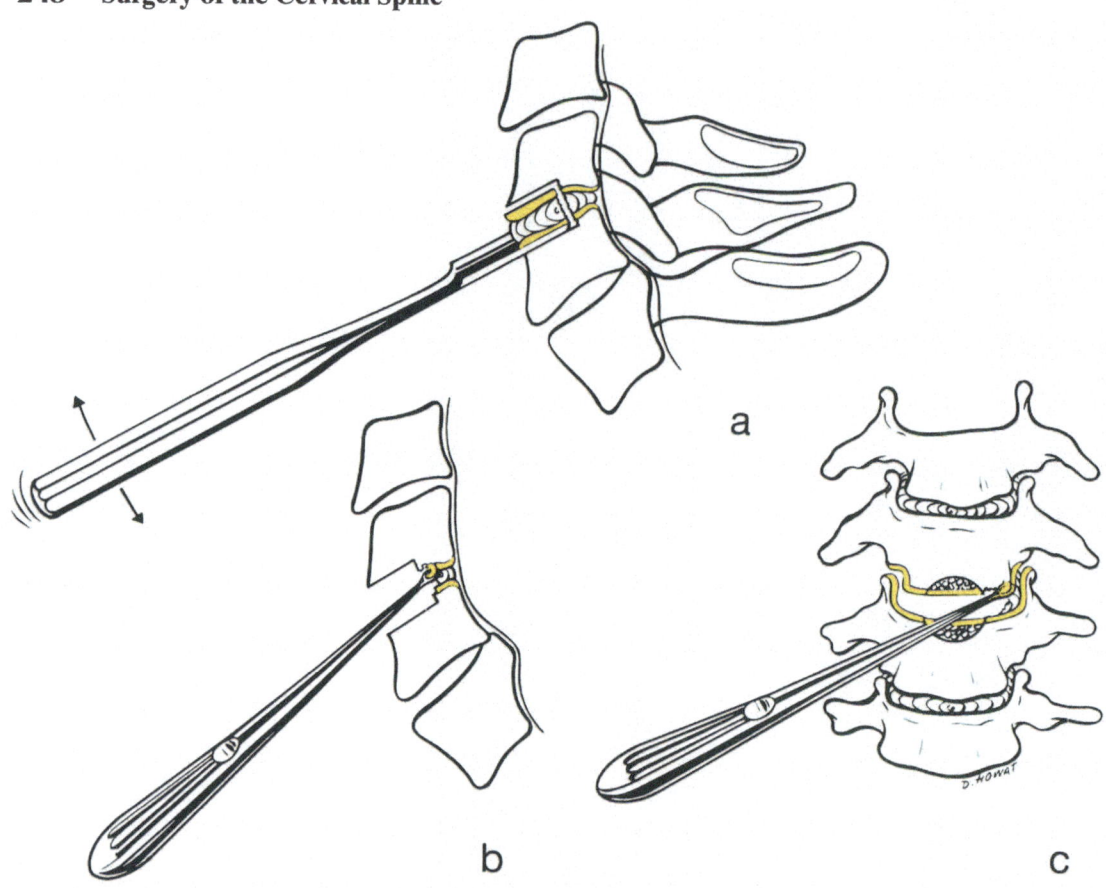

Figures 7.28 a–c. a A drawing to show the method of use of the tooled gouge for removal of the plug of the vertebral bodies and disc following the use of the cutter as depicted in Figs. 7.26 a,b. **b** A drawing to illustrate the use of a fine curette (2 mm cup) for removal of the vertebral end-plate remnants shown in yellow, after the plug of disc tissue sandwiched between vertebral end-plate margins has been displaced with the gouge and removed with a straight pituitary rongeur. **c** A drawing depicting the use of the fine curette (2 mm cup) showing the prepared dowel cavity from in front with the curette removing remnants of vertebral end-plate cartilage and disc tissue in the region of the left-sided unco-vertebral joint. It is possible to remove virtually all disc tissue and vertebral end-plate remnants in this manner

The fourth and final stage of preparation of the intervertebral space now commences, leading up to the actual impaction of the bone graft. Vertebral end-plate cartilage remnants are removed with a fine curette (1 or 2 mm cup), disc remnants attached, as illustrated in Figs. 7.28 b,c. Care is taken to avoid damaging the vertebral arteries (Figs. 7.1 a, b).

Longitudinal traction applied to the skull by the anaesthetist will result in opening up of the intervertebral space, allowing the surgeon to see the posterior longitudinal ligament in the depths of the dowel cavity. Through visible defects in this ligament in cases of sequestration of disc fragments into the cervical spinal canal, it is possible to remove the displaced disc tissue from the canal.

Excision of osteophytic bars of bone from the anterior aspect of the cervical spinal canal may be required in cases of cervical myelopathy. Depending on the transverse width of the disc, two overlapping dowel cavities may be cut, allowing a wider exposure for this delicate, and potentially dangerous, task.

The use of a high-speed drill with rounded diamond-tipped burrs is essential and facilities for good lighting, suction, irrigation and magnification are required. A small piece of plastic catheter should be fixed to the tip of the sucker to prevent it being damaged by the drill burr. Two or three vertebral levels are often involved and the decision needs to be made either to decompress and fuse individual levels or to excise intervening vertebral bodies and insert a strut graft (Fig. 7.29). In either case, the use of autogenous grafts cut from the iliac crest can be recommended. Fibular strut grafts are used by some authors but they are slow to vascularize.

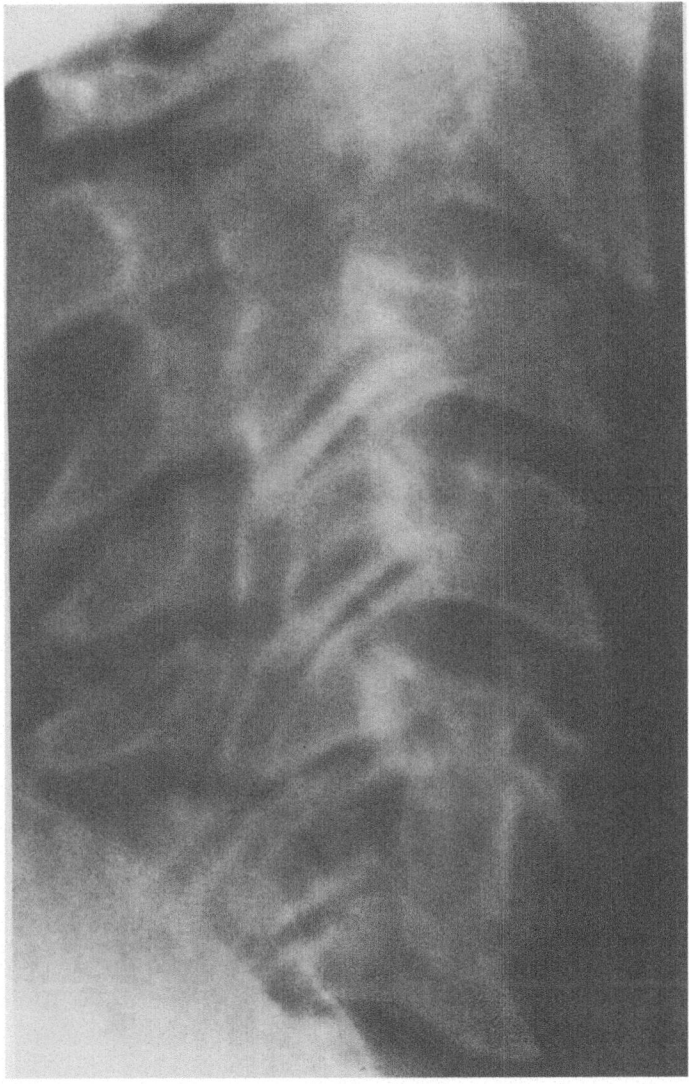

Figure 7.29. A lateral radiograph of the spine of the patient whose pre-operative films are illustrated in Figs. 7.4a,b. This patient had clinical evidence of cervical myelopathy with a spastic gait and weak upper extremities. Note the positioning of the interbody graft which is already incorporating. Note also that the large osteophyte has been excised completely from the front of the cervical vertebral column

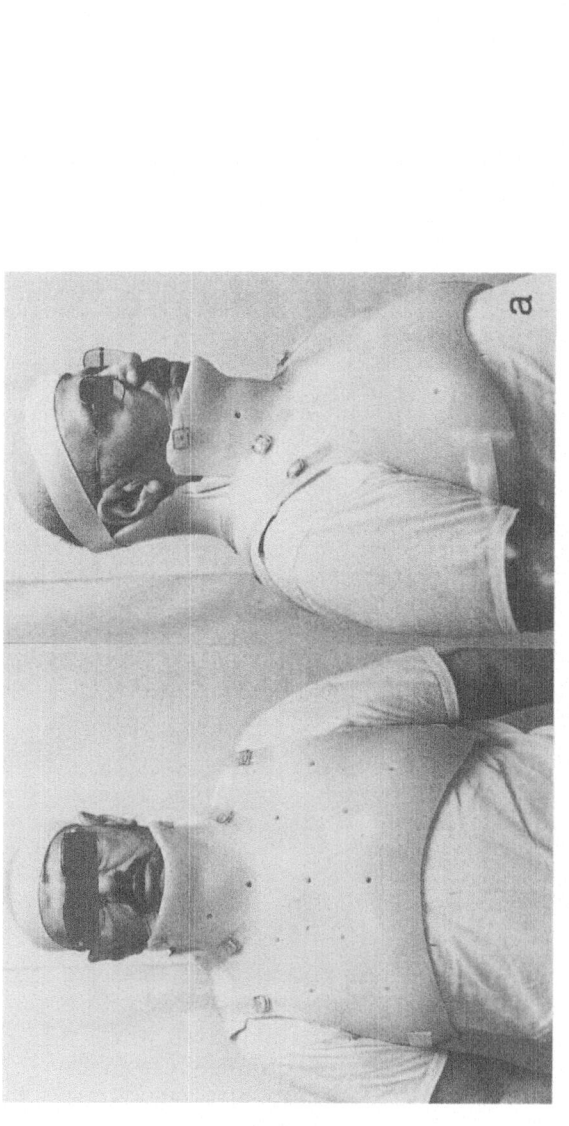

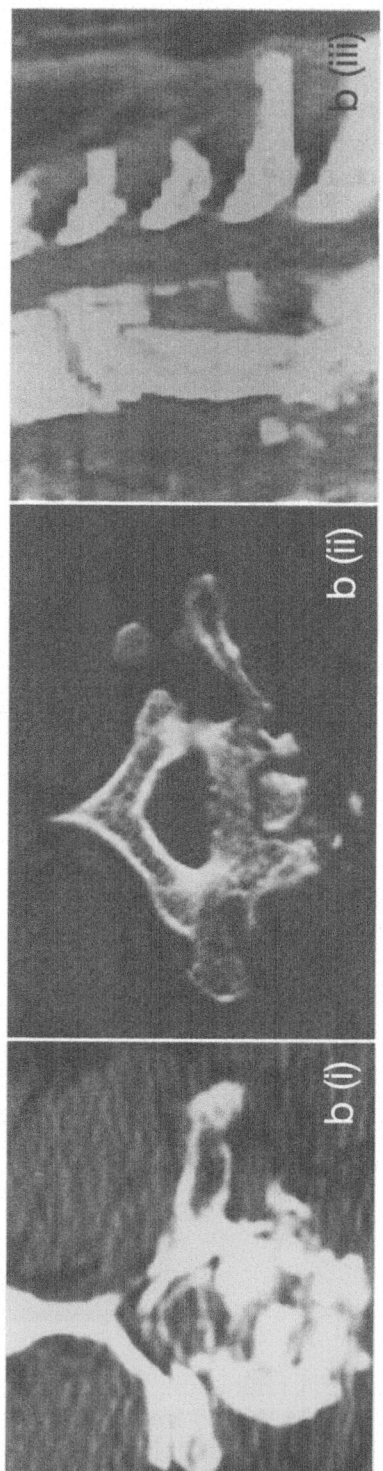

Figures 7.30 a, b. a Photographs of a 62 year old man showing the type of custom-made plastic thoraco-cervico-cranial corset suitable for use after decompression and anterior cervical interbody fusions at multiple levels. **b** (i) An axial CT radiculogram of this man's spine following inadequate surgery, with *bone cement* supplementing grafted bone. He presented with quadriparesis. (ii) Centre – a post-operative axial CT scan showing the upper end of the autogenous cortico-cancellous graft cut from his iliac crest – six weeks after revision surgery. (iii) A mid-sagittal reconstruction showing the strut graft in situ, with adequate decompression of the anterior wall of the cervical spinal canal. Reviewed one year after this operation, his quadriparesis had recovered fully

The vertebral osteophytes which project into the cervical canal are often surprisingly hard and thick. They can be drilled to egg-shell thinness before being removed from the dural surface with fine angled curettes. Occasionally ossified remnants of the posterior longitudinal ligament are adherent to the dura. They should not be removed for fear of producing dural injury and CSF leakage, problems not easily dealt with in this location. Recovery of neurological function in many of these cases is often gratifying though, in severely disabled patients, degrees of recovery vary and may be delayed for upwards of two years after operation.

Internal fixation is rarely indicated when strut grafts are used. However, special corsets or braces should be fitted (Figs. 7.30–32).

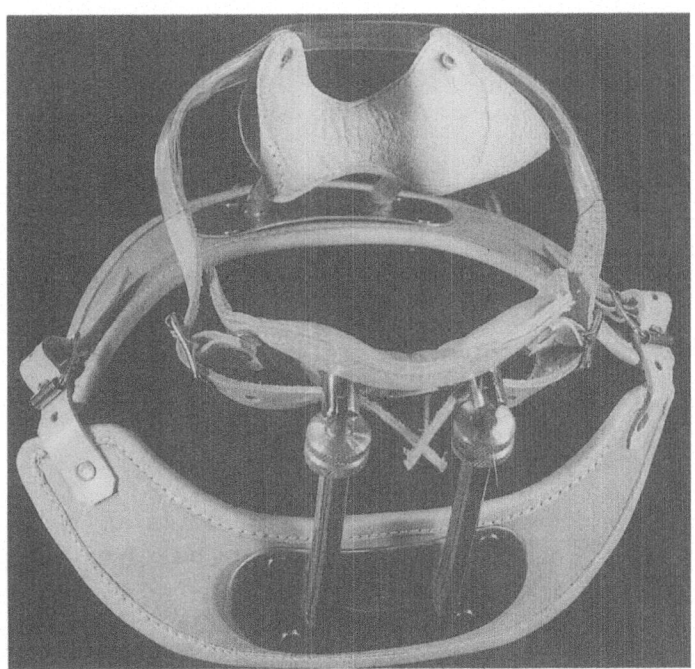

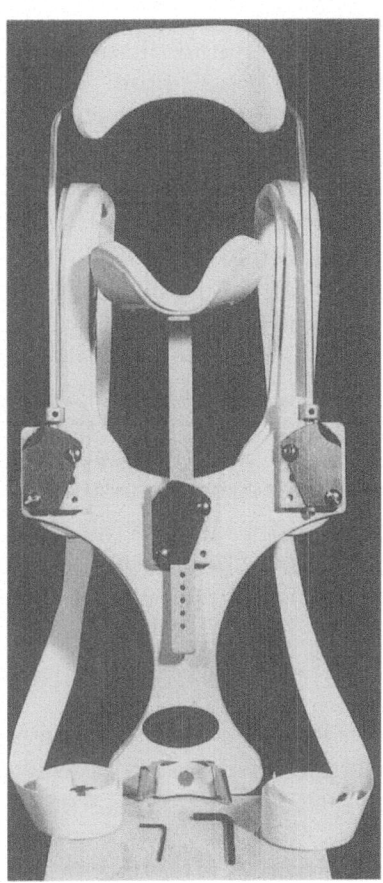

Figure 7.31   **Figure 7.32**

Figure 7.31. A photograph of an adjustable cervical collar of the Zimmer type, which can provide effective immobilization following multi-level cervical fusions and which may be used later in C1/2 fusions following removal of halo jackets or Minerva jackets

Figure 7.32. A photograph of a SOMI brace which provides an adjustable occipital support and an adjustable mental support fitted to a sternal plate. It is suspended over the shoulder and fixed firmly to the trunk with adjustable straps. On cine-radiography this has been shown to be one of the most effective devices for immobilizing the cervical spine. However, there are problems with its management as it tends to ride up when the patient lies in bed.

g) Graft Preparation

i) Autogenous Grafts

Autogenous grafts should be cut from the anterior third of the iliac crest. If only a single graft is required, this may be cut through a small vertical skin incision placed 2 or 3 cm behind the anterior superior iliac spine, splitting the fibres of tensor fascia lata in the line of the skin cut. The cutting cylinder must be one size larger than that used to prepare the dowel cavity in the neck.

Alternatively, using a short incision along the line of the inner margin of the anterior third of the iliac crest, a limited sub-periosteal exposure of the inner table of the iliac crest can be made, the cutter then being inserted to cut a bone plug extending from the inner to outer table of the ilium.

When more than one graft is required, the skin incision should run parallel to the iliac crest about 1 cm below it. The fascia lata is cut 1 cm below its upper attachment to the iliac crest and the muscles of the outer table of the ilium stripped down sufficiently to allow easy access for removal of the desired number of grafts. During wound closure, a suction drain tube should be inserted. The sutures should be placed deeply into the muscle mass from within-out, allowing the fibres of the tensor fascia lata muscle to be pulled up towards its former site of attachment on the outer wall of the iliac crest. If the sutures approximate only the fascial coverings near the margins of the incision, a noticeably ugly defect results in the zone of attachment of the tensor fascia lata below the iliac crest.

For rare indications, long strut grafts may be required to bridge multiple vertebral levels, where, for example, a cervical kyphotic deformity is being corrected (Fig. 7.11), or after excision of vertebral bodies for tumour or infection. Fibular grafts have been advocated for use in such circumstances. In my view, it is preferable to use long grafts cut from the ilium, to include both cortical surfaces, with cancellous bone between. These grafts will vascularize more rapidly than fibular grafts, the latter being useful only in exceptional circumstances.

ii) Bone Graft Substitutes

Ceramic dowels constructed of a "cancellous core" (pore size in excess of 100 u) capped on either end by dense "cortical" ceramic plates, have been used successfully in man[1] (Figs. 7.33, 7.34).

Titanium mesh implants have given rise to serious problems due to collapse, extrusion and fragmentation in some cases. They cannot therefore be confidently recommended for use in vertebral interbody fusion operations either in the neck or other areas of the spine (Figs. 7.35, 7.36).

Figure 7.33. A detailed lateral radiograph showing a "cortico-cancellous" ceramic dowel 6 months after insertion.

Figure 7.34. An axial CT image showing a "cortico-cancellous" ceramic dowel covered anteriorly by a thin operculum of bone, well incorporated in the vertebral body

---

[1] Manufactured by Kyocera Corporation, Kyoto, Japan.

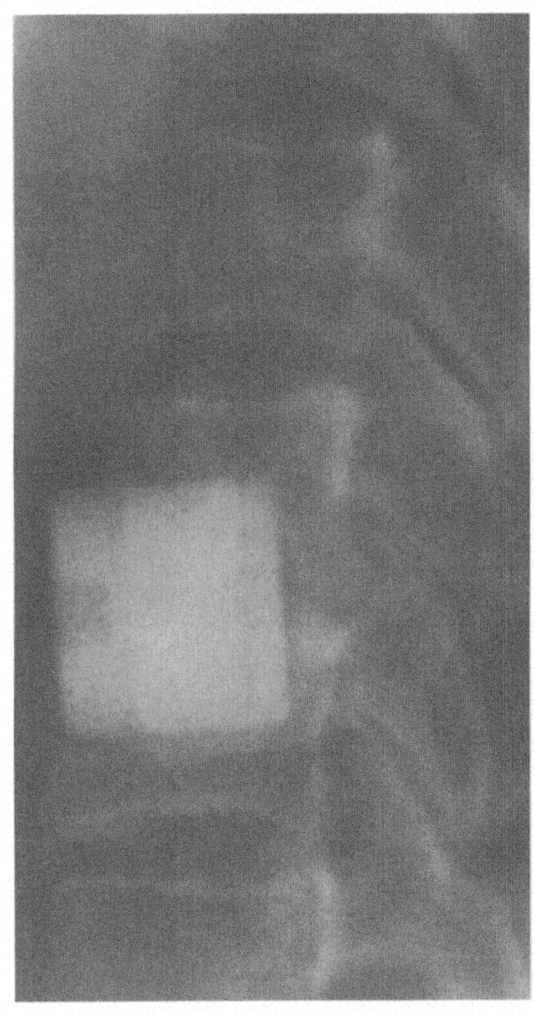

Figure 7.33

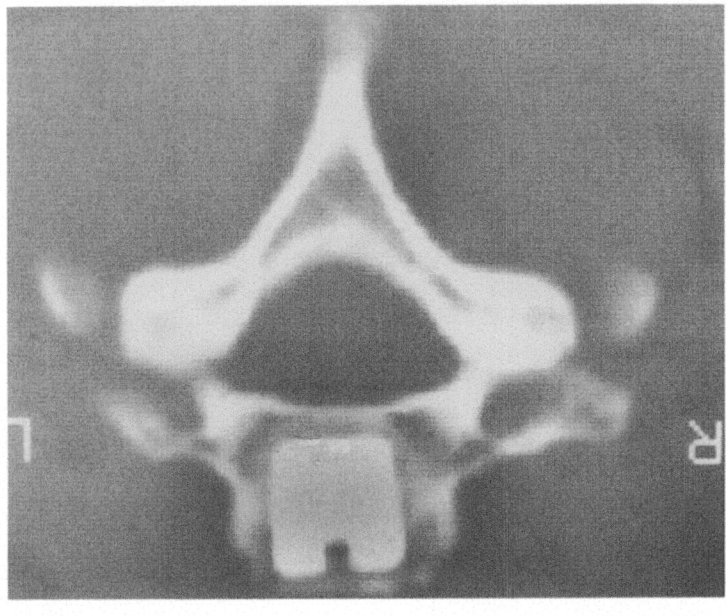

Figure 7.34

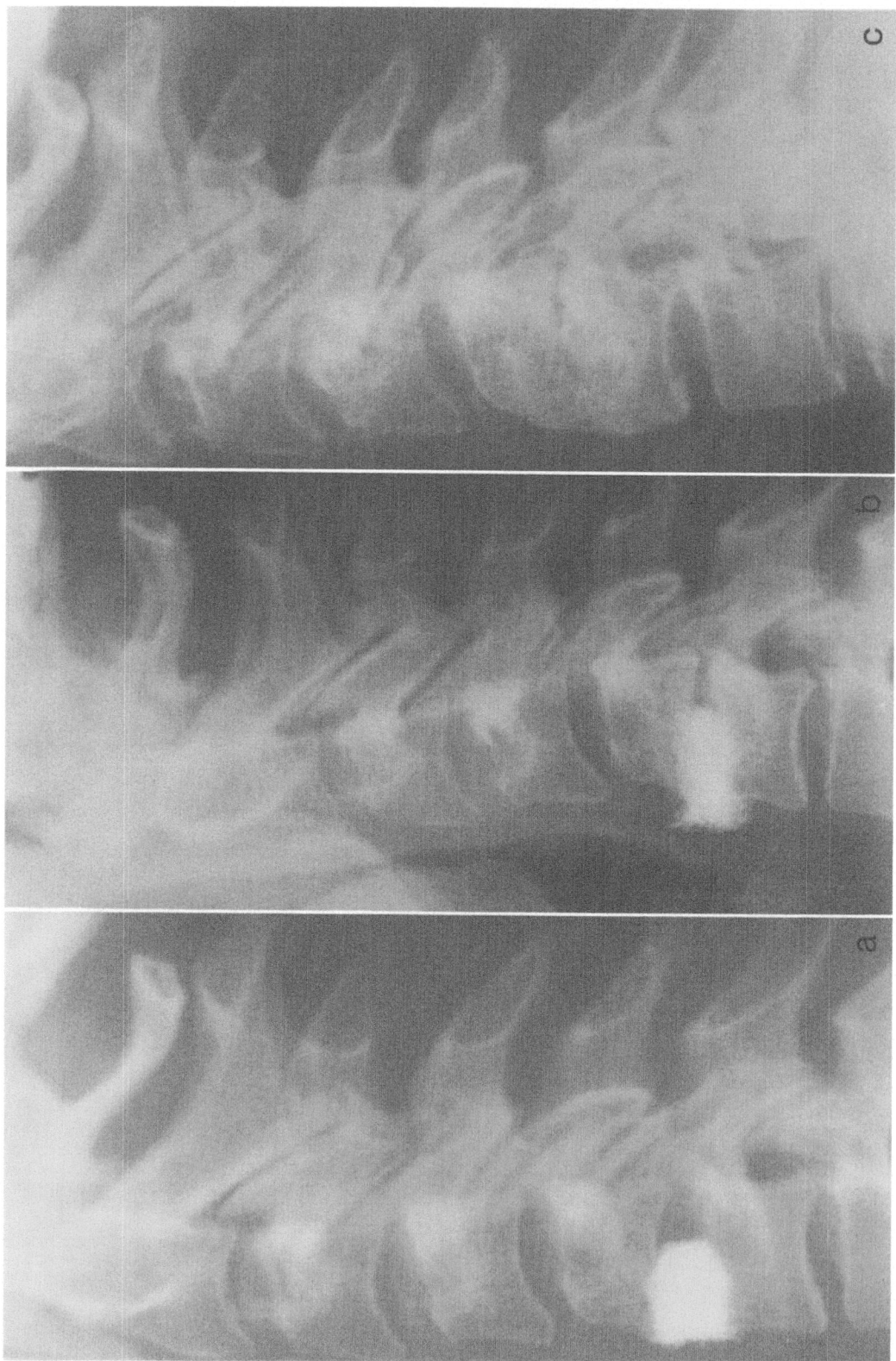

Figures 7.35a–c

h) Graft Impaction

The final critical manoeuvres required to seat the graft in the dowel cavity are illustrated in Figs. 7.37 a–d. Before insertion of the graft, the surgeon must always measure the depth of the dowel cavity and the depth of the graft. Great force is never required during their impaction. Soft tissues should be carefully retracted from the margins of the cavity and the neck should be gently elongated by traction applied to the skull before the graft is inserted.

i) Wound Closure

After the grafts have been inserted, a careful inspection should be made of the anterior aspect of the vertebrae; any bleeding points should be coagulated, especially along the medial margins of the longus colli muscles.

The neck wound may be closed, without drainage, except after multi-level fusions or in rare circumstances after associated thyroid surgery.

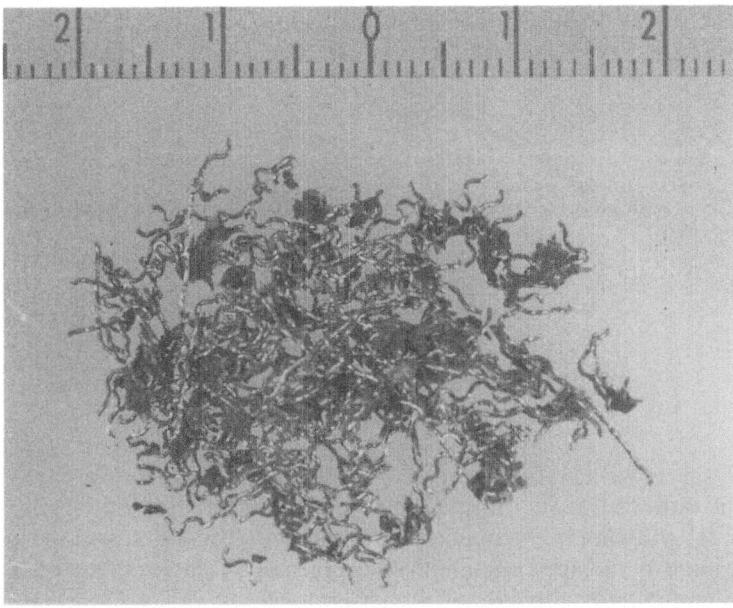

Figure 7.36. A photograph of the fragmented titanium mesh graft removed from the cervical spine of the patient whose X-rays are shown in Figs. 35 a–c. Soft tissues stained an intense black colour were mingled with the titanium strands

Figures 7.35 a–c. a A lateral X-ray of the cervical spine of a female patient aged 42 years showing a titanium mesh implant approximately 3 months after insertion. **b** Six months after insertion, the implant has collapsed and partially extruded anteriorly. The patient's symptoms of neck pain and brachial neuralgia had recurred. **c** A lateral X-ray of the same patient's cervical spine following removal of the titanium mesh implant, showing successful interbody fusion with an autogenous bone graft

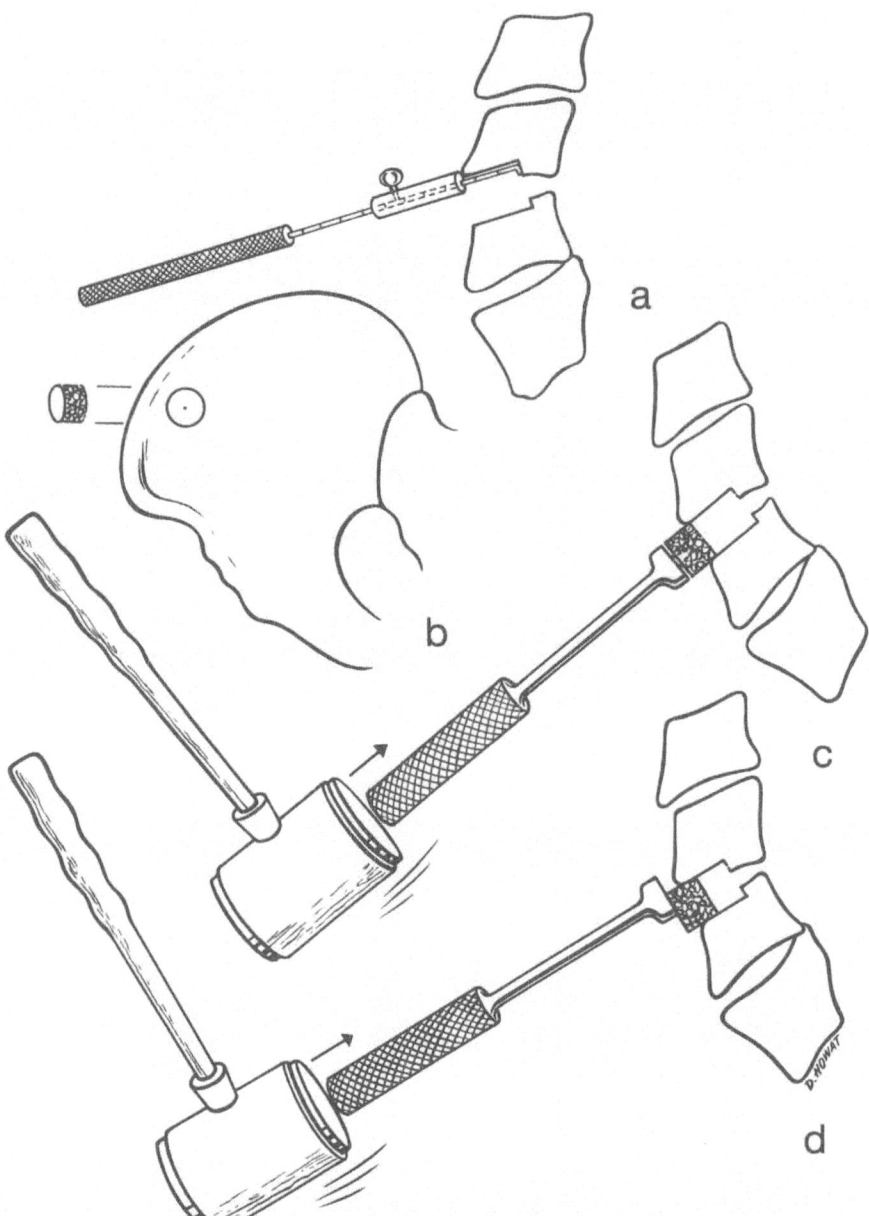

Figures 7.37 a–d. a A drawing of the cervical spine, viewed from the side, showing a prepared dowel cavity between two vertebral bodies with a depth gauge inserted to measure the depth of the cavity before the graft is inserted. **b** A drawing of the pelvic crest to show the site of removal of a plug of bone which is cut from the inner to the outer table. The measurement of this graft between the two cortical surfaces varies, depending on the size of the patient's pelvis. Grafts should be trimmed so that the anterior and posterior margins are parallel. The depth of the anterior iliac crest between the inner and outer cortical tables varies between 5 and 15 mm. In patients in whom the pelvis is thin (3–5 mm between outer and inner cortices), it may be necessary to cut grafts vertically downwards from the top of the crest, by the method used in lumbar interbody fusions. **c** A drawing to show the initial stages of impaction of the graft, the measurement of which has been checked carefully with the measurement of the prepared dowel cavity. At this stage the anaesthetist is asked to elongate the neck by applying traction under the angles of the mandible. **d** Final seating of the graft is sometimes necessary if the anterior margin is not flush with the anterior vertebral margins after use of the initial impactor which has a central nipple on it, as illustrated in (**c**) above. The manoeuvre shown is performed with a plain-ended impactor and it *is important to note the impactor is placed half-way across the graft and half-way across the adjacent vertebral body so that when a blow is struck with the hammer it is impossible to drive the graft too deeply* into the dowel cavity, the impactor coming to rest on the anterior vertebral margin. Accurate seating of the graft is essential if the complications of graft rotation or post-operative prolapse are to be avoided

j) Post-Operative Management

Patients complain of little pain after this operation, in contrast to those who have had cervical laminectomies.

Nursed with the head raised on two or three pillows, they should have collars fitted in the operating room (Fig. 7.38, 7.39). Patients are more comfortable when they wear an appropriate neck support after cervical fusion.

Dysphagia is common in the first few days after surgery; restriction of the intake of solid foods is advisable, but special measures in management are rarely required. During an anterior cervical interbody fusion at the C2/3 level, in one case, a small pharyngeal laceration occurred. This was sutured. Nothing was given to the patient by mouth for three days, intravenous fluid replacement being administered during that time, with prophylactic chemotherapy and no ill-effects resulted.

Within twenty-four hours of operation, patients should be encouraged to get out of bed and to walk short distances. Their stay in hospital averages 5 days.

Travel by car should be avoided for six weeks and then allowed only in vehicles fitted with head rests. Until the graft or grafts have incorporated with the vertebrae, a collar should be worn at all times when travelling.

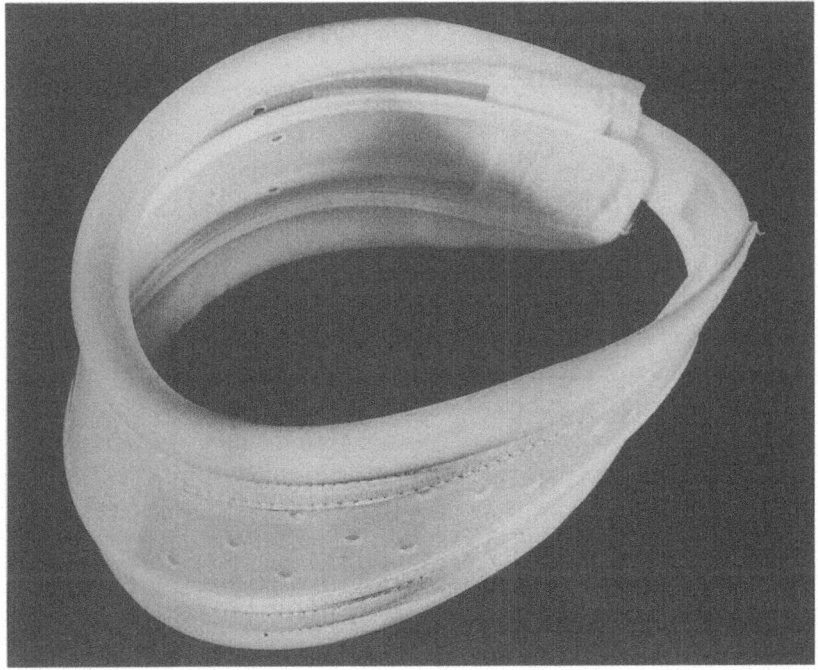

Figure 7.38. A photograph of a light plastic collar of adjustable height suitable for use in the post-operative period after single level anterior fusion operations. This type of collar is also suitable for use in the conservative management of patients with neck pain after neck injuries, or for the treatment of recurring symptoms of neck pain and occipital headache due to cervical spondylosis

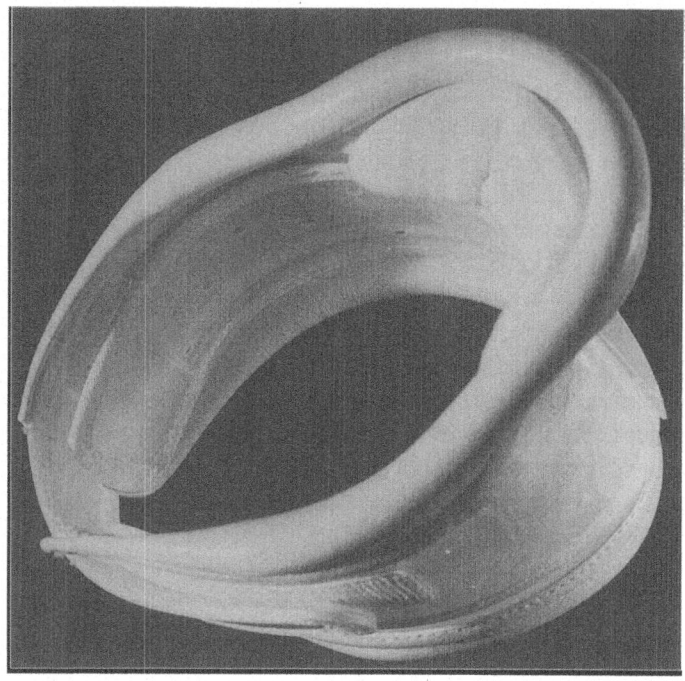

Figure 7.39. A photograph of an adjustable plastic cervical collar with supporting chin piece suitable for use after multi-level cervical fusions

7.5. *Radiological Changes After Interbody Fusion*

Autogenous grafts, even when they fill less than 50% of the dowel cavity into which they have been impacted, will fuse imperceptibly with the adjacent vertebral bodies and within a few years the whole of the vertebral interspace will ossify and consolidate. The capacity for remoulding of protruding graft margins and for *resorption of immature osteophytes* surrounding the vertebral margins is remarkable once interbody fusion has occurred. Lateral tomography is still the best method of assessing union of cervical interbody grafts (Figs. 7.40–42)

MRI now provides the most reliable information on changes in the dural sac and its contents in cases of cervical spinal canal stenosis with myelopathy, both before and after operation (Figs. 43a,b), while CT images, using "bone windows" with axial slices and sagittal reconstructions are best for measuring the dimensions of the canal.

Union with this method can be expected in about 96% of cases. Mal-union with kyphosis may occur, if the shape of the grafts at the time of operation was unsatisfactory because of the size and contour of the pelvis at the donor site. In such cases, X-rays should be taken at intervals of one, two and four weeks post-operatively. If the grafts rotate during that time, with resultant kyphotic deformity of the neck, the patient should be re-admitted to hospital and nursed with the head in traction and the neck in extension for several weeks. An orthosis of the type illustrated in (Fig. 7.30 a) should be fitted thereafter, with the neck held in the corrected position, checked by lateral X-rays taken with the collar applied. Alternatively a Minerva jacket can be made more cheaply (Fig. 7.44).

In general, collars should be worn for two or three months, until union of the grafts has occurred. Instruction in the use of gentle mobilizing neck exercises should be given at that time. Should restriction of neck movements persist beyond six months after fusion, the neck may be gently manipulated with gentle longitudinal traction and rotatory motions to right and left, under a short-acting general anaesthetic.

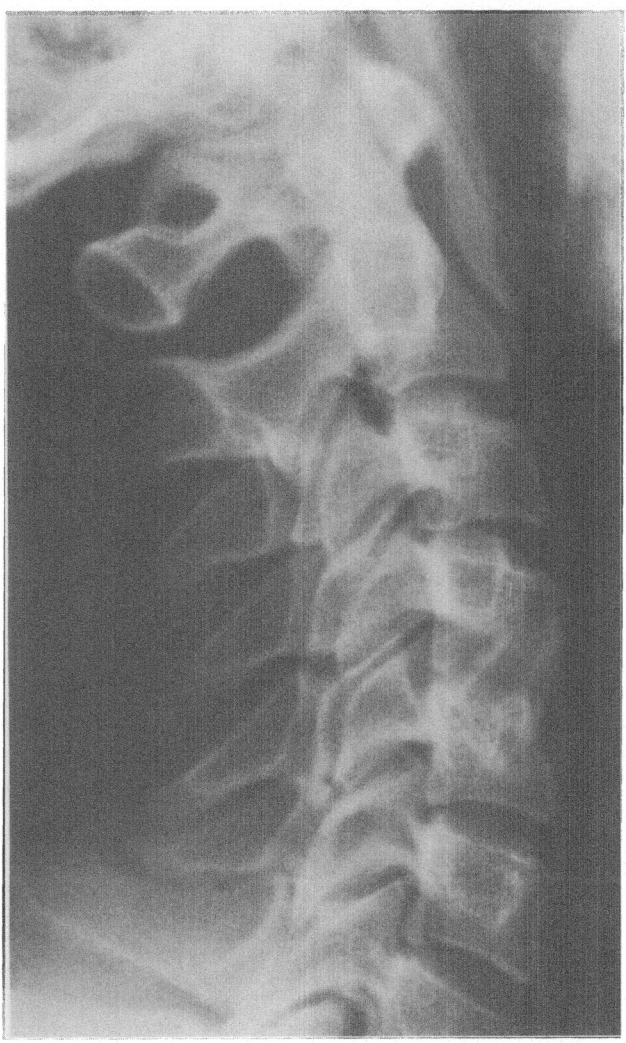

Figure 7.40. A lateral radiograph of the cervical spine of a man aged 24 years taken five months after an anterior cervical fusion performed at the C4/5 level for post-traumatic internal disc disruption. The fusion is solid and union has occurred without spinal deformity

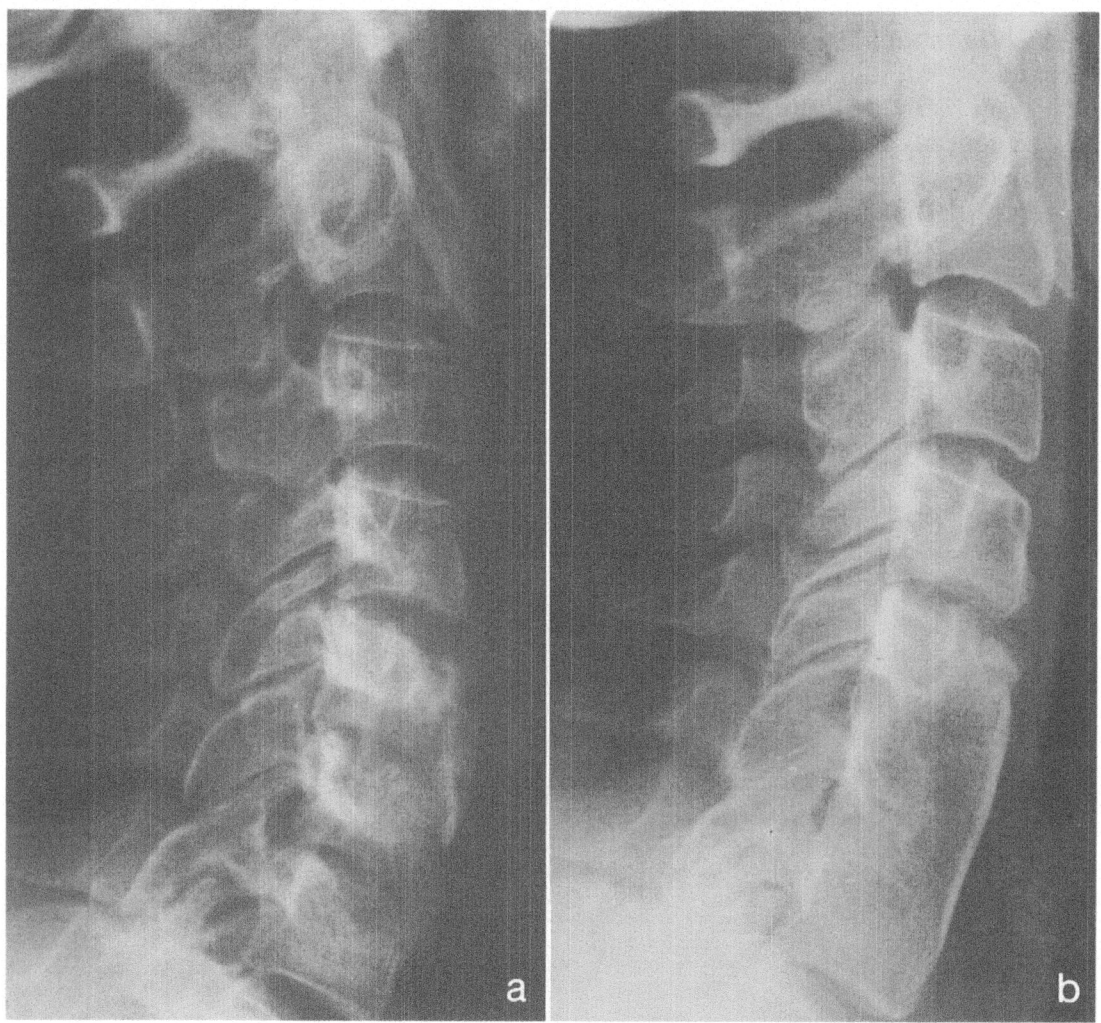

Figures 7.41 a, b. a A lateral radiograph of the cervical spine of a man aged 34 showing the appearance at three months following anterior interbody fusions at C5/6 and C6/7. Early incorporation of the grafts in satisfactory position is evident. The indication for the operation in this case was to control intractable neck pain and headache with some referred shoulder pain following post-traumatic internal disc disruption demonstrated by discography. **b** A radiograph of the same spine taken five years later showing complete remodelling of the fused segments between the vertebral bodies at C5/6 and C6/7

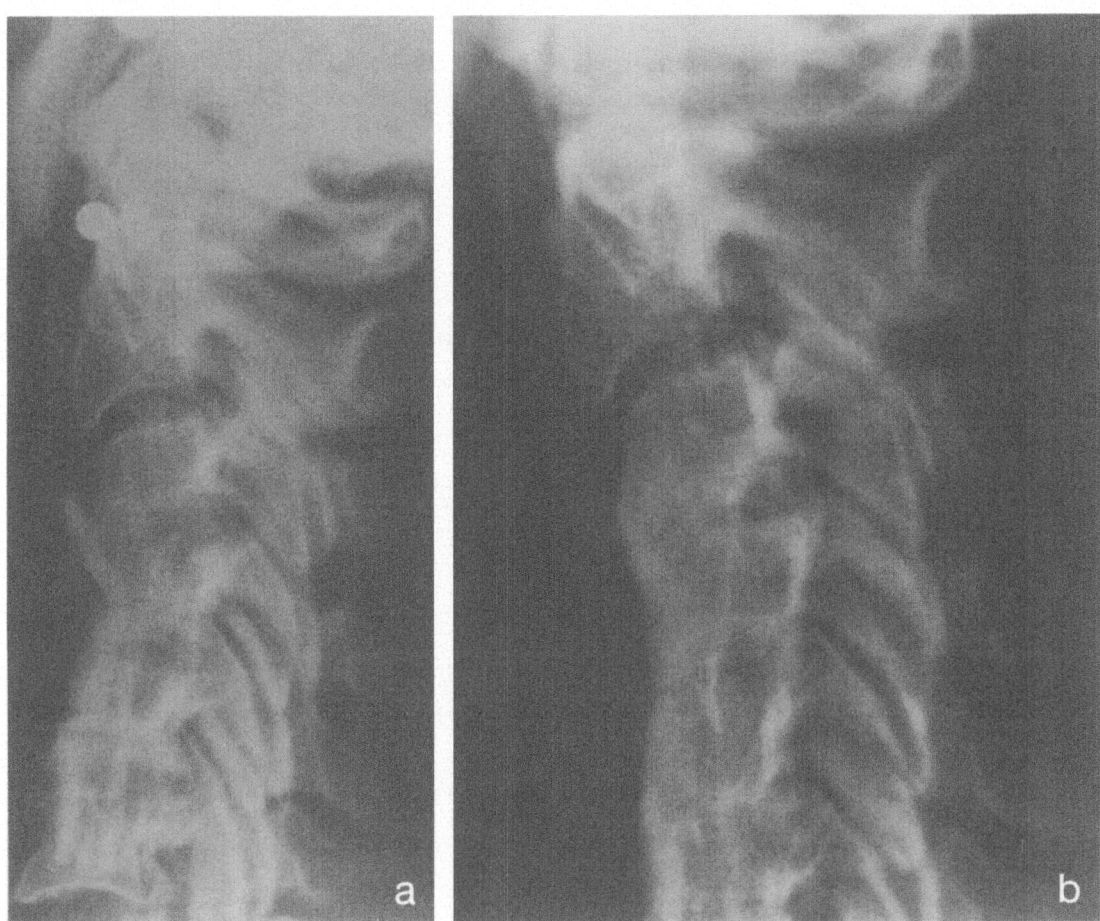

Figures 7.42 a, b. **a** A lateral radiograph of the cervical spine of a female aged 46 years taken 3 months after operation showing interbody grafts at C3/4, C4/5 and C5/6. This patient presented with symptoms and signs of cervical myelopathy. The lower two grafts have united in good position with the vertebral bodies. The graft at C3/4 has tilted and its upper anterior cortical edge is prominent in the retropharyngeal space. **b** A lateral radiograph of the same person's cervical spine 18 months after operation. Note the remoulding of the graft at C3/4

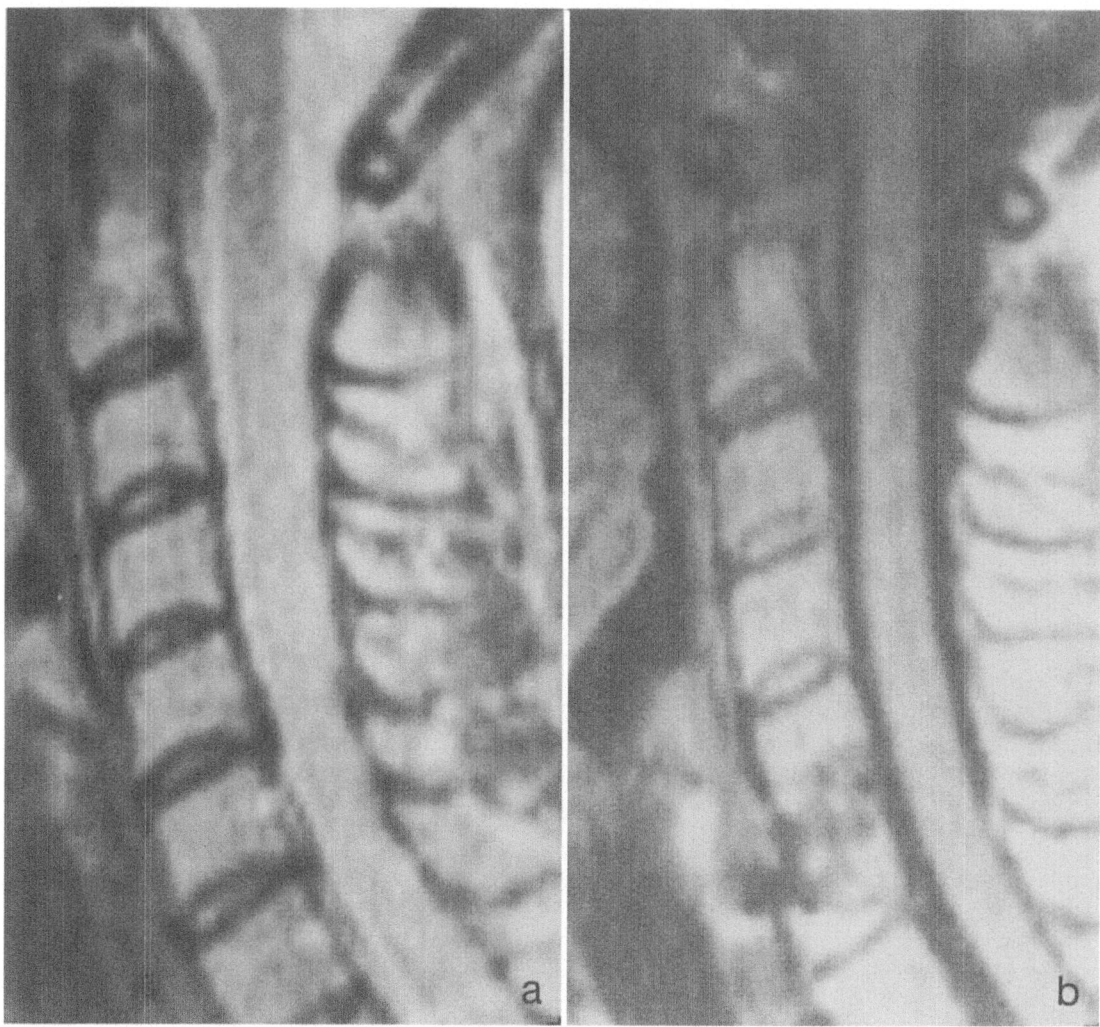

Figures 7.43 a,b. a A sagittal T2 weighted sequence MRI of a female aged 42 years presenting with signs of cervical myelopathy, with lower limb spasticity, showing constriction of the cervical canal at C5/6. **b** An MRI of the same patient one year after anterior cervical canal decompression, using a diamond tipped high speed drill. Sound interbody fusion has occurred and the normal dimensions of the spinal canal have been restored at the C5/6 level

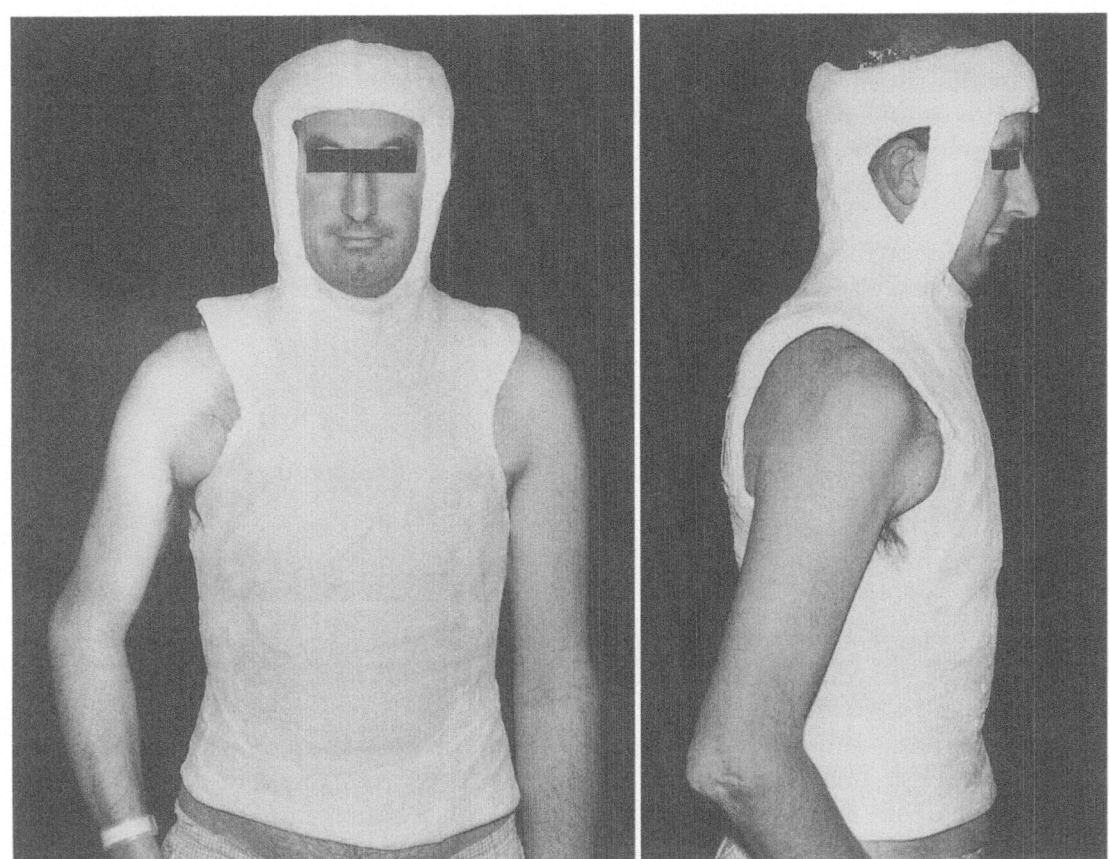

Figure 7.44. A photograph showing a patient viewed from in front and from the side, fitted with a Minerva jacket for immobilization of the upper cervical spine following occipito-cervical fusion. Although variations of halojackets are available, this useful method of spinal immobilization is illustrated for the benefit of surgeons who do not have access to more expensive commercially available braces such as the halo with thoracic jacket and pillar supports. Before the Minerva jacket is fitted, the patient should be placed on a tilting bed so that he is used to standing in a vertical position, and then the jacket can be put on when he is able to stand without dizziness for periods in excess of 30 minutes

7.6. Complications

The list of potential complications following anterior cervical interbody fusion operations includes:

1. Quadriplegia.
2. Unilateral blindness produced by the pressure of an assistant's hand resting on the globe.
3. Vascular catastrophe involving the vertebral or carotid arteries.
4. Severe venous haemorrhage following damage to the jugular vein.
5. Oesophageal laceration.
6. Horner's syndrome.

Reviewing my own experience with the use of this operation during the past thirty years, I have had to deal with a range of minor problems and with only a few serious complications.

a) Minor

These have included dysphagia and transient Horner's syndrome.

b) Major

In one case, a large haematoma in the neck required re-exploration for evacuation of the blood clot and coagulation of a small bleeding vessel in the margin of the longus colli muscle on one side.

In one case, the lady was very thin, and troublesome venous haemorrhage occurred when a small un-named vein was avulsed from the wall of the internal jugular vein. This was controlled with the use of a 6/0 atraumatic vascular stitch inserted into the medial wall of the internal jugular vein at the site of avulsion of the venule. This incident is mentioned because there is an important lesson to be learned from it. Anterior approaches to the cervical spine can be very difficult and time-consuming in heavily built patients with short thick necks. In very thin patients, however, it is often possible to complete an anterior cervical interbody fusion at a single disc level within one hour. *The case just cited shows that caution and vigilance must be exercised at all times.* A surgeon can never afford to approach this particular operation lightly, as problems may arise unexpectedly in any patient.

In one case, already referred to in the text above, a small pharyngeal laceration occurred.

Graft rotation with resultant acute cervical kyphosis has required surgical treatment in only four cases. However, unrecognized mal-union, with minor degrees of cervical kyphosis has been identified on X-rays taken three or four months after operation in a small number of cases.

Infection of neck wounds, with vertebral osteomyelitis occurred in six patients. One patient was diabetic, two others were heavy smokers with bronchitis, in the fourth, infection arose apparently spontaneously early after operation, while the fifth and sixth followed trans-oral C2–3 fusions.

These cases all resulted from infections with staphylococcus aureus organisms. All required drainage of pre-vertebral abscesses. Use of chemotherapeutic agents was determined on the results of sensitivity tests following culture of the organisms. Chemotherapy was used for at least three months, and in two of these patients its use was continued for one year after operation. Recurrent septicaemic episodes occurred in both when the use of Cloxacillin was discontinued after three months. Each of these patients recovered without disability – see Chapter 10.

Finally, I have had experience with the management of one referred case of quadriparesis resulting from neglect in treatment of a chronic wound infection in the neck. This patient presented with a small discharging sinus in the line of the neck incision which had been made at the time of anterior cervical fusion four months earlier. He was unable to stand or walk and had also severe paresis of both upper limbs. Lateral X-rays revealed a large pre-vertebral abscess, with a severe kyphotic deformity at the site of bone grafting.

The abscess was drained under general anaesthesia. Long-term chemotherapy was administered. The patient was nursed with skull traction with his neck extended over a rolled towel. See Chapter 8, p. 278 for further details. The quadriparesis recovered and spontaneous interbody fusion followed, with correction of the kyphotic deformity. Supplementary bone grafting was not required.

7.7. Results of Operation

Technically, excellent results can be achieved using this technique for anterior cervical interbody fusion. Non-union of grafts may occur in about 4% of patients.

Return to work is usual between four to six months following operation. I believe that it is unwise to persuade patients to return to work within one or two weeks of this operation – a claim made by some of its proponents – but foreign to my experience.

Neck motion is slightly restricted after multi-level fusion (Figs. 7.45 a, b), though normally full after single level grafting.

7.8. Posterior Cervical Spinal Fusion

The indications for these procedures have been set out above. Details of surgical technique will not be discussed as they involve simple manoeuvres which are in common use. However, radiographs showing the appearance of conditions requiring these procedures, with post-operative X-rays are found in Figs. 7.2 a, b, together with photographs of suitable braces and a Minerva jacket which may be used post-operatively (Figs. 7.30–32, 7.39, 7.40) if facilities are not available for obtaining expensive orthoses.

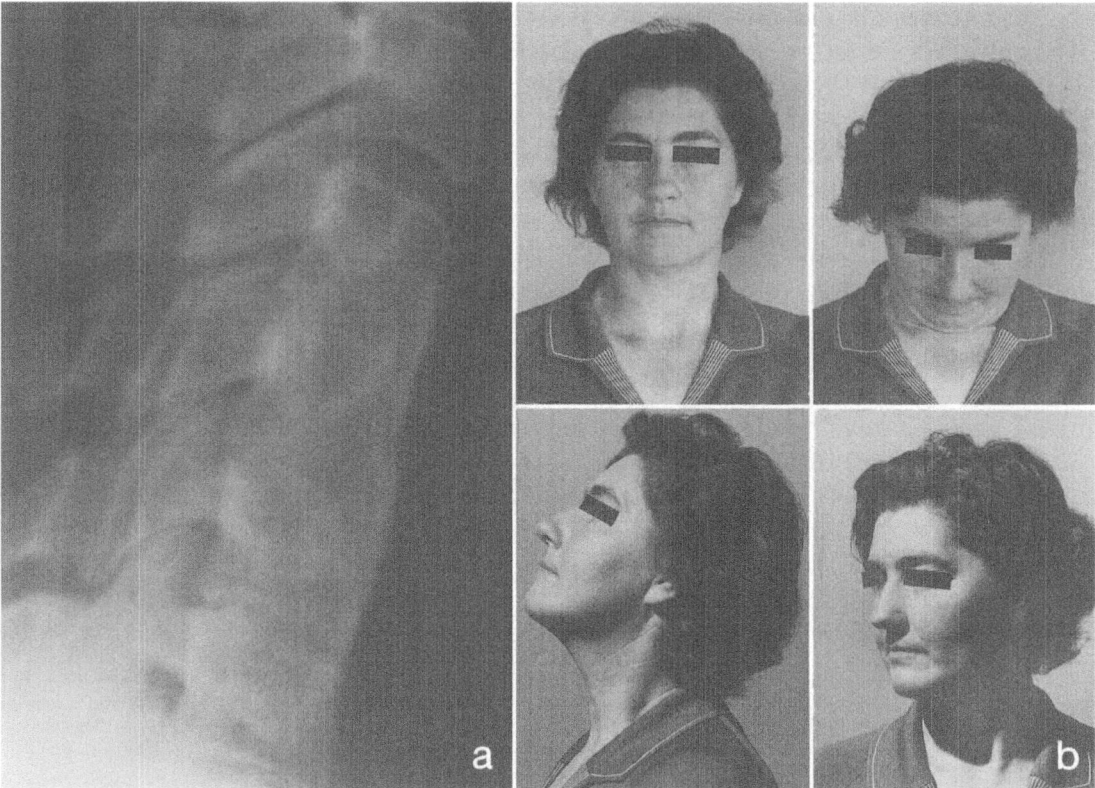

Figures 7.45 a,b. a A lateral radiograph of the cervical spine of a woman aged 46 showing a three-level anterior cervical fusion between the bodies of C4/5, C5/6 and C6/7 taken five years after operation for the relief of intractable neck pain and occipital headache with some referred arm pain, in the absence of neurological signs. This patient had post-traumatic multi-level disc disruption following a high speed rear-end collision which had inflicted a whiplash mechanism of injury on her cervical spine. **b** Four photographs of the patient whose X-ray showing multi-level cervical fusion is reproduced alongside, to demonstrate the ranges of motion of the neck after a fusion of this extent. Flexion and extension movements and the range of lateral rotation are all restricted. However, the functional result is regarded as satisfactory by the patient who has remained symptom-free for 15 years since this operation

Figure 7.46. A photograph to show the arrangements for posturing the patient on an operating table for posterior approaches to the cervical spine. When the patient is in the prone position for operations on the cervical spine, precautions must be taken to ensure that the anaesthetic tubes and airways are securely fastened, with all their linkage points strapped to prevent accidental separation during the surgery. When the patient is in this position, the skin of the neck is often lax. Strapping should be applied across the hairline transversely and fixed to the head support. Further strapping is then attached across the vertex of the skull running from the transverse strapping to the front of the headrest. In addition, long strips of strapping should be applied just lateral to the spinous process of C7 on both sides, running down the back to the buttocks. This will ensure that the skin of the neck is tightly stretched, making the incision and its subsequent closure much easier. Note also the inclination of the table. If the head is raised any further, then the potential risk of air embolism is increased

7.9. Cervical Laminectomy

a) Positioning (Fig. 7.46)

The prone position, using a neurosurgical headrest, provides satisfactory conditions for operation.

b) Exposure

The techniques used in this approach to the laminae are identical to those described for exposure of the lumbar spine, except that the scale and mobility of the bones is different, the cervical spine being small and very mobile. Smaller instruments are therefore required for use in this area.

The knowledge of applied anatomy assumes great importance because disastrous complications may occur as a result of uncontrolled haemorrhage, particularly in approaches to the occipito-cervical junction. Damage to the vertebral arteries may lead to catastrophic neurological complications following the resultant interference with cerebral circulation. In addition the sub-occipital veins are very large with

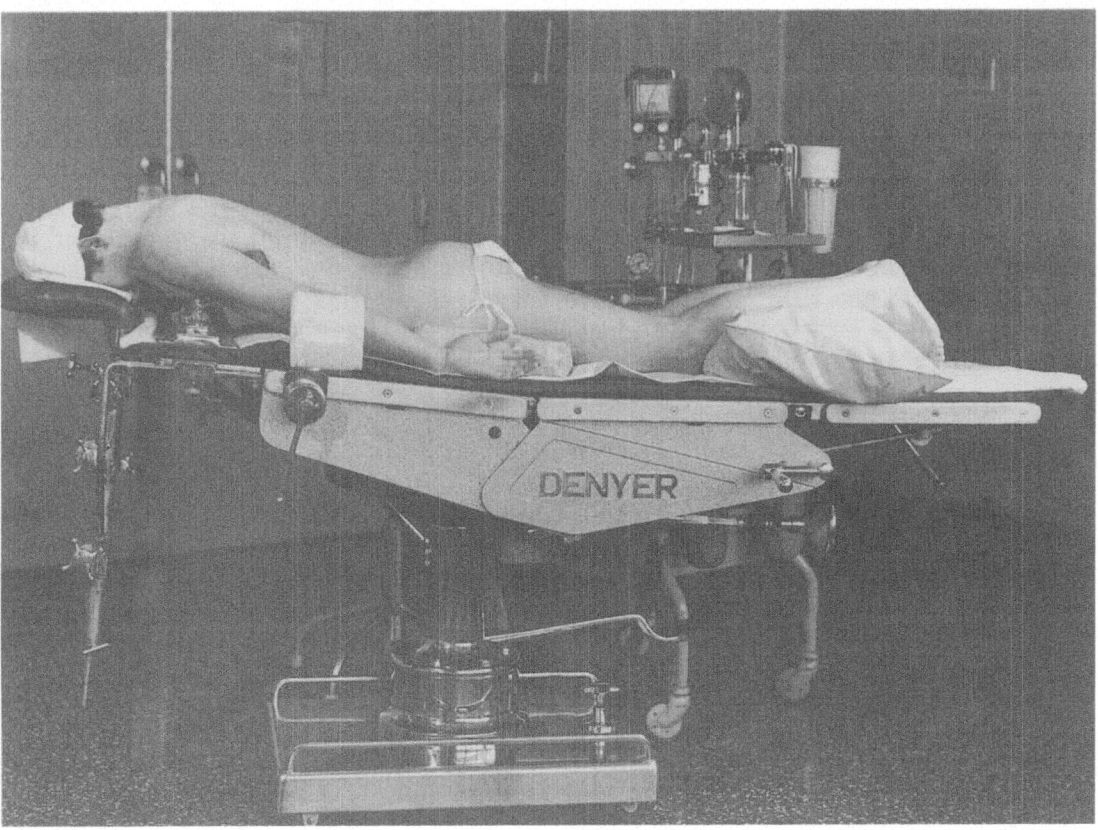

Figure 7.46

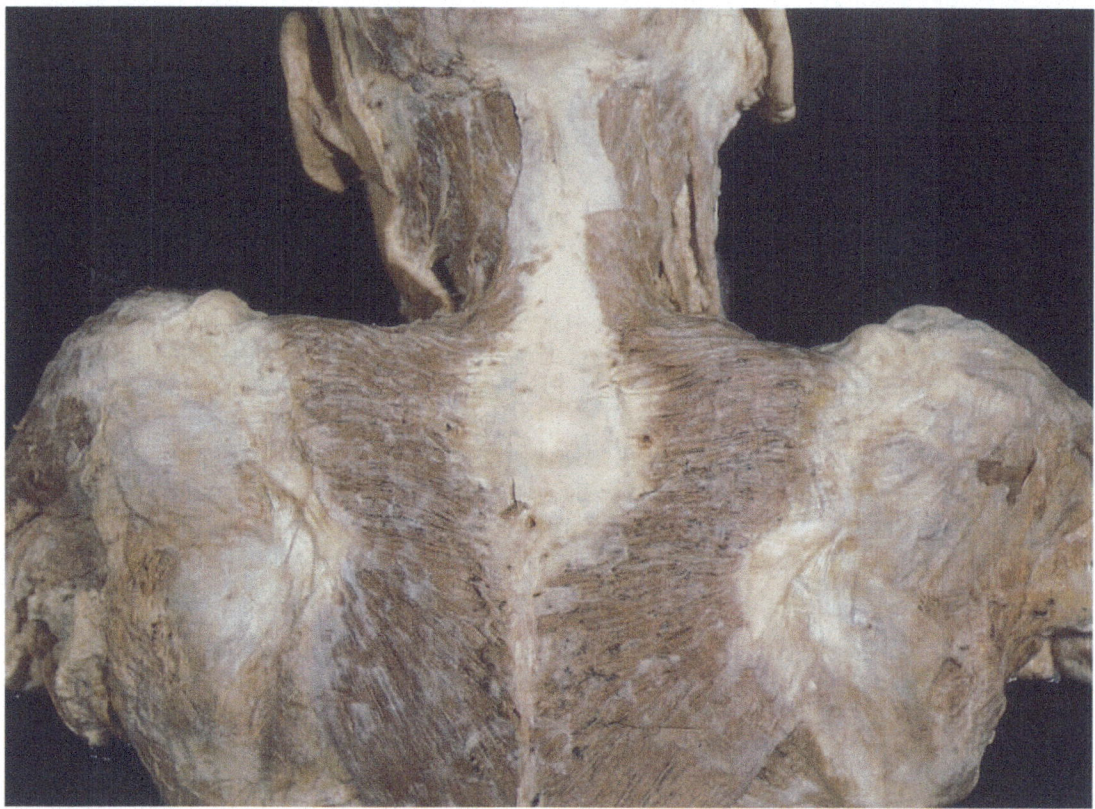

Figure 7.47. A photograph of a dissection of the posterior muscles of the neck and of the upper part of the trapezii. Note the central diamond shaped area of glistening white aponeurotic fibres from which the middle part of the trapezii arise on either side, the muscle fibres passing horizontally laterally. The investing layer of deep cervical fascia covers the trapezii and the splenius capitis muscles on both sides. On the left side of the specimen it has been largely removed while on the right side it has been left in situ covering the upper portion of the trapezius muscle to the level of its attachment to the skull. Note the large vascular channels which perforate the trapezius aponeurosis around its margins

delicate walls. If breached under certain conditions, air embolism becomes a potential hazard.

When internal fixation devices are to be used in the neck, a sound working knowledge of the applied anatomy of cervical osteology is essential. Developments in this area of instrumentation have led to the introduction of excellent devices for interlaminar fixation such as the Halifax interlaminar clamp (Figs. 7.47–50).

The use of sub-laminar wires should only be considered when the dimensions of the cervical spinal canal are within normal limits. When the C1/C2 vertebrae are fixed with trans-articular screws, the graft between the laminae is best held in place with sub-laminar braided nylon threads rather than with sub-laminar wires (Figs. 7.9 a,b).

Inter-segmental stabilization can also be obtained using plates and screws. In the anatomical position, the cervical facet joints from C2 distally lie in the coronal

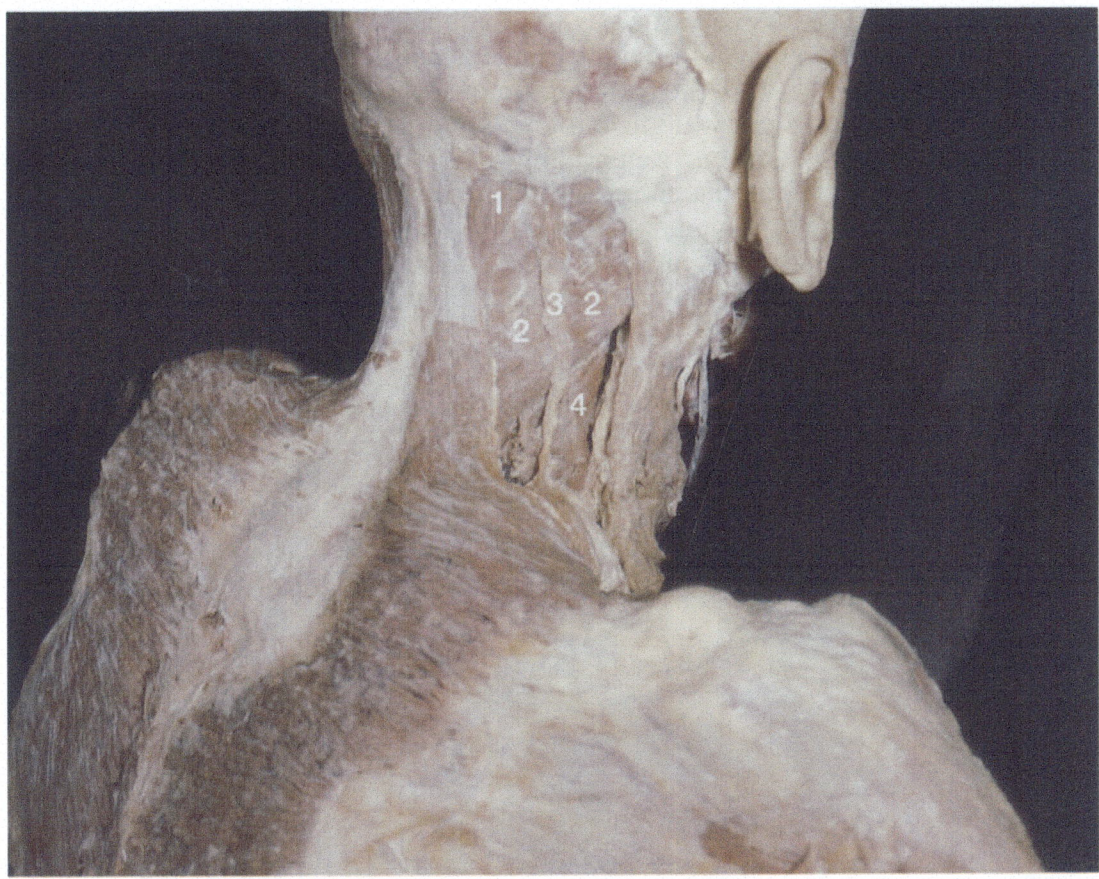

Figure 7.48. A photograph of the same specimen viewed from the right side. The encircling layer of deep cervical fascia has been removed along with a section of the trapezius muscle, to show the underlying muscles from left to right *1* the semispinalis capitis, *2* the splenius capitis, *3* the lateral edge of the trapezius and *4* the longissimus capitis

plane. Screws should be placed above and below the level of the facet joint in the sagittal plane and angled 10 degrees laterally (Fig. 7.7).

Having identified the lamina or laminae to be removed, the spinous processes should be excised. Then, using a Leksell-type rongeur, with thin cutting blades, the inferior surface of the superior lamina at the interspace can be removed piece-meal, while the thin ligamentum flavum is still intact. Having enlarged the inter-laminar space, the ligamentum flavum can be reflected and excised, after passing a small moistened patty beneath it, propelled gently laterally on the tip of the curved end of a Watson-Cheyne dissector. This done, on both sides of the canal, preparation is then made to perform foraminotomies. The soft tissues and veins are separated carefully from the remnants of the roof of the spinal canal, one side at a time. The pedicles can be identified using the curved tip of the Watson-Cheyne probe. Venous bleeding should not obstruct the surgeon's view, unless the manoeuvres just described have been carried out carelessly or too quickly.

Using a forward-angled 45 degree rongeur with a 1 or 2 mm cup, it is then possible to open the roof of the intervertebral foramen, protecting the dura and nerve root sleeve with a patty on the end of a fine sucker. When this has been done, the regional veins will distend remarkably if a stenosis in the region has been relieved. Some brisk venous haemorrhage may then occur. This is best controlled by the application of small fragments of gelfoam (or its equivalent) packed lightly in place with an overlying moist patty. The use of coagulating currents, through low voltage diathermy machines, is still widespread. However, I have not found it neces-

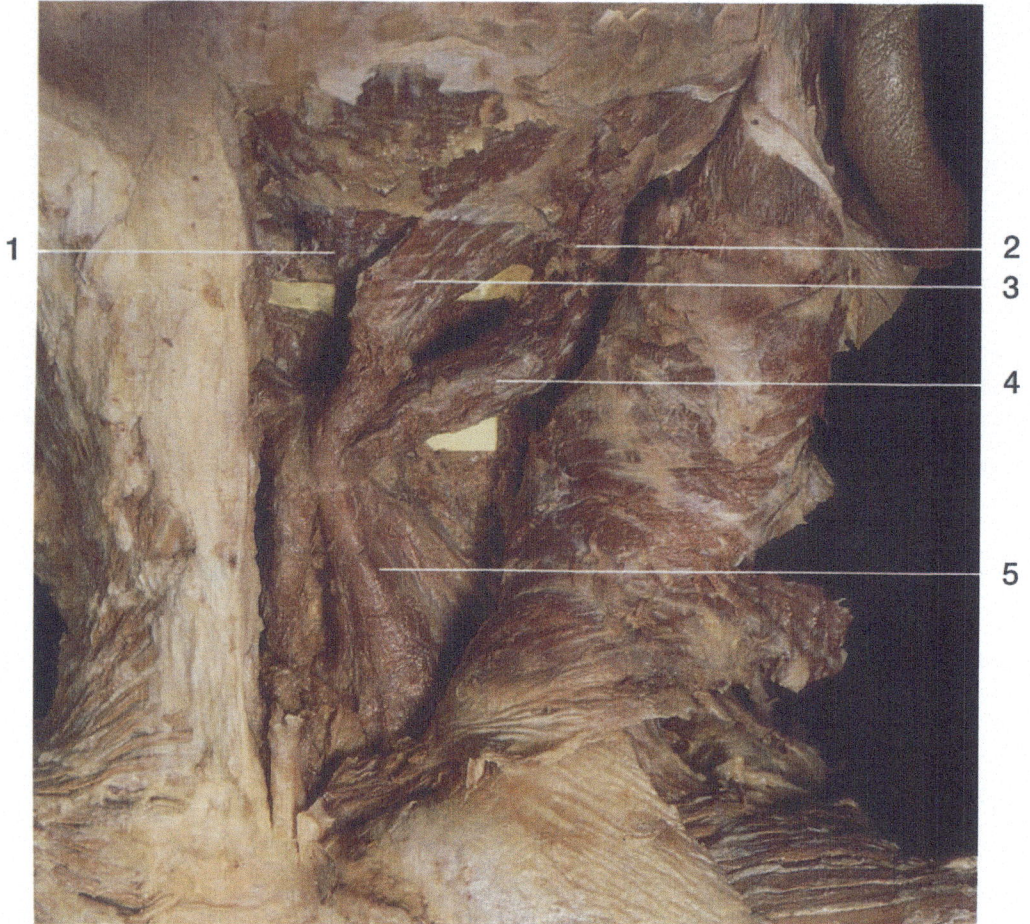

Figure 7.49. A photograph of the same specimen dissected to display the sub-occipital muscles. The upper yellow marker lies beneath the rectus capitis posterior major on the posterior arch of the atlas. The lower triangular shaped marker is placed on the lamina of C2. Lying between the margins of these individual muscles, large sub-occipital veins are found in life. The deep sub-occipital muscles are labelled below: *1* Rectus capitis posterior minor, *2* Obliquus capitis superior, *3* Rectus capitis posterior major, *4* Obliquus capitis inferior, *5* Multifidus cervicis. (Dissected by Doctors H. Nakamura and H. V. Crock and reproduced by kind permission of the President and Council of the Royal College of Surgeons of England. These dissections were prepared in the Anatomy Department with the permission of Professor S. Sinatamby)

sary to resort to this method of haemorrhage control, which I believe to be potentially dangerous if used at multiple levels in the cervical spine. There may be a significant risk of damaging the fine segmental arteries which join the anterior median longitudinal arterial channel of the cervical spinal cord if diathermy is used to excess in the region of the intervertebral foramina within the cervical canal (Crock and Yoshizawa, 1977).

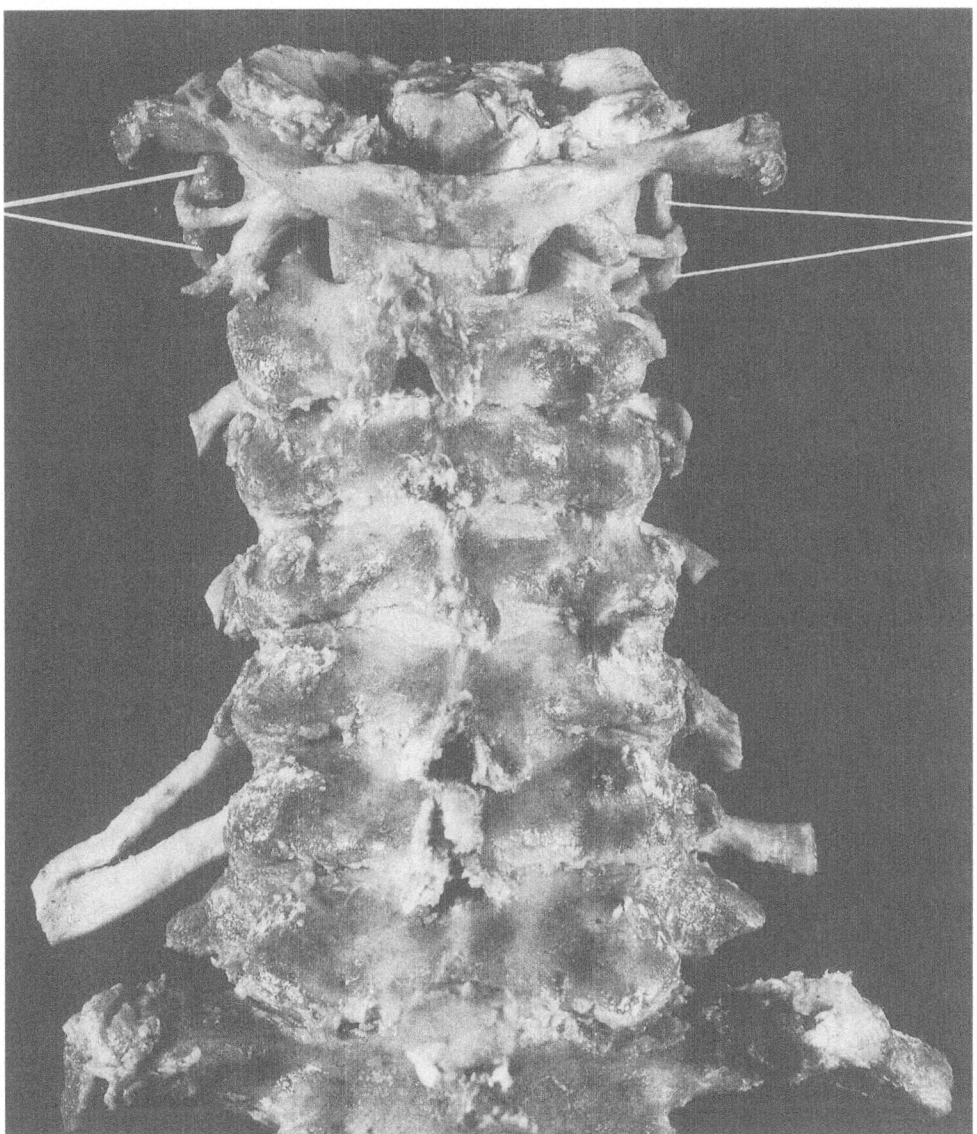

Figure 7.50. A photograph of a dissection of the cervical spine viewed from behind. All the soft tissues have been removed except the ligamenta flava, the dural sac and the emerging nerve roots. At the level of C1 and C2, note the relationships of the emerging nerve roots to the vertebral arteries on both sides (white arrows). The facet joints from C2 distally can be seen orientated in the coronal plain. In the cervical spine the interlaminar spaces are very narrow at all levels and only a few millimetres of ligamentum flavum can be seen in the normal state. (Dissected by Dr. M. C. Crock)

On completion of the "laminectomy" and foraminotomies, the partes inter-articulares of the laminae being preserved, along with the bulk of the facet joints, the wound should be closed with suction drainage. Before this is done, haemorrhage should be controlled, using haemostatic agents in the cervical canal as described, and diathermy in the muscle layer.

Facets should be preserved, except in cases of trauma, when facetectomy may be required to allow reduction of a fracture-dislocation. Localized inter-laminar posterior cervical fusion should be performed then, using either laminar clamps or screws inserted into the lateral masses.

In patients with multi-level cervical canal stenosis, due either to cervical spondylosis, or to ossification of the posterior longitudinal ligament (OPLL), various forms of laminoplasty have been in use in Japan for more than ten years. The method described by Hirabyashi *et al.* (1989) involves the use of a high speed drill to create parallel channels at the junctions of the laminae with the lateral masses, over the desired number of vertebral segments to be decompressed. The dissection enters the epidural space on one side, allowing the laminal segments to be elevated, thus enlarging the cervical spinal canal.

c) *Post-Operative Care*

Patients complain of severe pain after posterior cervical spinal operations. Adequate analgesia should therefore be ordered.

The use of soft collars for short periods can be recommended after de-compressions of the cervical canal.

8

Spinal Infections

8.1. Acute Vertebral Osteomyelitis

a) Introduction

In clinical practice, acute inflammatory lesions of the spine are relatively uncommon. For this reason alone, diagnosis of vertebral osteomyelitis is often delayed, so that patients may not receive specific treatment for the disease until they present with major complications.

The virtues of specialist hospitals are often hailed but cogent arguments favour the retention of specialist units in large general hospitals, where orthopaedic surgeons and neurosurgeons can be consulted readily about the surgical problems relevant to bone disease, not the least important of which are infective lesions of the spine.

Most referred cases of vertebral osteomyelitis will come from physicians. Vertebral infections follow repeated episodes of bacteraemia or septicaemia which may occur in many debilitating medical diseases such as pneumonia, chronic bronchitis and diabetes mellitus (Figs. 8.1a,b). One of the most elusive causes of pyrexia of unknown origin is sub-acute bacterial endocarditis. Acute vertebral osteomyelitis may complicate the course of this disease before the underlying pathology of the cardiac valvular disease is recognized and even before positive blood cultures have been obtained.

Some cases will be referred from general surgical wards, having been admitted with abdominal pain and fever (Fig. 8.2).

A third significant source of referred cases in general hospitals is from the urology department. Following urethral or bladder surgery, some patients will present with spinal pain due to vertebral osteomyelitis following gram-negative septicemia.

Some general hospitals in particular localities in large cities often admit many drug addicts and alcoholics, in whom complaints of severe spinal pain should raise the suspicion of underlying vertebral infection. A wide range of organisms, including fungi, may be identified either in blood cultures or from needle biopsy specimens in the drug-addicted patient.

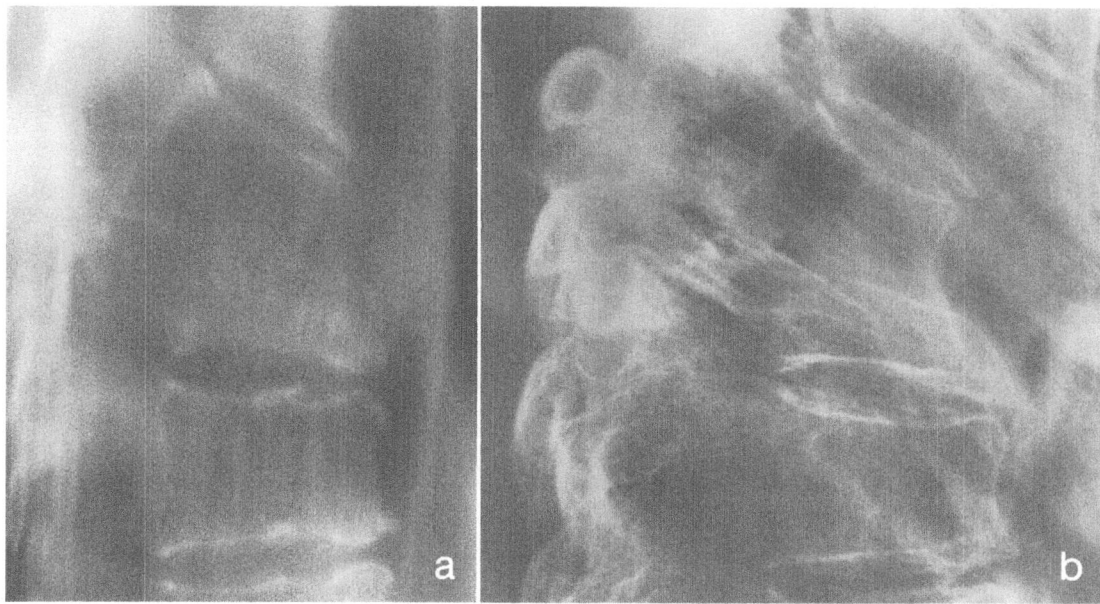

Figures 8.1 a, b. **a** A lateral tomogram of the mid-thoracic spine of a woman aged 66 who had been under treatment for chronic bronchitis for three months prior to her presentation with back pain and paraplegia. Gross destruction of the vertebral body of T7 is noted with pathological fracture-dislocation. **b** A lateral X-ray of the same area taken four years after conservative treatment of this lesion with long-term chemotherapy. Considerable remoulding of the vertebrae at the site of the dislocation had occurred and the paraplegia had recovered in part

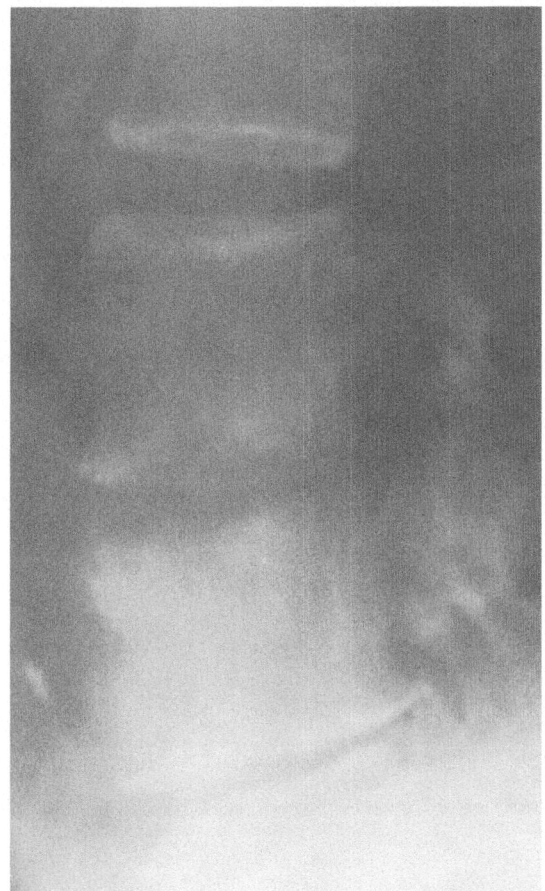

Figure 8.2. A lateral tomogram of the lower lumbar spine of a woman aged 59. Note the changes in the upper half of the body of the 5th lumbar vertebra in the region of the vertebral end-plate, with erosion and narrowing of the intervertebral disc space. The patient presented with acute abdominal pain, overshadowing back pain. The lesion was due to an acute osteomyelitis of the body of L5 complicating bronchitis.

Organisms lodge in the complex vascular bed, in the region of the vertebral end-plates, in children and adults (Crock and Yoshizawa, 1977). The pathological changes induced vary enormously depending on the bacteriological characteristics of different organisms.

Although the radiological appearances may be similar, in the case of staphylococcal infections chondrolytic activity destroys cartilage and disc tissue, whereas in tuberculous disease these tissues are not destroyed. The loss of disc height shown on X-rays in cases of spinal tuberculosis is due to osteitis with pathological fracture, the disc tissue simply collapsing into the adjacent carious vertebral bodies (Figs. 8.3 a, b).

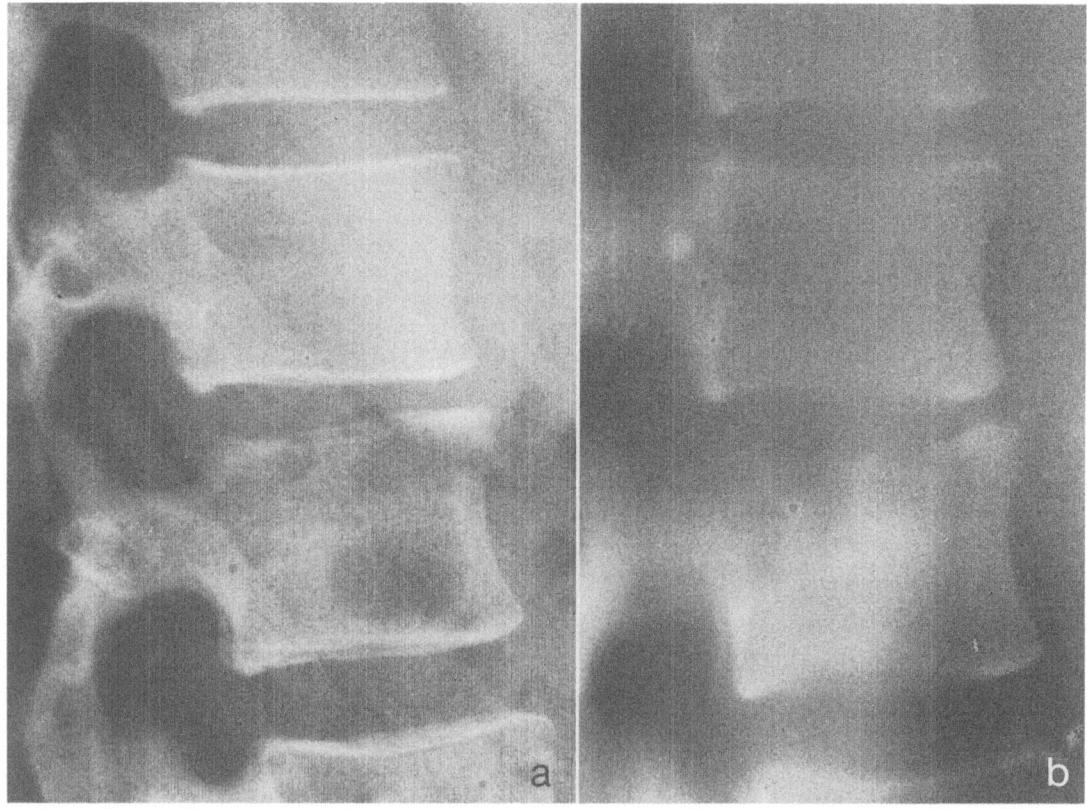

Figures 8.3a,b. **a** A lateral radiograph of the lumbar spine of a 32 year old lady who presented with a history of low back pain and weight loss. She had not complained of pain in the region of this lesion. The film is centred on the disc between T12 and L1 at the thoraco-lumbar junction. Note the narrowing of the disc space. **b** A lateral tomogram of the same area of the spine. Note the extensive erosive changes in the upper vertebral end-plate of the lower vertebra at the level of the narrowed disc space. This lesion was tuberculous and, at operation, intact disc tissue was found within the cavities of the lower vertebral body

b) Clinical Findings

The sudden onset of excruciating spinal pain in a febrile patient, should immediately arouse the suspicion of the diagnosis of vertebral osteomyelitis. Physical signs include:

– marked local tenderness in the spine;
– paraspinal spasm and rigidity, or psoas spasm causing fixed flexion deformity of the hip;
– local spinal deformity;
– rapidly advancing neurological deficits in cases with spinal epidural abscesses (Figs. 8.4 a–c).

c) Investigations

Full blood examination should be carried out urgently, and repeated samples of blood taken for bacteriological cultures, both aerobic and anaerobic. The diagnosis of spondylodiscitis is still made with difficulty. In a recent study the mean duration of symptoms before recognition was 6.4 month, Zilkens *et al.* (1991). These workers found estimations of the ESR, CRP and Neopterin (a marker of activated macrophages) very useful in helping to identify vertebral infections.

Other cultures may be taken from infected skin lesions, sputum, urine or faeces, depending on their predicted relevance on clinical grounds.

The significance of the results of many of these tests is that they may form the basis for decisions in the differential diagnosis between infections, acute and chronic, and neoplastic diseases. In addition, the critical choice of appropriate chemotherapeutic agents will depend on some of them.

d) Radiological Examinations

i) Plain X-Ray

Plain X-rays and tomograms will demonstrate a variety of changes in the bones and soft tissues, pointing to their likely inflammatory basis.

ii) Computerized Axial Tomography

C.T. scanning has been of inestimable value in demonstrating the relationships between pathological changes in the vertebrae and in the related soft tissue structures. Paravertebral and spinal epidural abscesses may be mapped accurately using this technique.

iii) Myelography

Myelography may be essential to identify the level of obstruction in the spinal canal caused by vertebral collapse or epidural abscess.

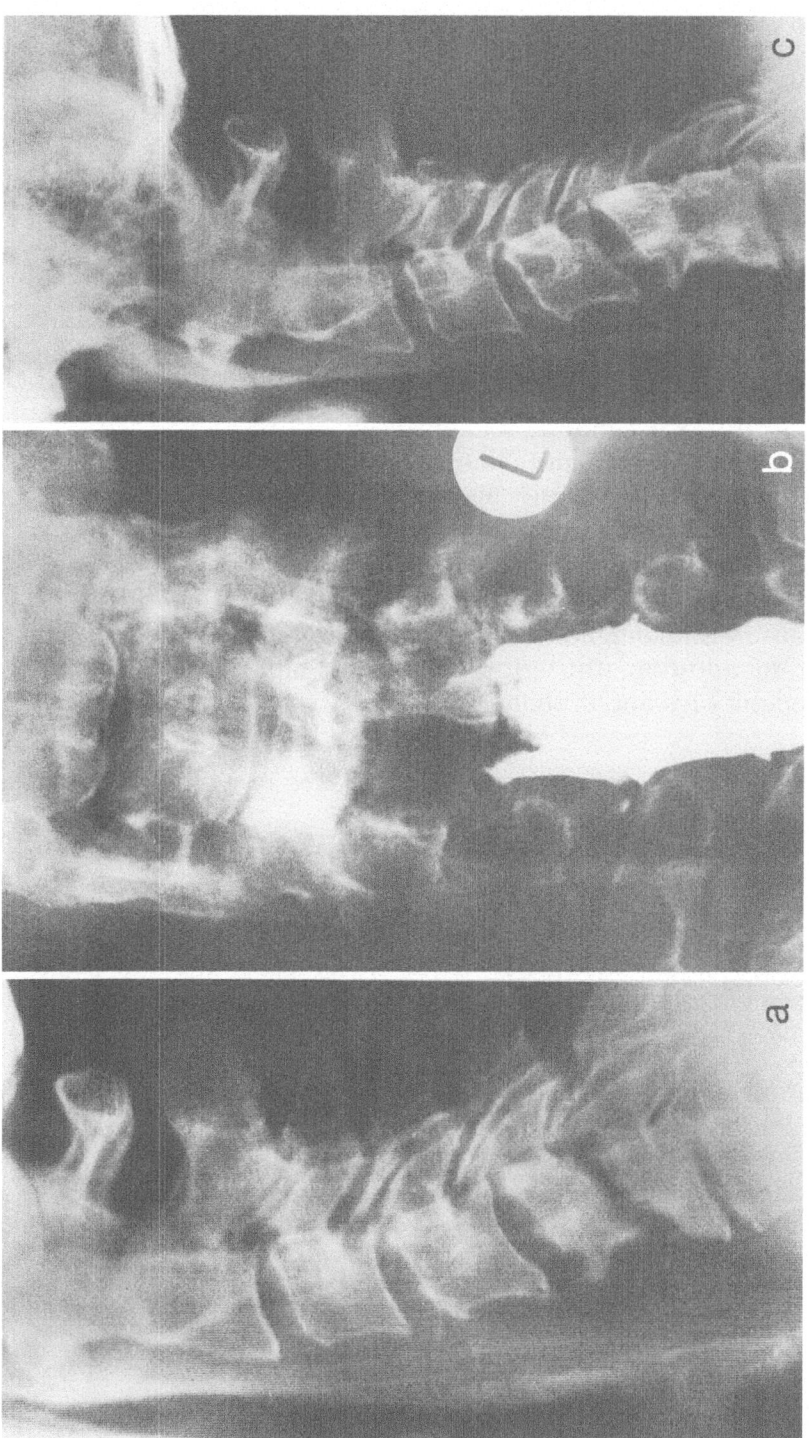

Figures 8.4a–c. **a** A lateral radiograph of the cervical spine of an alcoholic male patient aged 54 years who presented with severe neck pain of subacute onset. Note the extensive changes in the vertebral bodies of C5 and C6 with vertebral end-plate erosion in the adjacent vertebral margins of these vertebrae; the disc space is also reduced in height. Note in particular the wide separation of the gas shadow in the pharynx and oesophagus from the anterior aspects of the cervical vertebral bodies, indicating the presence of a pre-vertebral abscess. This patient became quadriplegic within 48 hours of presentation. (By courtesy of Mr B. J. Dooley and Mr J. K. Henderson.) **b** An antero-posterior radiograph of the spine of the same patient showing complete obstruction to the flow of a Myodil column upwards at the level of C6 and C7. **c** A lateral radiograph of the spine of the same patient taken 15 months after operation. The spinal canal was decompressed from behind and a large epidural abscess aspirated. Treatment then consisted of splinting the neck in traction with hyperextension; chemotherapy was administered for twelve months. Note the restoration of the normal relationships between the pharynx and oesophagus and the anterior surfaces of the vertebral bodies

iv) MRI

MRI with gadolinium enhancement has become extremely useful in diagnosing inflammatory lesions of the spine, though it is not always possible to distinguish between neoplastic and inflammatory tissues with this examination (Figs. 8.5 a, b).

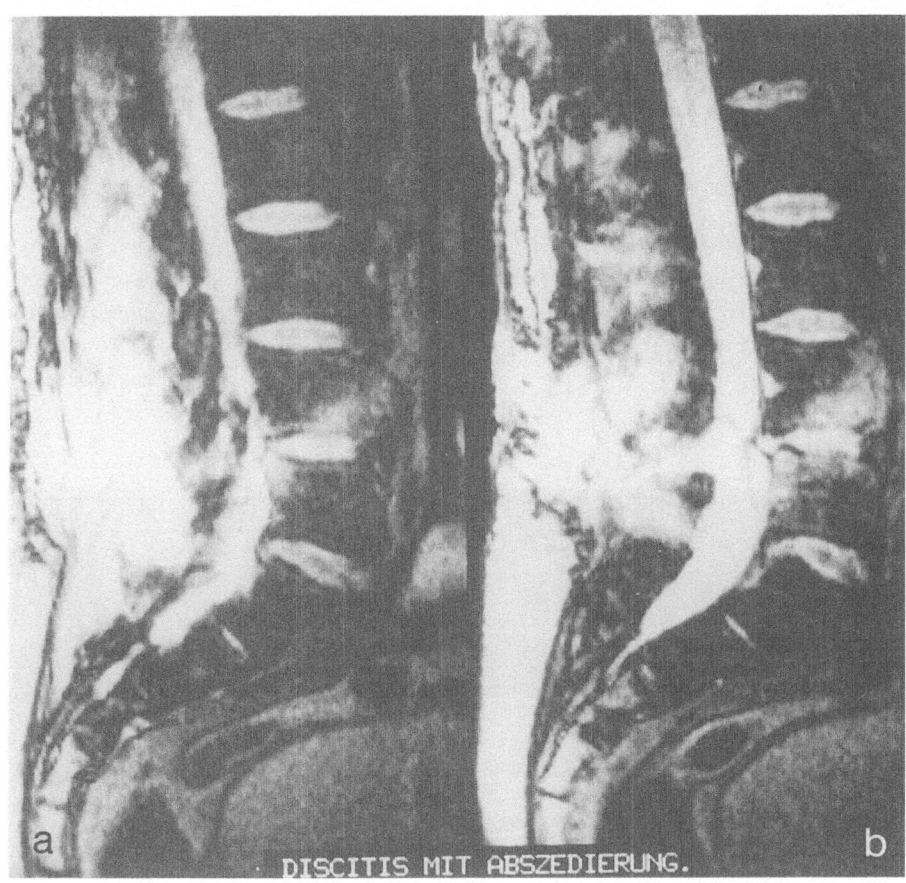

Figures 8.5 a, b. MR images with gadolinium enhancement showing extensive abscess formation involving the paraspinal muscles, epidural space and vertebral bodies following infection at an operation site

e) Needle Biopsy

The use of needles or small trephines inserted into vertebrae under X-ray or CT control represents one of the most significant advances in management of patients with neoplastic or inflammatory lesions. In parts of Asia, where infective lesions of bone are still common, the use of this method to obtain samples both for histological and bacteriological examination has proved the accuracy of diagnosis in many cases of non-tuberculous spinal infections which would have been classified previously as tuberculous (Chari, 1979).

f) Bed Rest and Chemotherapy

i) Conservative Treatment

Many patients will respond satisfactorily to conservative treatment. Spontaneous spinal fusion often follows healing of lesions in staphylococcal osteomyelitis.

Problems arising in cases of osteomyelitis due to staphylococcal infections vary with the virulence and sensitivity of the particular organisms. The use of chemotherapy continuously for more than six months may be necessary in patients who have developed multiple bone lesions complicating septicemia (Figs. 8.6a,b).

ii) Drainage of Abscesses

Emergency surgery is required for decompression of the spinal canal in cases developing tetraplegia or paraplegia due to the formation of epidural abscesses.

Occasionally drainage of psoas abscesses may be required, even in cases of non-tuberculous infections (Figs. 8.6a,b).

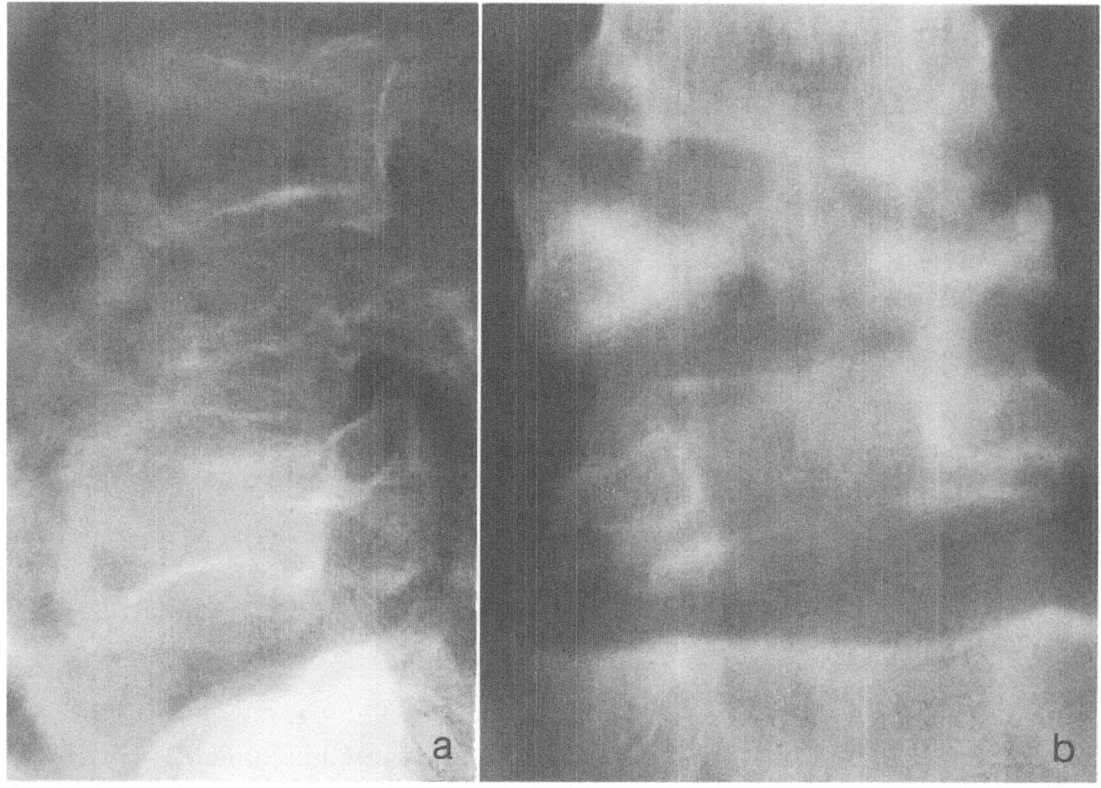

Figures 8.6a,b. a A lateral radiograph of the lower lumbar spine of a boy aged 14 years. Extensive destruction of the vertebral body of L4 is noted. This lesion developed in the spine twelve months after he had been treated for acute osteomyelitis affecting his upper tibia. **b** An antero-posterior tomogram. A large para-vertebral abscess required extra peritoneal drainage. Staphylococcus aureus organisms were cultured and found to be Penicillin sensitive

Surgical treatment of this type is recommended early in the management of vertebral osteomyelitis in drug addicts, because of the high resistance of organisms in these cases to chemotherapy alone (Hartman, 1978).

Even after extensive destruction of vertebral bodies due to staphylococcal infection, spontaneous spinal fusion usually occurs. Supplementary bone graft operations should not be required, providing sharp contrast with the requirements in the surgical management of Pott's disease.

8.2. *Tuberculous Disease of the Spine*

The surgical treatment of tuberculosis of the spine has attracted widespread interest in the past twenty years. During that time, the most authoritative accounts of the various surgical procedures which may be required in dealing with the spinal complications of this disease have come from the East, especially from Hong Kong (Hodgson, 1956).

Tuberculosis is now re-emerging in Western communities.

The illustrations in this chapter have been chosen simply to draw attention to some of the outstanding features of this disease as it affects the spine (Figs. 8.7–10).

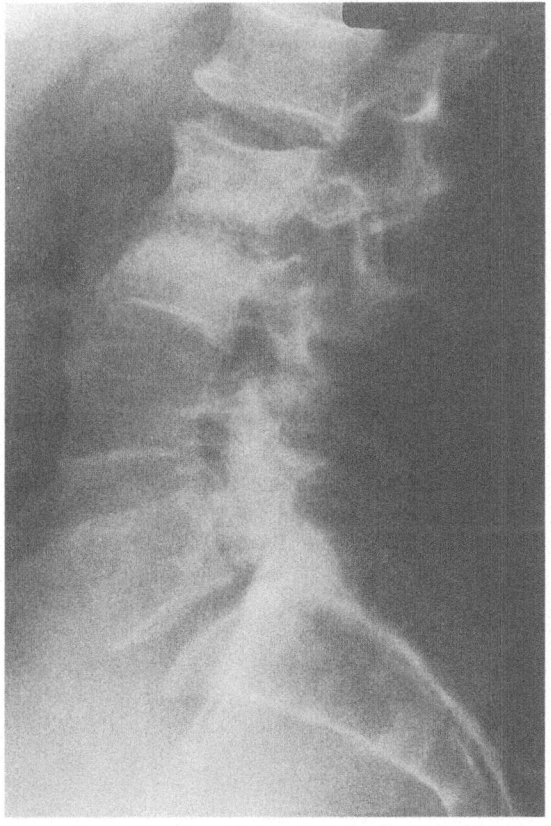

Figure 8.7. A lateral radiograph of the lumbar spine of a man aged 54 who presented with severe low back pain. Note the loss of disc space with erosive changes in the adjacent vertebral bodies at the level of the disc between L2 and L3. The body of L4 is somewhat osteoporotic. In the antero-posterior view the classic deformity of the psoas shadows indicated the presence of bilateral psoas abscesses. This is an example of relatively localized tuberculous disease with minimal spinal deformity at the time of presentation

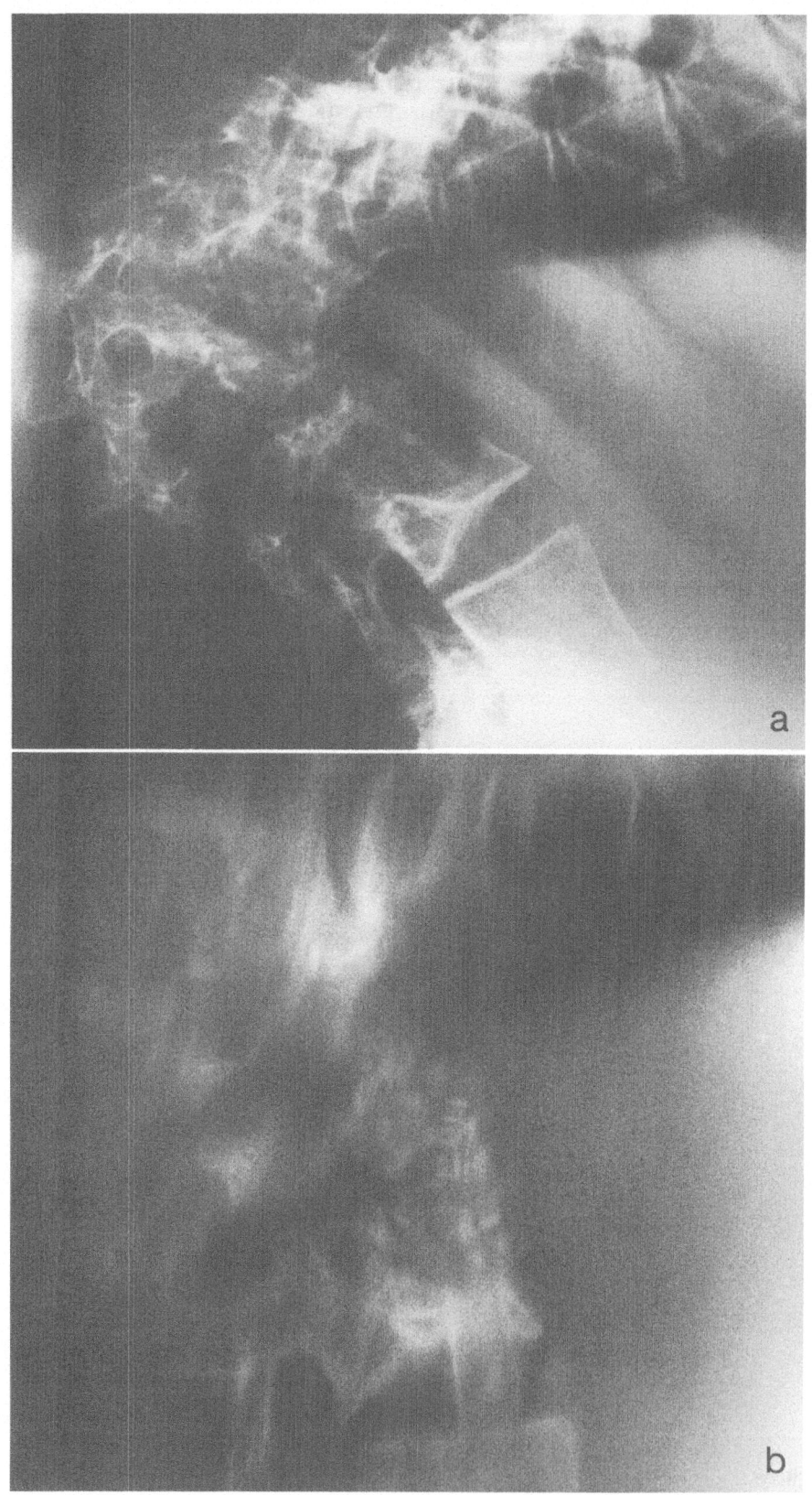

Figures 8.8 a, b

Publication of these records may serve a useful purpose for those readers whose experience of this disease has been limited, reminding them of the magnitude of the problems which may occur in spinal tuberculosis.

Surgical treatment has been dominated by the use of interbody fusion operations, performed through anterior approaches at every level of the vertebral column, allowing debridement of carious debris and necrotic bone fragments before the insertion of strut grafts (Fig. 8.14).

Correction of kyphotic deformities of the spine due to Pott's disease has been undertaken with considerable success in a limited number of special centres in the world.

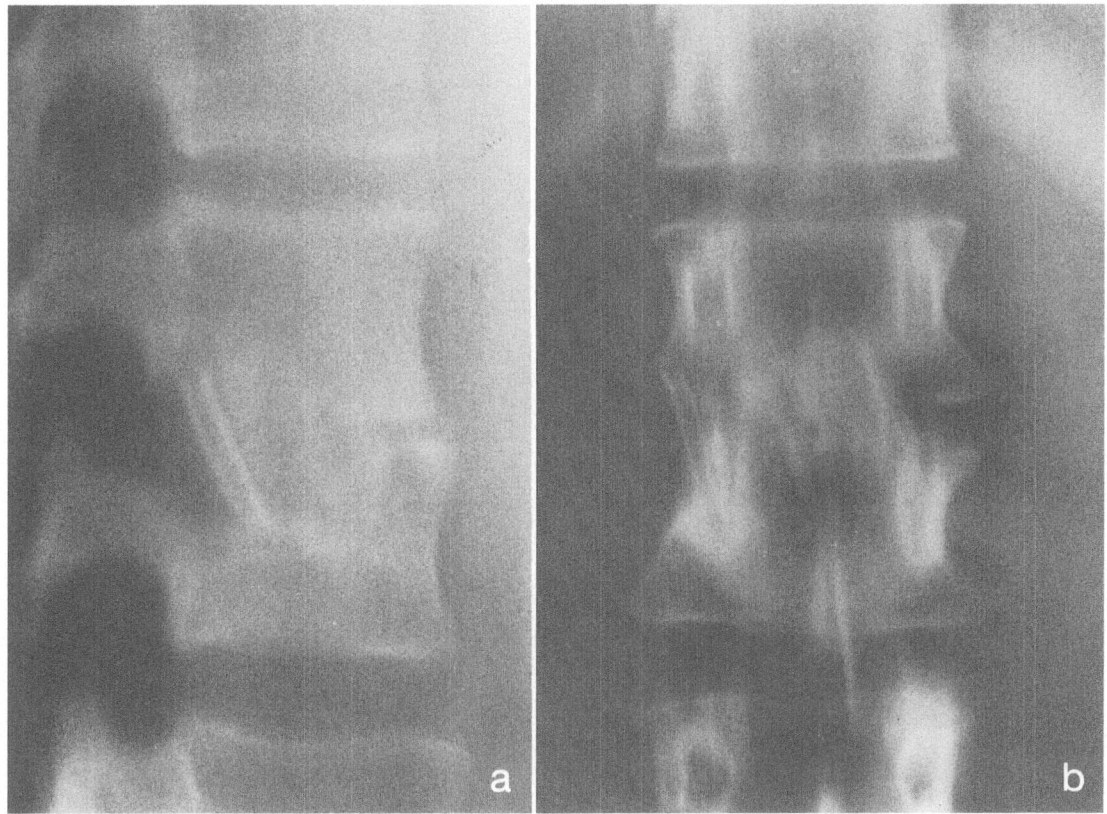

Figures 8.9 a, b. **a** A lateral tomogram taken four months after operation showing the incorporation of grafts inserted for the treatment of tuberculous disease in the patient whose preoperative films are illustrated in Figs. 8.3 a, b. Note the fragment of rib graft adjacent to the spinal canal. **b** An antero-posterior tomogram of the same spine showing sound interbody fusion with no lateral deformity of the spine

---

Figures 8.8 a, b. **a** A lateral radiograph of the thoraco-lumbar junction of the spine of a man aged 24 years who presented with complaints of spinal pain and increasing weakness of the lower extremities. **b** A lateral tomogram of the same area of this patient's spine following debridement and bone grafting of the bone of the area for active Pott's disease. No attempt was made to correct the deformity. The patient was managed post-operatively in a plaster bed and anti-tuberculous chemotherapy administered

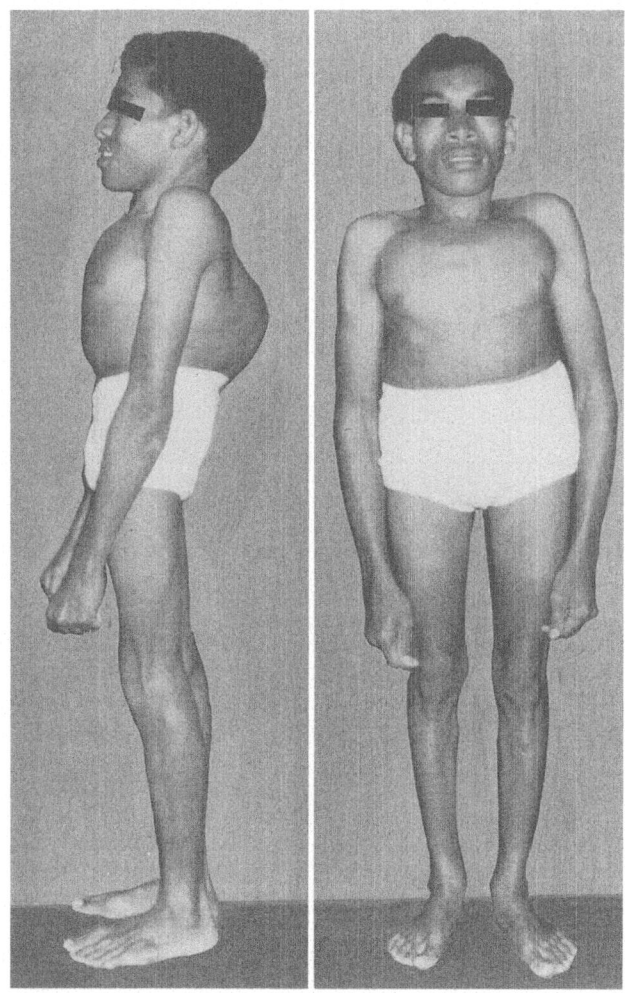

Figure 8.10. Lateral and anterior photographs showing the gross deformity of the spine resulting from Pott's disease at the thoraco-lumbar junction. The X-rays of this patient are shown in Figs. 8.8 a,b, 8.9a,b

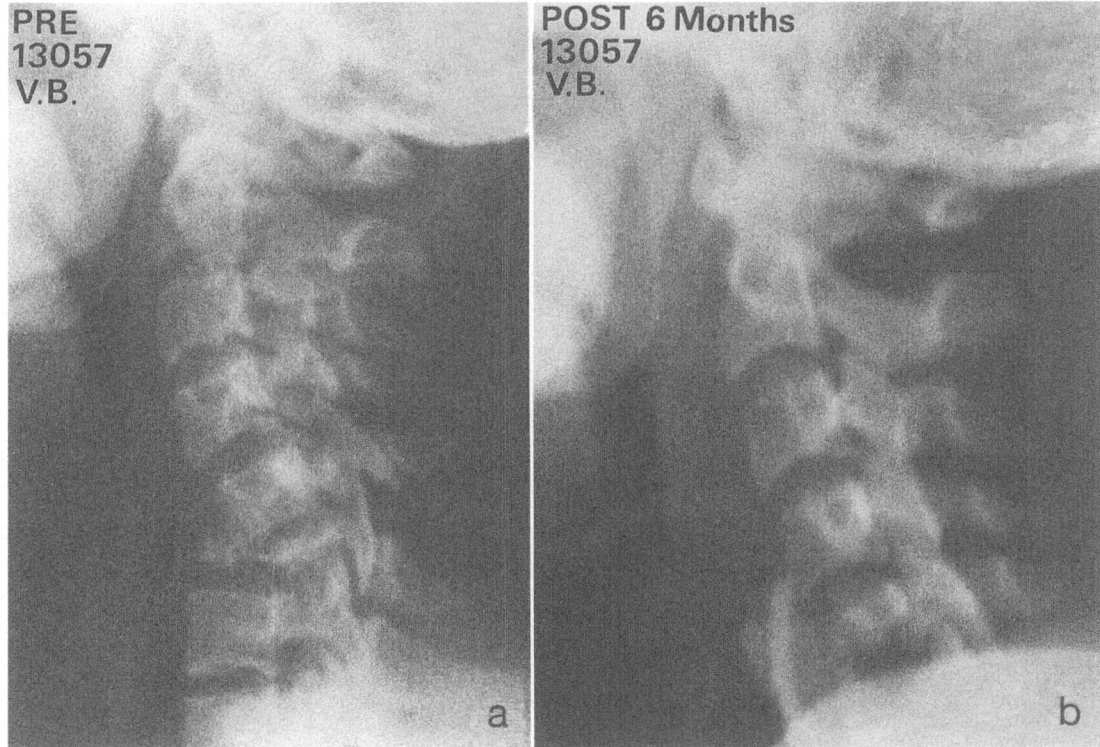

Figures 8.11a,b. a A lateral radiograph of the cervical spine showing gross vertebral destruction at C6 with subluxation of the spine complicating tuberculous infection. **b** A lateral radiograph of the same spine six months after operative treatment for debridement and anterior interbody fusion. Note the correction of the deformity and the presence of a uniting interbody fusion

A surgeon who has had no special experience in the management of post-infective kyphoses should avoid "trying his hand" on such cases. Should he be obliged to operate on a patient with a gross spinal kyphosis, with active tuberculous disease and clinical evidence of spinal cord dysfunction, he should treat the case by anterior decompression and anterior interbody fusion, making no attempt to correct the deformity. The patient should be nursed in a plaster bed for three months after surgery (Fig. 8.12).

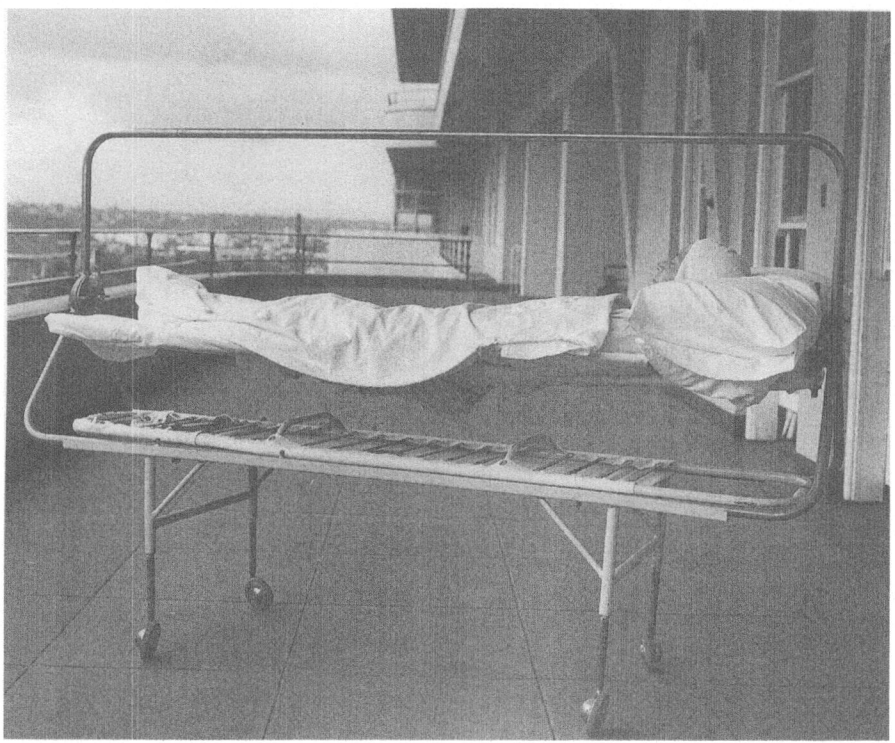

Figure 8.12. A photograph of a Stryker rotor bed suitable for nursing patients following spinal surgery for infective or neoplastic lesions

8.3. Post-Operative Infections

Some of the surgical aspects of the management of post-operative infections following spinal operations are discussed in Chapters 7 and 9.

Fortunately, serious infections are uncommon. Surgeons, therefore, have a natural tendency to hope that wound infections may subside with the use of chemotherapy alone. They may be reluctant to explore the wound early after the onset of infections.

Clinically, distinction should be drawn between superficial and deep wound infections. In patients with a thick layer of subcutaneous fat between skin and lumbo-dorsal fascia, fat necrosis and infections in the haematoma between the skin and the underlying paraspinal muscle layer will give rise to the appearance shown in Fig. 8.13. The patient's temperature will be only slightly elevated and local pain in the wound will not be severe. Although slow to heal, this type of infection is not serious. It will respond to limited local drainage, following removal of a few sutures, and the use of chemotherapy.

On the other hand, with deep infections, patients become febrile and ill, and they complain of extremely severe pain. Prompt surgical drainage should be carried out under anaesthesia. All sutures should be removed from the skin and deeper structures, so that the vertebral column can be re-explored. Infected blood clots and free pus should be aspirated, and material sent for further detailed bacteriological tests.

The whole wound should be washed out with a solution of hydrogen peroxide. Dry packing should then be inserted. Secondary suture of the wound can be performed when cultures from the granulating wound surfaces have become sterile.

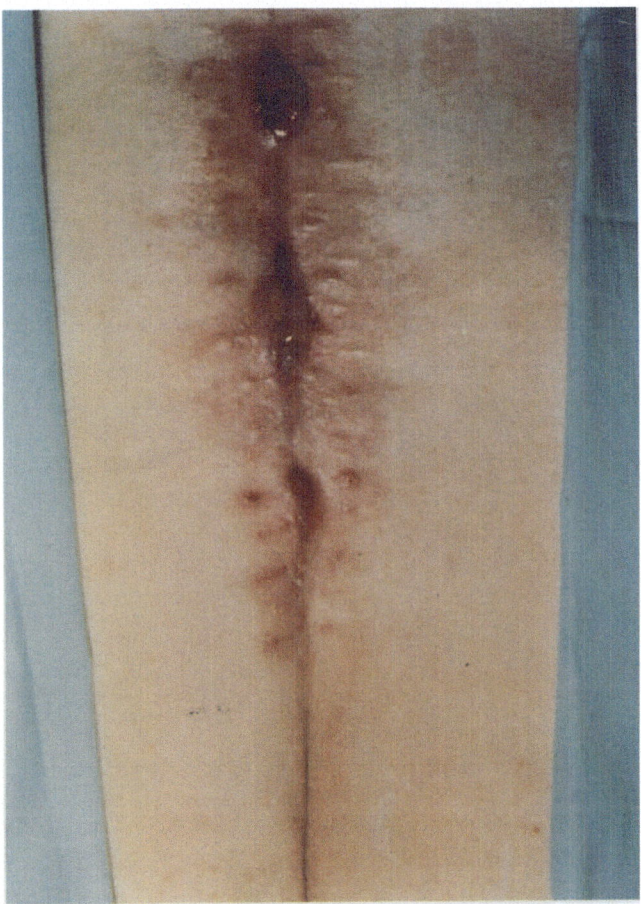

Figure 8.13. A photograph of the incision used for lumbar laminectomy in a young woman in whom the subcutaneous fat layer between skin and lumbo-dorsal fascia measured 9cms. Serous fluid containing fat droplets leaked from the wound. The incision was re-opened in the mid-line but extensive dissection was not necessary, the problem being confined to the subcutaneous layers of tissue superficial to the lumbo-dorsal fascia, as is usual in this type of wound infection

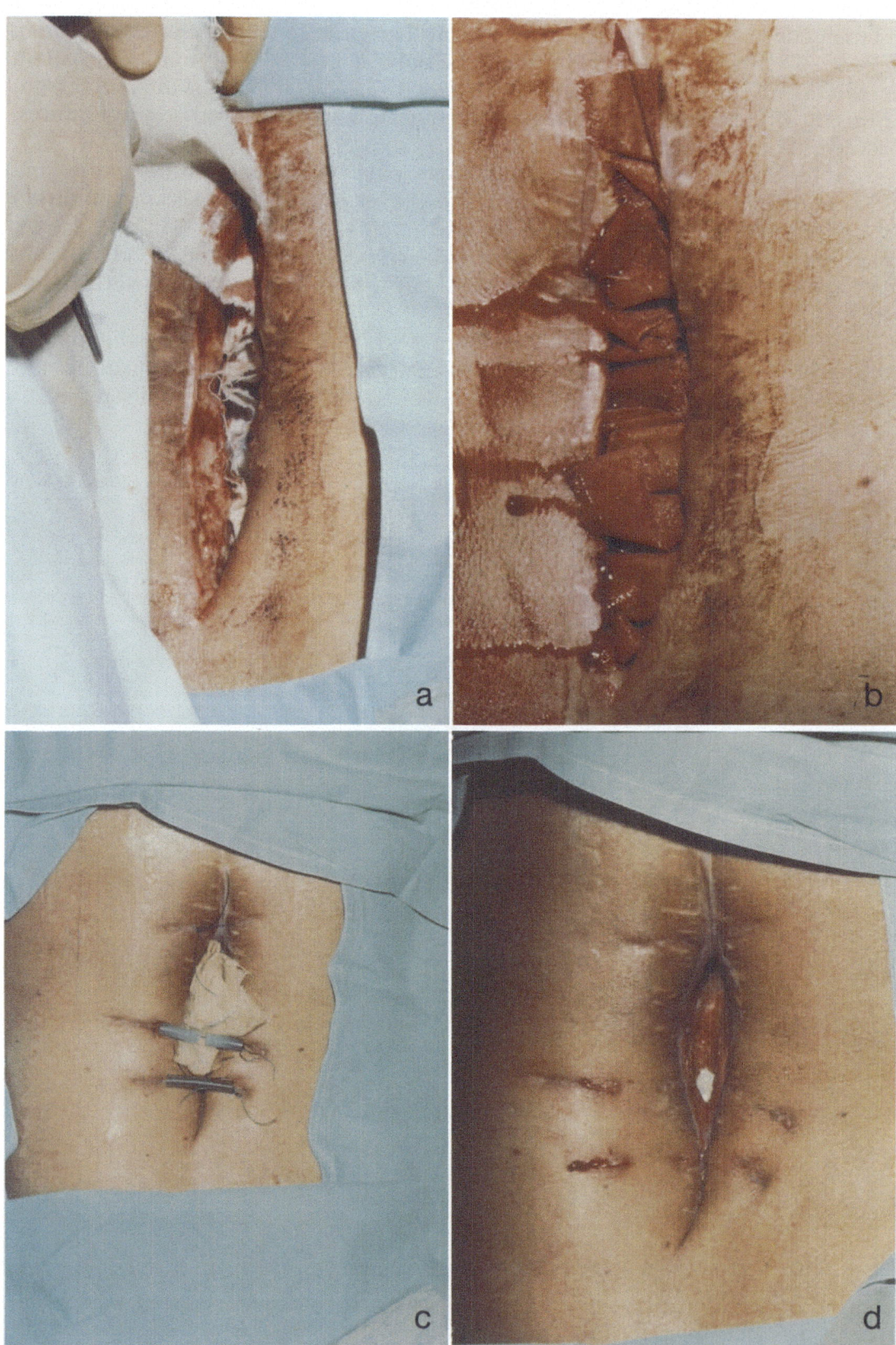

Figures 8.14 a–d

If deep infections, either in the neck or elsewhere in the spine, are treated promptly in this way, the dreaded complications of vertebral osteomyelitis, epidural abscess formation, or even meningitis should not develop (Figs. 8.14 a–d).

Patients who present with persistent severe spinal pain (with or without small discharging sinuses) some months after treatment for post-operative wound infections, will require very careful re-assessment. In this group, chronic osteomyelitis and chronic spinal epidural abscesses may be discovered resulting in crippling and prolonged illness (Fig. 8.15).

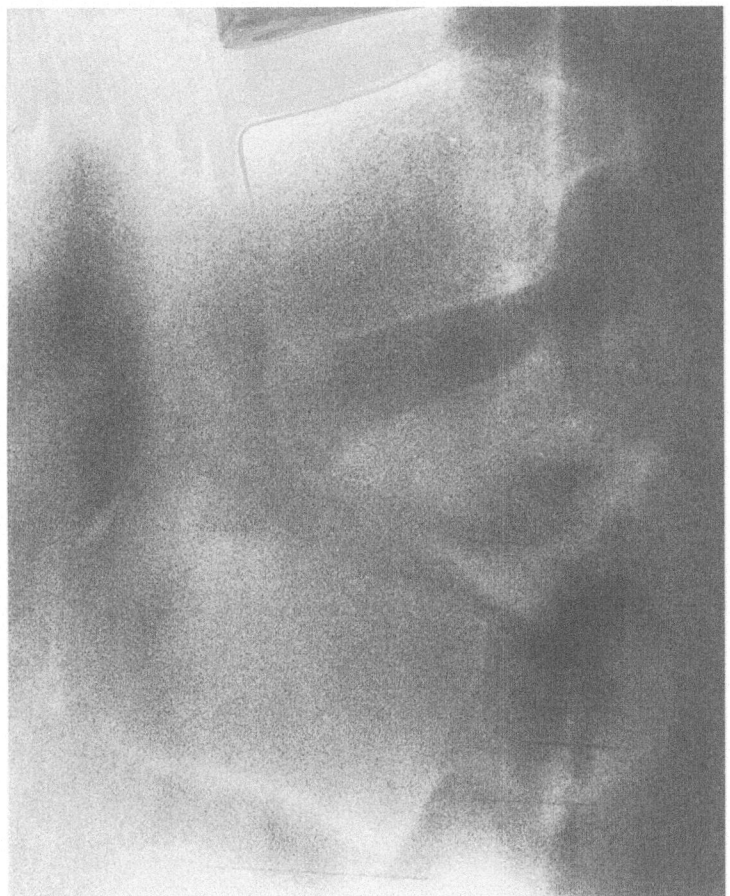

Figure 8.15. A lateral tomogram of the mid-lumbar spine of a woman aged 58 years. Note the gross destruction of two adjacent vertebral bodies and the resultant marked kyphotic deformity. This patient developed an epidural abscess and vertebral osteomyelitis following infection of a laminectomy wound

Figures 8.14a–d. Photographs illustrating progressive stages in the management of chronic osteomyelitis of the spine following posterior bone grafting for spondylolisthesis 15 years earlier. This patient had had a discharging sinus in his back with intractable back pain for many years. **a** The problem was treated by radical excision of the graft and packing of the cavity with calico. **b** The appearance of the wound three days after the operation for graft excision. **c** The appearance of the wound at the time of secondary suture when cultures from the granulating surfaces were sterile. **d** The appearance of the wound following removal of the tension sutures after secondary suture. Note the dural tissue in the base of the wound. The wound healed completely and epithelialized four weeks after this photograph was taken. The patient was treated with appropriate chemotherapeutic agents for more than one year

9

The Management of Failed Spinal Operations

9.1. Introduction

Waddell *et al.* (1980), painted a gloomy picture of the outcome for patients who have had multiple back operations. Little wonder that patients with persisting serious spinal problems are often given dire warnings about further operations, not only from non-medical sources but even from some specialist surgeons. There are certainly daunting problems in their management. These patients are often debilitated and demoralized. Family breakdown, financial stress, drug dependency and frank persecution by insurers, examining doctors and employers constitute some of their difficulties – leaving aside the question of the actual physical causes of their persisting disability.

This is one of the most challenging fields of spinal surgery and there is no place in it for a surgeon who is sceptical or suspicious of his patient or whose attitudes are in any way defeatist.

9.2. Investigation

The cornerstone of management is to investigate these problems with great care and with compassion, before recommending further surgery. The surgeon must establish a good working relationship with the patient's general practitioner and physical therapist and call upon the expertise of other specialists with declared interests in this type of work when indicated.

Before outlining a simple system for the analysis of failures after spinal operations, some general comments should be made on the subject of investigations.

Clinical neurological examination may be unrewarding in assessing the level or severity of nerve root or cauda equina lesions in patients who have had previous spinal surgery. This is especially true in those who have had multiple operations.

Radiological examinations which may be essential in helping to establish diagnoses and to plan further surgery in particular cases include:

a) Motion studies of the spine.Instability may require spinal fusion.

b) Oblique views of the facet joints and intervertebral foramina.Unrecognized foraminal stenosis may require decompression.

c) Antero-posterior and lateral tomograms in any case of failure following spinal fusion or canal exploration. Irregular laminal remnants or re-formed bone in scar tissue may require revision of canal decompression.

d) Repeat myelography to demonstrate space-occupying lesions or arachnoiditis.

e) Discography to plan the extent of spinal fusion.

f) Computerized tomography, especially if reconstructed scans in three planes can be obtained. Offers a wide range of diagnostic information but does not necessarily supersede the use of a–e.

g) MRI, especially with gadolinium enhancement, is probably the best investigation for demonstrating unrecognized disc lesions, epidural scarring or chronic inflammatory disorders.

The analysis of individual cases of failed spinal operations may be facilitated by using the following classification:

1. Outright Failure
   This group comprises patients who show no improvement or who become worse after the first operation.

2. Temporary Relief
   These patients may be free of symptoms for months or years after operation.

3. Failures in Spondylolisthesis
   These patients are considered separately because of special features of the pathological anatomy in this condition (see Chapter 5 and p. 305).

4. Infection

9.3. Outright Failure

Failure is usually related to wrong diagnosis. Some pain and discomfort are to be expected after any spinal operation. Pain protracted over weeks may follow some operations in which adherent root sleeves have been tediously separated from disc tissue, yet a successful outcome can be predicted. Such special circumstances excluded, patients in this group can usually be identified soon after operation. They complain of pain which is more severe than is normally expected. Those with infections will have elevated temperatures and altered blood counts.

The questions to be determined are simply these:

– Is the failure due to an unrecognized condition?
– Is it due to wrong diagnosis of the spinal lesion?
– Or finally, has it followed some technical failure?

a) Unrecognized Conditions

Investigations should begin as soon as possible, but several months may elapse before the correct diagnosis can be established. For example, a carcinoma involving the apex of the lung may be the cause of neck pain and brachial neuralgia persisting after anterior cervical fusion. Operation for lumbar spondylolisthesis may fail because the true cause of pain is a secondary prostatic carcinoma of the vertebra.

Rarely, infection after a spinal operation may be caused by tuberculosis or gonorrhoea.

Primary tumours in the spinal canal are relatively rare. They are usually diagnosed before operation by clinical examination and by myelography. However, in cases of failure, the possibility that such lesions may be the cause of continuing symptoms should be considered. Even MRI may fail to define some lesions such as intradural neurilemmomas unless gadolinium enhancement is used.

b) Error in Diagnosis of the Spinal Condition

Three questions must be answered:

1. What was the primary diagnosis?
2. What were the operative findings?
3. What was the nature of the operation?

Stenoses of the spinal canal or of a nerve root canal must be excluded as underlying causes of failure. The possibility that the symptoms are those of "claudication" of the cauda equina must be borne in mind. Under such circumstances, myelography with CT or MRI should be used to help clarify the diagnosis.

c) Technical Errors

i) In Operations for Disc Prolapse

Persistence of severe pain after operation is unusual if the diagnosis of disc prolapse has been confirmed at the time of surgery. If a considerable amount of fragmented and desiccated disc material has been removed, it is likely that a further fragment has been displaced beneath the root sleeve after operation, or that a migrating sequestrated fragment has not been removed.

If a pre-operative diagnosis of disc prolapse was made but no disc prolapse was found at operation, it is likely that the intervertebral space at the wrong level has been explored (Fig. 9.1). Removal of a disc prolapse or of sequestrated disc fragments occurring at the site of isolated disc resorption usually leads to failure unless bilateral foraminal and nerve root canal decompressions are performed at the same time. More commonly this diagnosis is simply overlooked and operation is performed at an adjacent level on the basis of a minor disc "bulge" seen on a myelogram (Figs. 9.2, 1.2).

Most failures in this group occur when no disc prolapse has been found at operation yet one or two discs have been incised in the attempt to locate a "prolapse". These patients are often subjected to further myelography even on two or three occasions and subsequently have further unsuccessful explorations of their spinal canals (Fig. 9.3a–c).

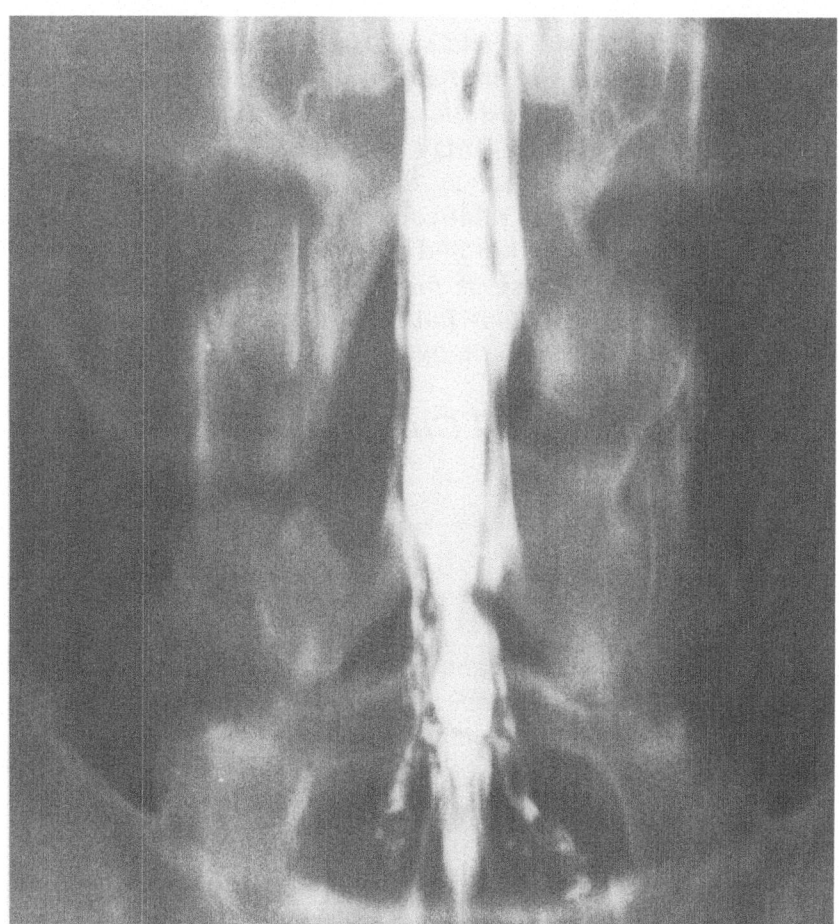

Figure 9.1. An antero-posterior tomograph of the lower lumbar spine in a patient aged 37 years, said to have undergone laminectomy for removal of a left-sided lumbo-sacral disc prolapse. Part of the upper margin of the lamina of the 4th lumbar vertebra has been removed, so that the space between the 3rd and 4th vertebrae was probably explored. The outline of the myodil shows that there is bilateral stenosis of root canals at the L4/5 level. This patient's symptoms were relieved by further decompression of the spinal canal, involving removal of the central segment of the arch of the 4th lumbar lamina, combined with bilateral nerve root canal decompression at that level

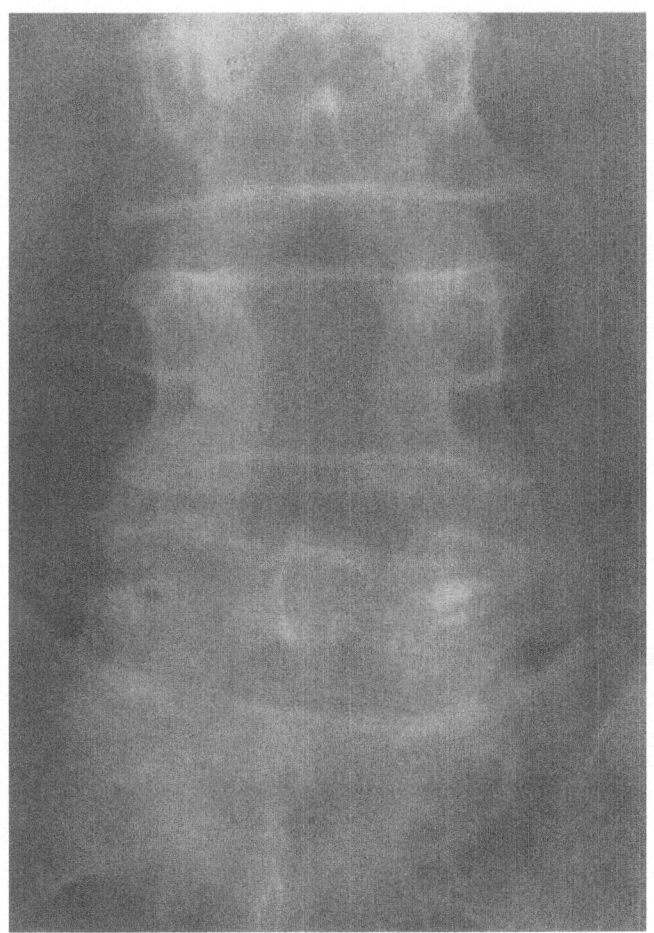

Figure 9.2. An antero-posterior radiograph of the lumbar spine of an 82 year old man showing the extent of decompression of the lumbar spinal canal at the L 4/5 level where no disc prolapse was found. The lesion was at L 5/S1 in the form of a well-established isolated disc resorption which responded very satisfactorily to bilateral foraminal and nerve root canal decompressions subsequently (see Fig. 1.2 which shows a lateral radiograph of this patient's spine)

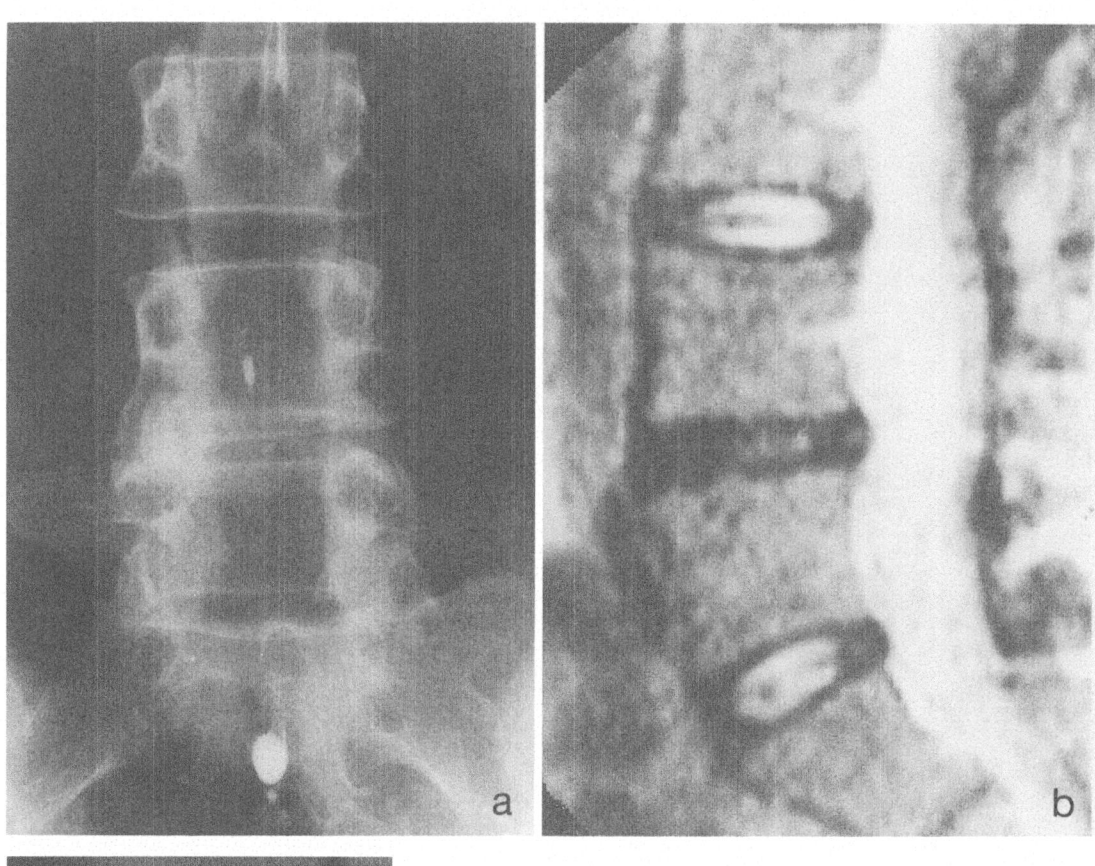

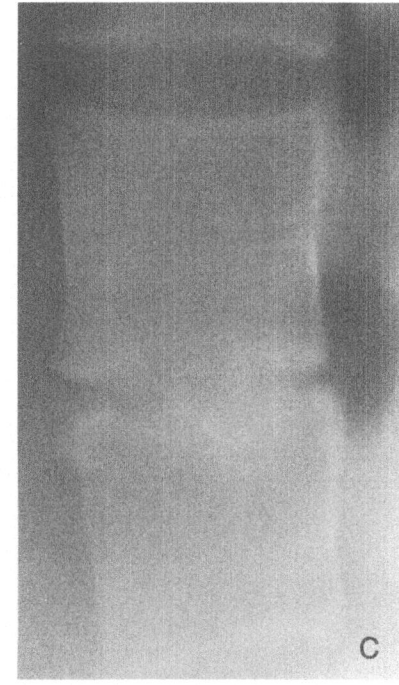

Figures 9.3a–c

ii) In Operations for Internal Disc Disruption

If this diagnosis has been established by discography and disc excision and interbody fusion has been done, early failure may indicate that the wrong level has been fused. In the neck particularly, levels should always be identified by radiographs taken during operation. The injection of methylene blue at the time of discography is an unreliable method of identifying the level of an affected disc. Even in the lumbar spine, levels may be wrongly identified, especially if there are segmentation anomalies.

9.4. Temporary Relief

In this group initial relief of pain after operation may last for weeks or months before the recurrence of disabling pain. The largest number of cases fall into this category.

a) Failure After Operation for Disc Prolapse

Recurrence of pain is usually caused by further prolapse at the level operated on, especially if a large volume of disc material was removed at the original operation, or by a fresh prolapse at another level.

Recurrent but contra-lateral sciatica occurs after asymmetrical settling of the vertebrae when several grams of disc material have been removed at the initial operation. Radiographs show collapse of one side of the intervertebral space. Recurrence of pain is caused by a fresh prolapse of disc material or by stenosis of the nerve root canal following its deformation due to the reduction in height of the intervertebral disc space.

The commonest cause of late recurrence of symptoms after initial successful excision of a disc prolapse is stenosis of the spinal and nerve root canals, secondary to degenerative changes (Figs. 9.4a–c). Ectopic ossification or calcification in the remnants of ligamentum flavum may be found at the site of re-exploration in such cases.

Another cause of late recurrence, often associated with secondary canal stenosis but contributing to the overall problem, is the presence of a meningocoele caused by damage to the dural sac at the time of the original operation.

Figures 9.3a–c. a An antero-posterior radiograph of the lumbar spine of a 27 year old female who had had two previous lumbar laminectomies involving excision of the L4 and L5 laminae and spinous processes. She presented with intractable pain and hysterical paraparesis. **b** A lateral sagittal MR image, T2 weighed sequence of this patient's spine showing isolated disc resorption at L4/5. **c** A post-operative tomogram showing sound interbody fusions at L4/5 in this patient's spine. Her gait returned to normal and she made a complete recovery

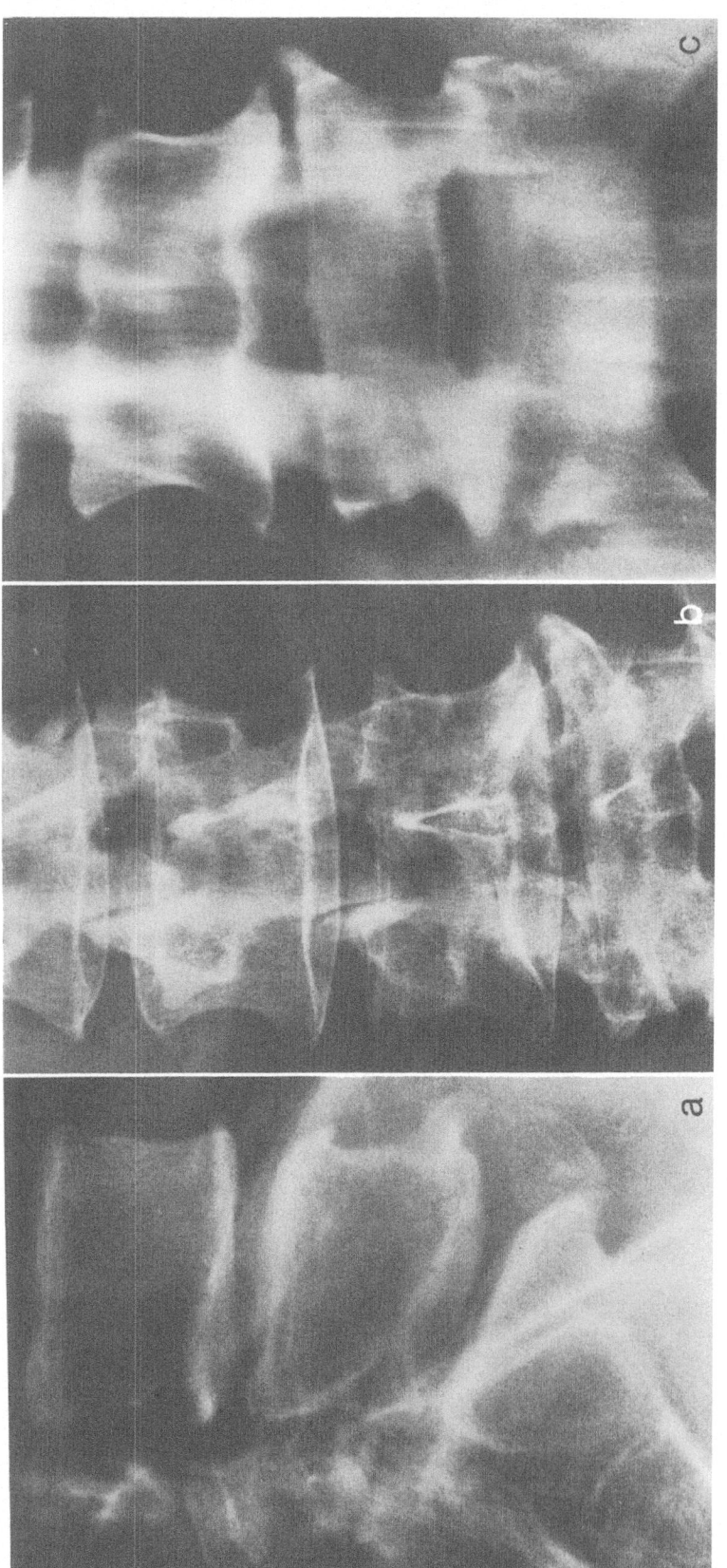

Figures 9.4a–c. Degenerative changes 30 years after removal of an intervertebral disc prolapse at L 4/5 level in a patient aged 61 years. Note the inter-laminar calcification in the antero-posterior view in **b**, **c**. A tomogram showing the extent of the decompression of the spinal canal and nerve root canals

b) Failure After Operation for Internal Disc Disruption

If interbody fusion has been performed for this lesion, early recurrence of severe symptoms within two or three months of operation may be due either to complications of the discography or to trouble arising at the site of grafting.

Severe pain occuring within six weeks of operation may be due to discitis in adjacent un-operated discs in which discograms had been performed. Erosion of the vertebral end-plates and bodies in the area of the nucleus pulposus occurs on either side of the disc, leading to gross narrowing of the intervertebral space at the level of the normal disc above or below the "fused disc". Histological examination of specimens removed at operation shows inflammatory changes with plasma cell infiltration. Cultures are sterile (see Chapter 2, Figs. 2.23, 2.48).

Non-union of grafts occurs in a few instances. These problems are discussed in detail on pp. 93, 96. The incidence of non-union of interbody grafts has been reduced in recent years following improvements in surgical technique reported by Crock (1976), by Crock (1982) and by Fujimaki, Crock and Bedbrook (1982). Grafts of cancellous bone were shown to have two disadvantages. They are prone to infiltration by disc remnants with subsequent non-union and graft resorption; secondly, even though union occurs, loss of intervertebral height may follow collapse of the cancellous graft and its settling into the vertebral bodies. Stenosis of the nerve root canal follows and may cause recurrence of pain in both lower limbs (Figs. 9.5 a, b).

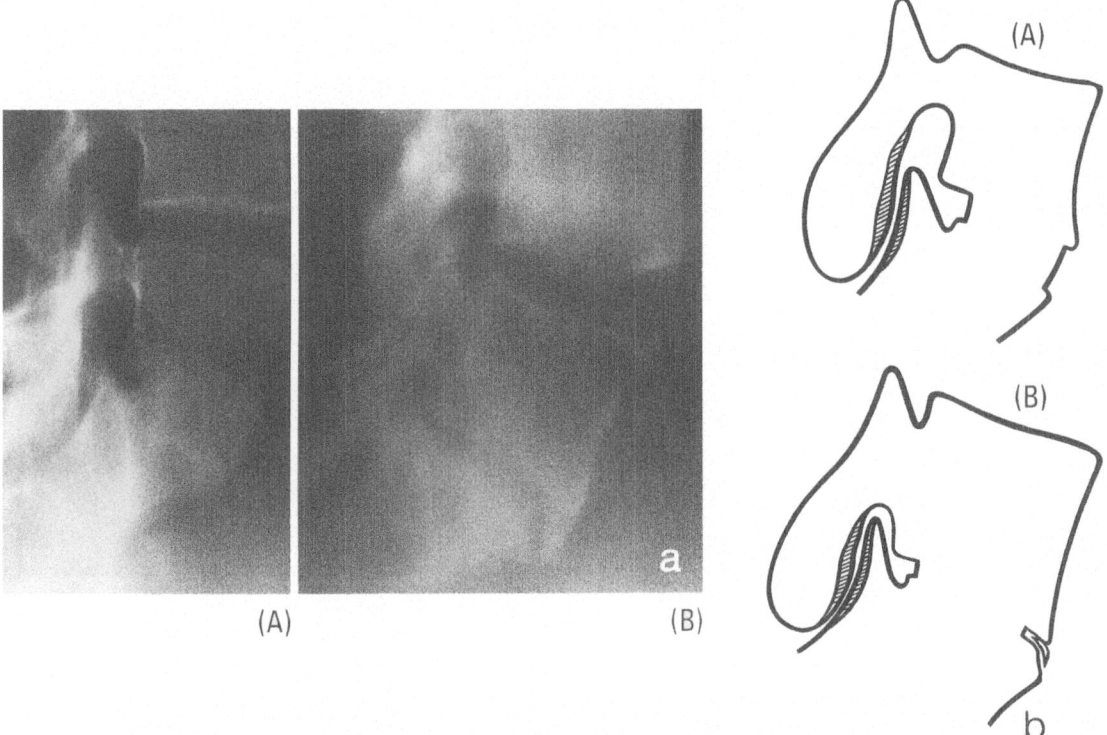

Figures 9.5 a, b. Lateral tomographs of the lumbo-sacral junction in a man aged 46 years. (**A**) is taken four months after operation, (**B**) is taken 18 months after operation. The graft has incorporated but secondary disc space collapse has occurred with resultant nerve root canal and intervertebral foraminal stenosis. The diagrams (**A**) and (**B**) alongside depict the evolution of the foraminal stenosis

Block or dowel grafts cut from the anterior half of the iliac crest provide grafts which are rapidly revascularized, usually maintain height and always resist infiltration by disc remnants (see Chapter 2, Figs. 2.26, 4–8).

Following successful interbody fusions, the ligamentum flavum related to the fused segment will atrophy, adhering then to the dura and nerve root sleeves. With vertebral column movements above the fused segment, stretching of the dural root sleeves may occur and cause pain. Relief follows total laminectomy and excision of the ligamentum flavum over the area of the fused spinal segment or segments, leaving intact the facet joints between the fused and mobile segments of the column. In the cervical spine, the relevant root canals should also be decompressed, using a very fine forward-angled rongeur.

c) *Failure After Operation for Isolated Disc Resorption*

This condition has been discussed in detail in Chapter 1. Acquired disc resorption may follow partial disc excision or intradiscal injections of chymopapain. In such cases symptoms usually recur or persist after a second exploration of the disc space with hemi-laminectomy and removal of more disc material (Figs. 9.6 a, b). The appropriate surgical treatment of bilateral nerve root canal decompression is discussed

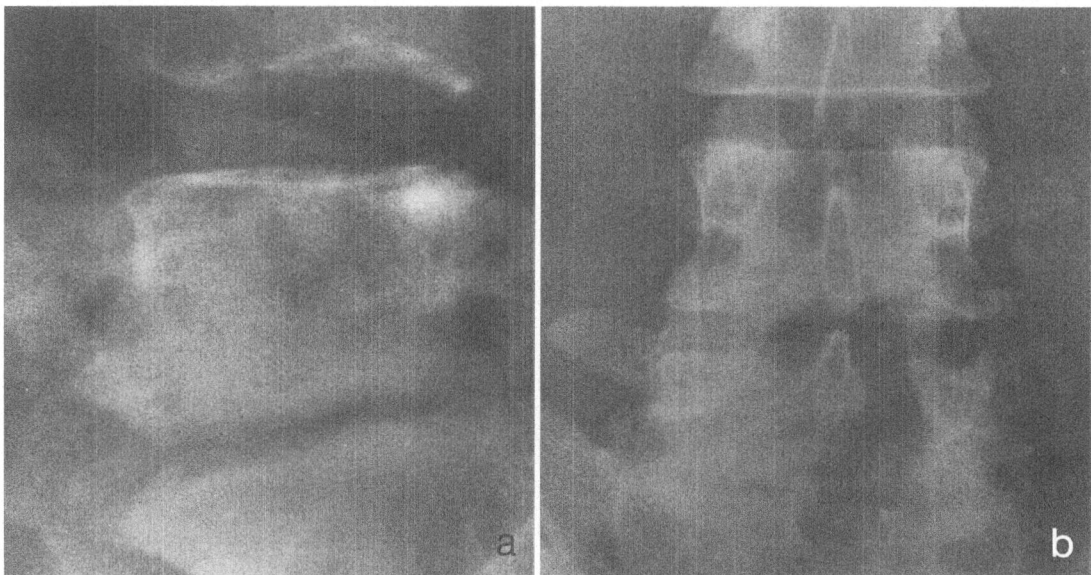

Figures 9.6 a, b. **a** A lateral radiograph of the lower lumbar spine of a woman aged 37 years with persistent pain in the back and lower limbs. Note the narrowing of the lumbo-sacral intervertebral disc space, with minimal osteophyte formation and marked sclerosis of the adjacent vertebral body. **b** The antero-posterior radiograph shows the amount of residual laminal bone after two previous operations. This patient's problem was due to acquired disc space narrowing following intervertebral disc surgery, with resultant bilateral nerve root canal stenosis. The second operation had been inadequate, the remnants of the central portion of the 5th lumbar lamina should have been removed, and bilateral nerve root canal decompression performed as described in Chapter 1, pp 30–35, 127–138

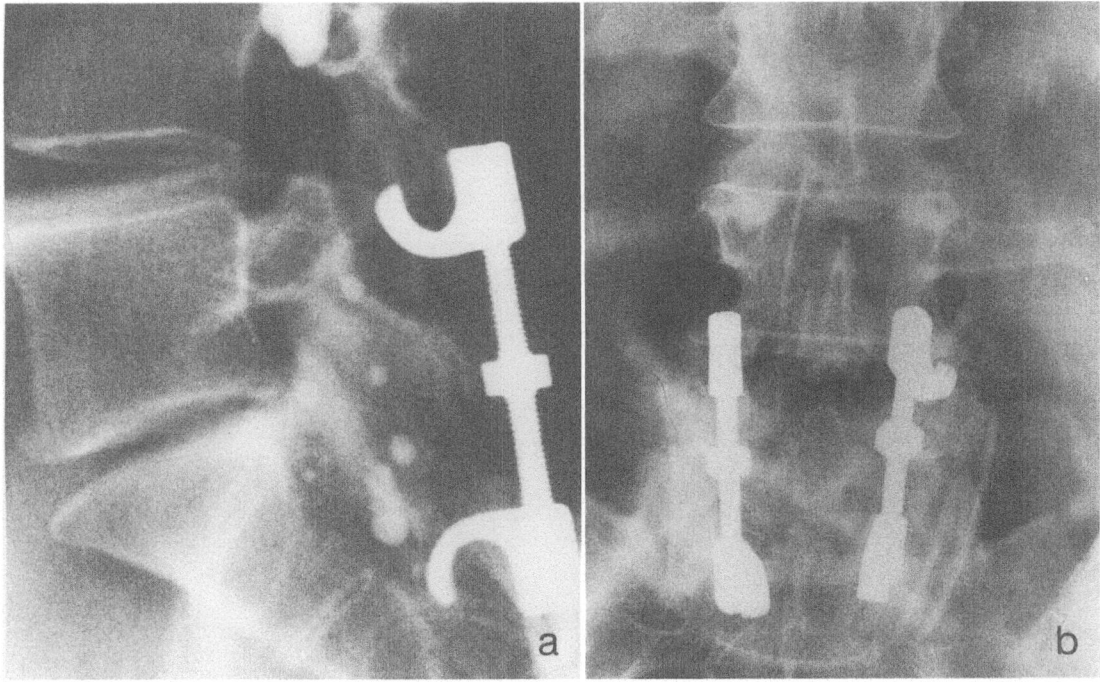

Figures 9.7a,b. a A lateral radiograph of the lower lumbar spine. Isolated disc resorption is noted at the lumbo-sacral junction with a degree of retrolisthesis of L5 on S1 and a positive Knuttson sign. The L4/5 disc space is normal. Knodt's rods have been inserted beneath the lamina of L4 above and into the sacrum below. **b** An antero-posterior radiograph of the same spine. Note the bilateral Knodt rods and the segments of graft, some of which extend upwards to lie against the left side of the spinous process of L3. The pathology in this case was present only at the L5/S1 level. In this patient, two other normal spinal segments have been operated upon unnecessarily. Supplementary treatment in this case involved removal of the Knodt rods, excision of the unwanted bone at L3/4 and L4/5, and bilateral nerve root canal decompression at L5/S1 level

in detail on pp. 30, 127–138. If the true significance of the pathology of isolated disc resorption is not appreciated, the patient may be subjected to further major surgery, involving adjacent normal segments of the spine (Figs. 9.7a and 1.2).

9.5. Surgical Techniques for Re-Exploring the Spinal Canal

a) Preparation

These procedures are often time-consuming and may be associated with considerable blood loss. Blood transfusion facilities must be available. Adequate supplies of bone wax, gelfoam or equivalent haemostatic agents should be ready for use.

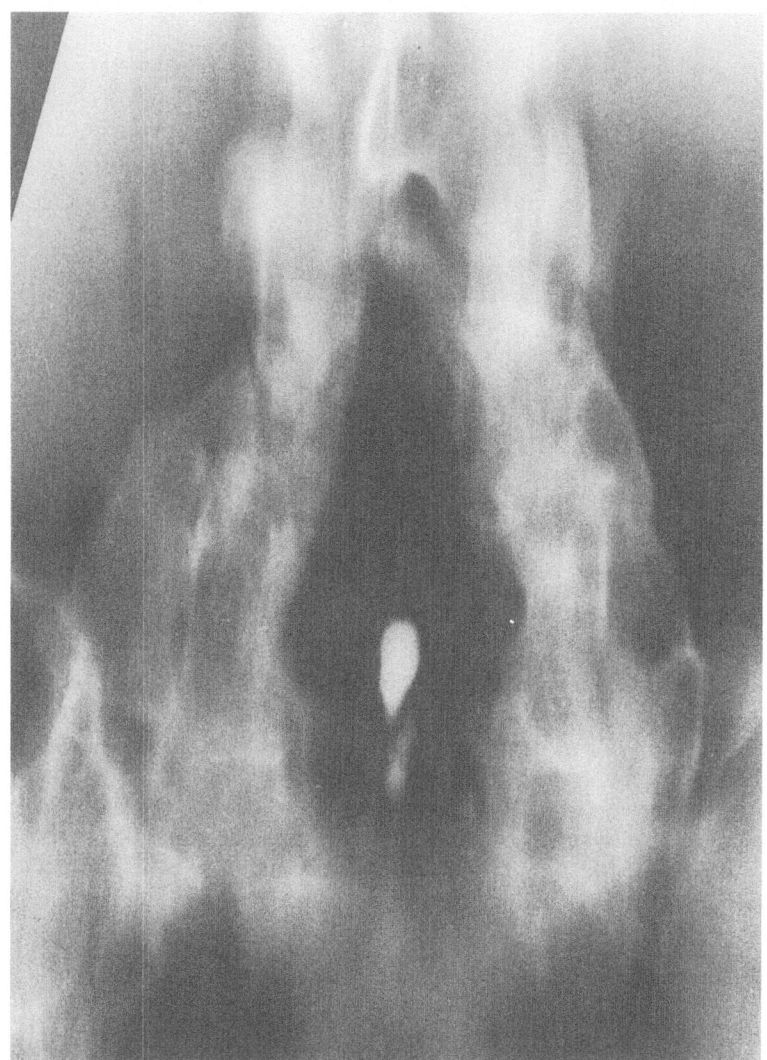

Figure 9.8. An antero-posterior tomogram of the lower lumbar spine of a man aged 52 years who complained of recurrent back and leg pain following two previous spinal operations, including spinal canal decompression and postero-lateral inter-transverse-alar fusion. Note the reformation of the laminal remnant near the top of the picture on the right side at the upper extremity of the previous exploration

b) Radiology

Radiographs of the patient's spine should be displayed on a viewing box in the theatre. The most valuable information for the operation of re-exploring the spinal canal is usually provided in antero-posterior views, including tomograms which show the anatomy of the roof of the spinal canal or its remnants most clearly (Fig. 9.8).

c) Positioning

Positioning on the operating table is important and use of the prone position on a suitable frame is recommended.

d) Instruments

Opening of the dural sac may be indicated if arachnoiditis of the cauda equina is recognized during operation. Dural tears may occur accidentally in the course of dissection, especially at the junction of previously operated and non-operated areas. If the dural sac and nerve root sheaths are tethered to the floor of the spinal canal by dense adhesions, it may be necessary to open the dural sac to gain access for removal of prolapsed disc fragments. On rare occasions meningocoeles may be encountered unexpectedly. An adequate array of instruments, including a fine sucker, long handled fine toothed forceps, long handled fine needle holder and long fine "atraumatic sutures" on fine needles (4.0 or 6.0 sizes) should therefore be readily available so that any of these problems may be dealt with promptly during the operation.

Dense laminal bone is likely to be encountered in some cases. A high-speed drill with diamond-tipped burr should be available for use. Debris dispersed in a fine spray from the tip of the drill may be the source of spread of the HIV virus. *Theatre staff should nowadays wear suitable protective masks for the face and eyes to avoid contamination.*

e) Exposure

A mid-line incision should be used. Bony landmarks at the extremities of the incision should be palpated with the aim of exposing intact spinous processes and laminae above and below the area to be re-explored.

f) Orientation

When the incision has been made over the desired length of the spine, the soft tissues are separated from the sides of the intact spinous processes at each end of the wound. The paraspinal muscles should be separated carefully from the lateral aspects of the spinous processes and the posterior surfaces of the laminae, leaving the periosteum intact and avoiding any disturbance of the capsules of the facet joints. At the upper end of the incision the intact lamina and its inferior facets should be clearly defined, as should the posterior surface of the sacrum below, to the level of its superior laminal edge. Self-retaining retractors should then be inserted before any effort is made to expose the actual area to be re-explored.

The surgeon must re-assess the patient's X-rays at this stage, to be certain of the location of laminal remnants in the dense scar tissue which has usually formed between the paraspinal muscles and the roof of the spinal canal following previous surgery.

Using a sharp scalpel, an oblique incision is made into this scar tissue, starting in the mid-line at the upper extremity of the wound on one side, the direction and depth of the cut being gauged by the orientation of the cleared lamina and its inferior facet joint, laterally and inferiorly to the level of the next joint. The extent of muscle damage resulting from the previous surgical procedure or procedures will be variable. Where it has been slight, there will be a clearly defined fatty layer between the anterior surface of the paraspinal muscles and the bony canal. Through this soft tissue the surgeon can easily palpate the facet joint with the tip of his/her index finger, thereby determining the plane of dissection. In cases where very dense scar tissue has invaded the paraspinal muscles at the site to be re-explored – a likely finding after multiple explorations – identification of the lateral edge of the pars interarticularis of the lamina and its inferior facet joint is difficult. The site of the pars interarticularis below the normal facet joint at the upper end of the incision can be identified either by removing the extra-synovial fat pad from this facet joint or by locating the main stem of the posterior branch of the lumbar artery which is a constant lateral relation of the pars interarticularis. Using either or both of these guidelines, one can determine the direction of the incision which will lead safely to the exposure of the outer edge of the lamina and its related facet joint. Depending on the findings in particular cases, one may proceed to expose the entire area to be re-explored on one side between the sacrum below and the normal spinous process and lamina above, then repeat the procedure on the opposite side. Where there have been multiple previous operations, it is often wiser to make limited exposures, one level at a time, on the right and left sides alternately, moving the self-retaining retractors progressively as required.

If a meningocoele is present, it will be identified early. Cerebrospinal fluid will fill the wound when the scalpel is used to cut obliquely into the scarred tissue after preliminary exposure of the normal bony segments of the canal, as described above. The inexperienced surgeon will be shaken by the appearance of C.S.F. so early in the operation. The meningocoele should be identified as such and thereafter ignored until the formal exposure of the roof of the spinal canal or its remnants has been completed.

Once the lateral bony margins of the laminae and the facet joints have been exposed on both sides, the self-retaining retractors are positioned definitively.

g) *Timing of Retractor Application*

The time of their application should be noted because re-exploration operations may last more than two hours. The retractors should be removed at intervals of 45-60 minutes for 5 minutes, to restore circulation in the paraspinal muscles. During these rest periods the wound may be irrigated with Ringer's solution.

At this stage of the procedure, a bulky mass of scar tissue of variable depth remains in the mid-line between the lumbar spinous process above and the back of the sacrum below. Its relationship to the underlying dura will vary depending on the amount of laminal bone remaining or reformed after the previous operation or operations. The surgeon should now strip all soft tissues from the outer surface of each lamina or laminal remnants, referring once again to the patient's X-rays. Identification of laminal levels can be very difficult, particularly in cases with anomalies at the lumbo-sacral junction or in spondylolisthesis with the higher grades of slip of the vertebral body (Figs. 9.9, 9.10) so that it may be necessary to take control X-rays in the operating theatre in such cases. This done, the bulky mid-line scar tissue can be excised or thinned down to the level of the bony canal, at each level between

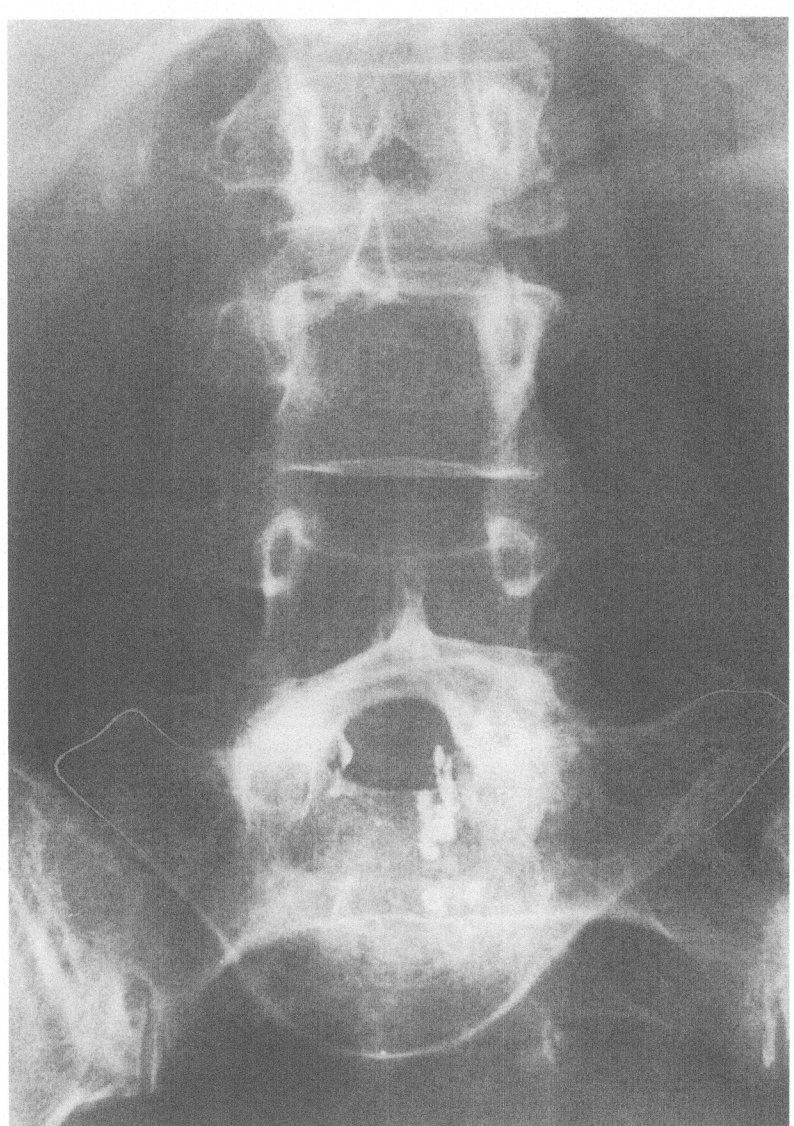

Figure 9.9. An antero-posterior radiograph of the lumbar spine of a woman aged 53, with spondyloptosis of L5. Note the classical radiological sign of "Napoleon's Hat". At operation, identification of vertebral levels can be difficult in such cases. Despite two operations aimed at decompressing the lumbar canal and nerve roots related to the spondyloptosis, the lamina of L5 remains intact. However, the laminae of L2 and L3 have been removed, along with some of their related facets

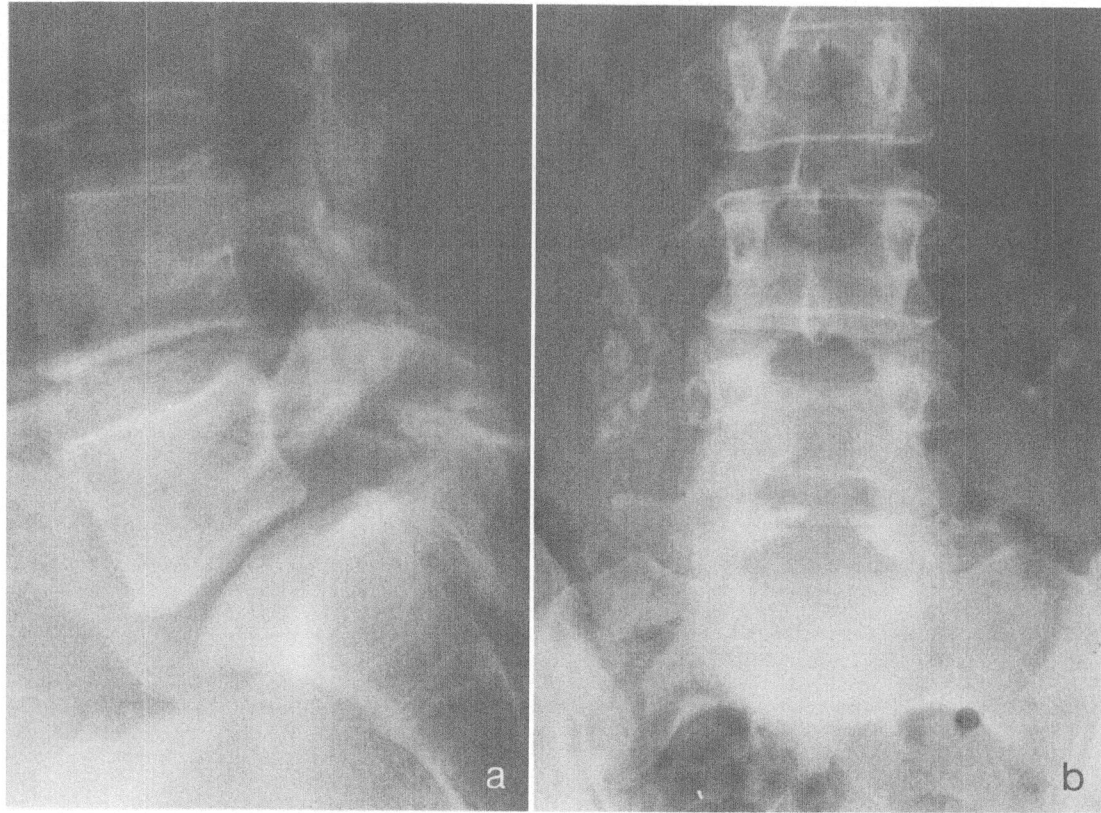

Figures 9.10 a,b. **a** A lateral radiograph of the lumbar spine of a 39 year old woman showing grade I spondylolytic spondylolisthesis with disc resorption at L5/S1. **b** An antero-posterior radiograph following operation which had aimed to produce lumbar canal decompression and inter-transverse-alar fusions. Scattered bony fragments unrelated to the spinous processes of L3 and L4 are seen on the right side. On the left side scattered fragments of graft bone are seen in the region of the transverse processes of L3 and L4, no bone graft material being visible at the L5/S1 interspace. A central portion of the lamina of L4 has been removed and a small portion of the lamina of L5, leaving a gaping defect in the spinal canal with ragged margins

the sacrum and the normal lamina and spinous process above, using either a large rongeur with sharp cutting edges or a sharp scalpel. *Forceful use of periosteal elevators should be avoided as scar tissue of the density frequently encountered in these cases can only be dissected with sharp instruments.*

h) Re-Opening the Spinal Canal

If the upper end of the sacral lamina is in the field of operation, the canal can be re-entered easily in the mid-line, even if the dural sac is covered with densely adherent scar tissue. This can be done by thinning the lamina in the mid-line and then stripping the scar tissue carefully away from its upper edge with a pointed probe (such as the Watson-Cheyne probe). Alternatively, when the bone is very thin, a small gouge directed proximally from a few millimetres distal to the free edge of the lamina can be used. A small plug of laminal bone is turned out, allowing the insertion of a blunt-ended probe into the canal. The dura is pushed away and a 2 or 3 mm sized cup of a 45 degree forward-angled rongeur then inserted to open the roof of the sacral canal, a few millimetres distal to its upper free edge, from the mid-line outward on both sides to the level of the medial margins of each S1 pedicle. Dural tearing may occur at this stage. It can be avoided by careful handling of the fragments of sacral bone created by the use of the angled rongeur. These fragments should not be pulled on forcibly. They are best left attached to the scar tissue, to be dissected free from it by sharp dissection after the canal has been exposed to the level of each S1 pedicle.

Should it be decided to commence the dissection for entry into the spinal canal at the upper end of the operation field, it may be easily done by removing the normal ligamentum flavum from the spinal segment immediately adjacent to the area to be re-explored. The central portion of the lamina on the inferior side of this vertebral interspace is then removed, using the same techniques described in dealing with the removal of the sacral laminal bone at its site of attachment to the scar tissue overlying the dura. Further dissection distally follows, using the landmarks of facet joints, medial pedicular margins and partes interarticulares, obtaining exposure one side at a time, with the careful technique outlined above.

Scar formation between the dura and nerve root sleeves and the paraspinal muscles is prevented by normal ligamentum flavum. This fact should be remembered when re-exploring a spinal interspace, which may have been opened previously on one side only as it may be put to good use, allowing safe entry into the spinal canal without risk of injuring the dural sac.

Regrettably, notes made at the time of the original surgery are rarely available to a surgeon when he is re-exploring a patient's spine. The identification of a segment of normal ligamentum flavum often assumes great importance. Although the outer surface of this ligamentum may be covered with dense white scar tissue arising from the deep surface of the paraspinal muscles, its presence can be determined most easily by removing the extra-synovial fat pad from the adjacent facet joint, and then defining its characteristic yellow colour, where it attaches to the medial edge of the superior facet at the interspace. Once its presence has been confirmed, the white scar tissue can be cut away, defining its full extent, before incising this ligamentum flavum to gain access to the spinal canal.

In the course of the dissection just described, root canal stenosis or foraminal stenosis can be identified and relieved easily (see pp. 30, 127–138). Once the lateral margins of the dural sac and the regional nerve root sleeves have been exposed on both sides over the whole area being re-explored, the surgeon is then in a position to assess the dural contents by digital palpation. If they are normal, the question of separating all the scar tissue from the dura should be addressed. It is not necessary to remove it entirely, but if scar tissue is left attached, it should be thin and should not contain any remnants of bony spicules. Bone left in scar tissue is likely to grow and it may lead to further canal stenosis after a few years, especially if a hemi-lamina is left nearby (Figs. 9.8).

With the canal thoroughly decompressed and any problems of root canal or foraminal stenosis already resolved, the regional intervertebral discs should be inspected, using digital palpation and probing with the Watson-Cheyne instrument. A nerve root may be bound to a recurrent disc prolapse by dense scar tissue. The use of an operating loop may be necessary to enable the separation of the root sleeve from prolapsed disc tissue, minimizing the risk of nerve injury. If recurrent disc prolapse is found, curettage of the intervertebral disc space may be indicated. The risk of penetration of the abdominal cavity may be high in these circumstances so that realization of this hazard should be uppermost in the surgeon's mind (see Chapter 3, Fig. 3.3 a).

i) Dural and Epidural Problems

i) Meningocoeles

These lesions are uncommon. They are often only recognized at operation and may be found early in the course of a re-exploration operation. When the spinal canal has been opened as described above, a meningocoele sac may then be dealt with quickly. It will usually have a single ostium which can be closed with a fine atraumatic suture after the bulk of the wall of the cystic cavity surrounding it has been separated from the dural sac and excised. In large long-standing meningocoeles, closure may require the use of tissue patches fixed to the ostium with biological adhesives such as Tisseel (Figs. 9.11 a–c).

With attention to the details of dissecting technique outlined above, the creation of dural tears can usually be avoided. They may occur inevitably in some patients in whom the dura is abnormally thin. In such patients multiple tears sometimes occur and closure of the dural defects becomes impracticable. The closure of the wound at the completion of the operation then becomes critical. Several layers of sutures should be used in the muscle and fascial layers rendering the wound watertight. Appropriate chemotherapy should be administered post-operatively until the surgical wound has healed, Penicillins and Sulphonamides being used together when applicable.

Small dural tears should be identified and closed with fine "atraumatic sutures", the area of the tear being kept dry with a fine low-pressure sucker and protective patty. Care should be taken to avoid trapping nerve root filaments in the sutures as they are passed through the dural margins.

The management of the dura in cases of arachnoiditis of the cauda equina is discussed on pp. 206, 213. The technique of transdural disc fragment excision is found on p. 141.

Figures 9.11 a–c. a A photograph of a large meningocoele extending from the back of the sacrum to the level of T12 spinous process. This sac contained about 2 litres of cerebrospinal fluid. It was subcutaneous and filled within a few minutes of the patient standing. This meningocoele had formed after dural injury ten years previously. **b** A photograph of the sac opened showing a single ostium in its base. The tip of the probe is pointing to a spinous process which has been eroded by the pressure of fluid over a period of ten years. **c** A photograph showing a patch of tissue cut from the wall of the sac applied to the ostium with Tisseel. The ostium could not be closed with sutures. The wall of the meningeal sac had been separated from all the surrounding soft tissues and its redundant tissue folded over the spinous processes and sutured in place, reinforcing the tissue patch which had been used to seal to the ostium

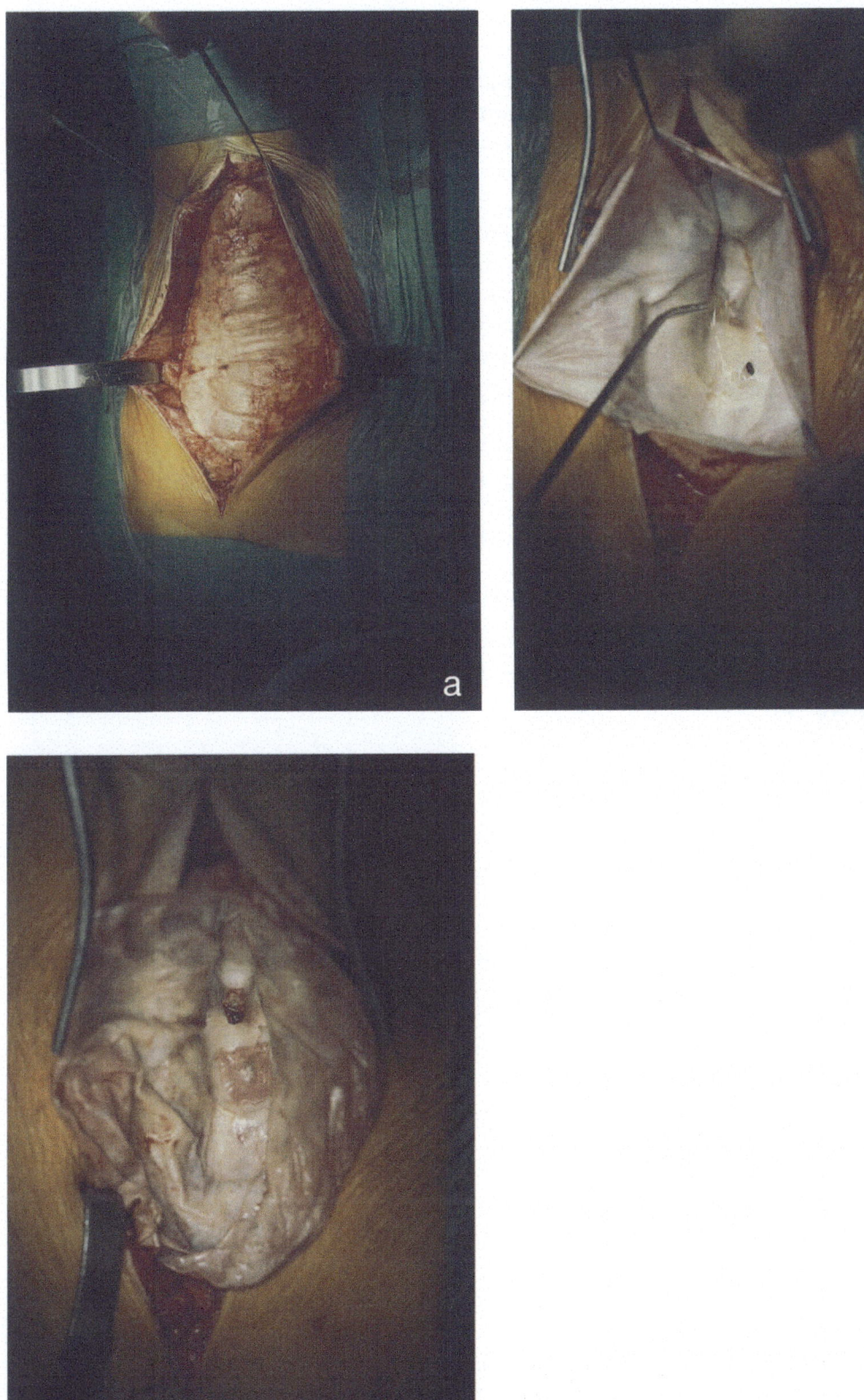

Figures 9.11 a–c

ii) Unrecognized Epidural Infection

Rarely, during re-exploration of the lumbar canal, previously unrecognized epidural or vertebral body infections may be found. The history of a superficial wound infection, followed by persistent spinal pain, out of proportion to what might have been expected post-operatively, should raise the possibility of this diagnosis. The planned operation of canal decompression should proceed, and intravenous chemo-therapy should be commenced. Special care should be taken to avoid dural injury though the dura in such cases is often thickened. The epidural abscess should be sucked out and its extent defined. If possible, pus in the intervertebral disc space should be aspirated and sent immediately for bacteriological examination.

The decision for primary or secondary wound closure should be resolved on the assessment of the extent and severity of the infection. It is better to pack the wound open with dry gauze where a large abscess cavity has been discovered, particulary if the vertebral bodies are infected. Secondary closure of the wound may be performed when cultures taken from the granulating surfaces become sterile (Chapter 8, Figs. 8.13, 8.14). Such wounds, even if they are extensive, will heal by secondary intention in 6–8 weeks. The first few post-operative weeks will be spent in hospital and thereafter daily wound care can be managed at home by visiting nurses.

j) Re-Exploration of the Spine Following Spinal Fusion Operations

The principal indications for these operations are for the treatment of the following complications:

a) Non-union.
b) Graft overgrowth.
c) Development of secondary stenosis.
d) Disc or facet joint lesions above or below fused spinal segments.
e) Fusion at the wrong level.
f) Infection.
g) Spondylosis acquisita.
h) Ligamentum flavum atrophy.

i) Non-Union of Spinal Grafts

The multiplicity of methods of spinal fusion underlines the fact that it is difficult to produce union of the grafts with the vertebral column. The success rate of the lengthy spinal fusions used with Harrington's or Luecke's rods in scoliotics has not been matched when applied to the treatment of degenerative disorders or spondylolisthesis in the lumbar spine.

Non-union of the various spinal grafts used in the lumbar area can be diagnosed usually with plain X-rays, motion X-rays or tomograms. Discography may have a special place in the assessment of persisting pain after posterior spinal fusion with pseudarthrosis, as advocated by MacNab (1977, p. 195), though MRI may provide sufficient evidence of the state of adjacent discs. Myelography may also be useful to demonstrate acquired canal stenosis.

Attempts at re-grafting in failed posterior fusions frequently fail. This problem may be managed most effectively in the majority of cases by a supplementary anterior interbody fusion.

Conversely, where an anterior interbody graft has failed, supplementary posterior inter-transverse grafting will often succeed, fusion of the anterior graft occurring pari-passu with the union of the posterior graft.

Particular problems may be encountered when attempting to repeat an anterior lumbar interbody grafting operation when no other method is applicable. The first is the identification of the vertebral interspace which will be obscured by extensive scarring. Facilities must be available for obtaining good quality radiographs in the operating room. The second problem of adherence of the great vessels to the vertebral column is always anticipated, so that a proper range of instruments and sutures should be available to deal with injuries to the great veins or their branches which may be inflicted on them inadvertently during dissection. Lumbar interbody fusion operations are usually performed through left-sided abdominal incisions. In the special circumstances of attempting to re-graft in the case of failure, the risks of ureteric injury or of damage to the left common iliac artery or vein are high. It may be safer to expose the lower lumbar vertebrae through a right-sided extra-peritoneal approach. Without doubt, attempted re-fusion of a failed anterior lumbar interbody graft should only be undertaken by a surgeon with special training in the use of these techniques of spinal fusion. Even equipped with the necessary training and with the help of skilled assistants, it may prove technically impossible to perform a re-fusion by this method. The patient should be informed in advance of the potential problems, including the possibility that the operation may need to be abandoned without completion of the re-grafting.

Non-union of cervical anterior interbody fusions is uncommon. Re-grafting is usually easy, though identification of the site of the pseudarthrosis can be difficult. Special care is needed when inserting the instruments to cut a new graft bed to ensure proper siting of the dowel cavity between the vertebral bodies, both in the longitudinal and transverse planes. In these cases it is potentially easy to expose and so to damage the vertebral artery and its venae comitantes if the cutter has been inserted too far laterally. The outlines of the inner margins of the longus colli muscles are usually obscured by the scar tissue formed following the previous surgery, so that the safety factor normally provided by the identification of these landmarks is lost. Damage to the vertebral artery and subsequent efforts to control the ensuing haemorrhage from it may lead to quadriparesis (Figs. 9.12 a–c), or to cerebro-vascular accidents.

ii) Graft Overgrowth After Posterior Spinal Fusion

Attention was drawn to this particular complication by Crock in 1976. It may occur following the use of techniques for posterior spinal fusions involving the use of fragments of cortico-cancellous bone. While every effort should be made to place the bone chips accurately at the time of performing inter-transverse, postero-lateral or Hibb's type posterior fusions, the movement of some of the graft fragments beyond the desired area of fusion may occur and these bony fragments may continue to grow. An extreme example of this problem was seen in an elderly lady who had

had multiple spinal operations performed for a lumbo-sacral disc lesion. A dense spicule of bone had extended to the level of the facet joints at L1/2 on one side where the point of this "unwanted graft" impinged upon the facet joint capsule causing chronic pain. Examples of this unwanted overgrowth of graft are shown in Figs. 9.13 a–d. Gratifying relief of intractable back pain can be obtained in these cases by simply excising the "unwanted bone", leaving the main body of the graft intact.

iii) Development of Secondary Stenosis Beneath the Graft

Hypertrophy of posterior fusions has been reported and may lead to secondary lumbar canal stenosis after many years. The complication is not common. Currently it is best assessed either by the use of MRI or by CT radiculography.

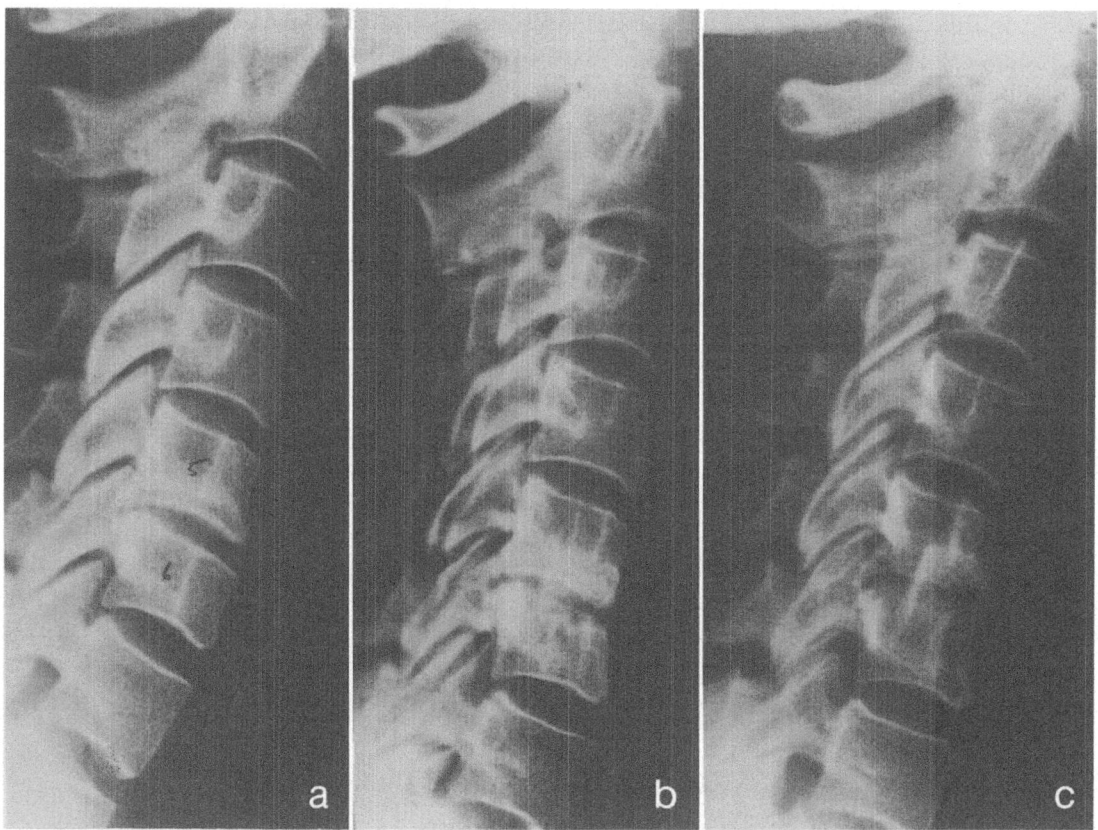

Figures 9.12 a–c. Lateral radiographs of the cervical spine of a man aged 39 years. **a** Shows an isolated spondylitic degenerative change between the vertebral bodies of C5 and C6, the cause of intractable neck pain, occipital headache and brachial neuralgia. **b** Is a lateral radiograph taken nine months after interbody fusion performed by the Cloward method, showing non-union of the graft with some kyphotic deformity. **c** A lateral radiograph taken six months after replacement of the graft using the technique described in Chapter 7, p. 237

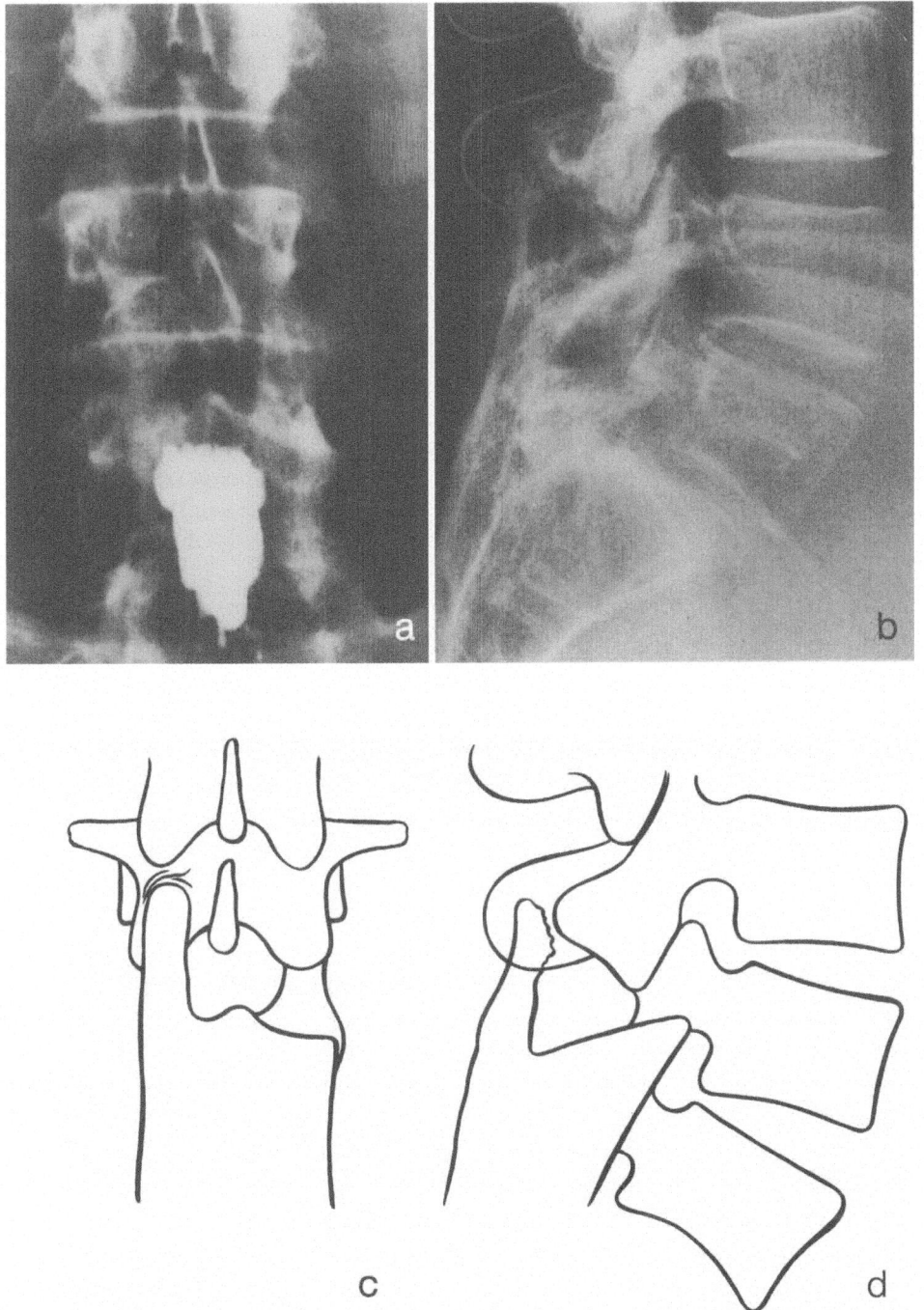

Figures 9.13a–d. a and **b** Antero-posterior and lateral radiographs of a posterior spinal fusion for spondylolisthesis in a woman aged 48 years. The prolongation of a bar of grafted bone can be seen on the left side overlying the lamina of L3 with reactive bone formation near the adjacent facet. **c** and **d** Explanatory drawings of the radiographs. **c** Shows solid fusion between the posterior elements of L4 and S2, with upward extension of the "unwanted graft"

Relief of this form of stenosis can be difficult technically because the graft may measure many centimetres in depth. Usually it is possible to relieve the stenosis without interfering with the stability of the graft. This is done by removing the central segment of the graft and exposing the dural sac beneath it, being guided by the principles of re-exploration of the spine which have been outlined above.

iv) Disc or Facet Joint Lesions Above or Below the Fused Spinal Segment

Disc prolapse above a fused spinal segment occurs in a few cases. It usually occurs some years after the fusion and its identification is easy on clinical grounds. MRI or CT radiculography scanning are useful investigations when the diagnosis is suspected.

Acute nucleus pulposus calcification may be seen in discs adjacent to a previously fused spinal segment (Chapter 4).

Secondary degenerative arthritic changes may affect the facet joints above and below fused spinal segments, leading to secondary root canal stenosis or even spinal canal stenosis. Limited root canal decompression operations are usually effective in relieving symptoms.

v) Fusion at the Wrong Level

Surgeons dread this problem which may occur either when anterior interbody or posterior fusion methods are used at any level in the vertebral column. Readers are referred again to the sections of this book dealing with the operative technique of anterior interbody fusion operations, Chapters 2 and 7 (Figs. 9.7, 9.9, 9.10 a, b).

vi) Infections

Fortunately, infection after most spinal fusions is uncommon, though it is usually chronic and often difficult to control. Its incidence after the combined use of grafting with internal fixation is, regrettably, high, averaging 4 to 5% of cases.

Early post-operative death from gas gangrene has been reported following inter-transverse-alar fusion.

Chronically infected posterior grafts can be treated successfully by open drainage and the use of long-term chemotherapy; that is, by the same methods which are usually effective in controlling chronic osteomyelitis in long bones.

Infection after anterior interbody grafting operations is rare but serious. Epidural abscess formation is likely and may lead to cervical cord compression or cauda equina compression. Urgent radical drainage is required, with special measures in the neck to prevent the development of secondary kyphotic deformities. Skull traction may be required for some weeks or some form of halo applied, fitted to a thoracic jacket.

If the infection is due to staphylococcal organisms, long-term chemotherapy for at least 6 months is recommended (Fig. 9.14).

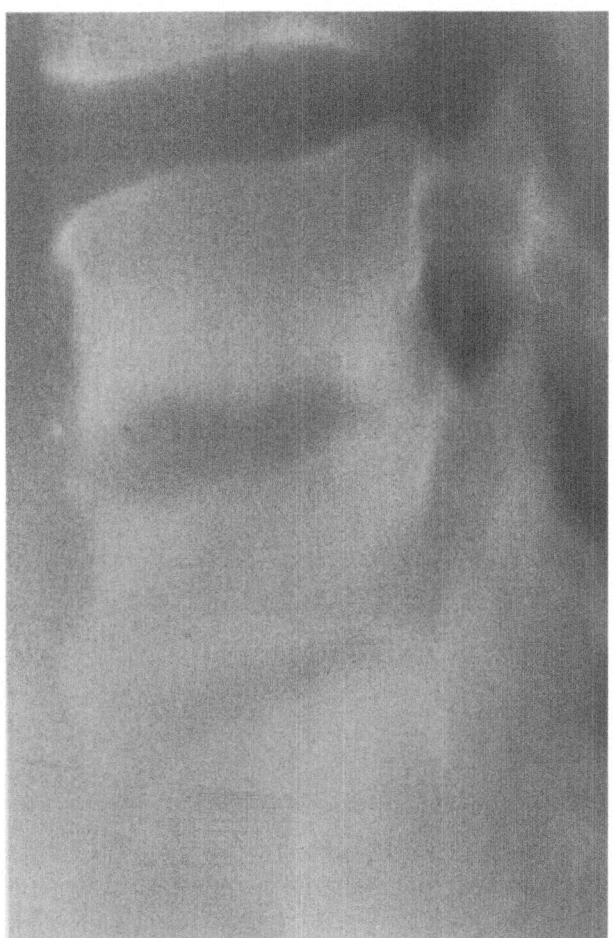

Figure 9.14. A lateral tomogram of the lower lumbar spine of a man aged 45 years. This film was taken more than twelve months after interbody fusions had been performed at L4/5 and L5/S1 levels, following which staphylococcal infection of the spine had occurred, leading to the development of an epidural abscess and to infection of the laminae and spinous processes at both levels. The infection was due to a staphylococcus aureus sensitive to Cloxacillin. The patient was treated by surgical drainage of the paravertebral abscess through the left loin and subsequently by extensive laminectomy for removal of infected laminal bone and for further drainage of an epidural abscess. Long-term chemotherapy was required over the course of 18 months and fibrous union followed

vii) Spondylolysis Acquisita

This is a well-recognized though uncommon complication of posterior spinal fusion, though as MacNab has pointed out (1977, p. 216) it does not complicate inter-transverse fusions in which the pars interarticularis of the proximal vertebral segment in the spinal fusion is supported by the graft.

Assuming that the disc at the level of the spondylolytic defect is intact, it may be satisfactory to perform a localized foraminal decompression, even on one side only.

viii) Ligamentum Flavum Atrophy

Atrophy of the ligamentum flavum occurs following interbody fusion operations, both in the lumbar and cervical regions. In some cases, this may lead to dural root sleeve tethering, so that, with normal movements at the first mobile segment above the fusion, the nerve roots at the level of the fusion may be stretched because the ligamentum flavum adheres to them. In the lumbar region, total laminectomy with excision of the ligamentum flavum over the area of the fused segment of the spine, leaving intact the facet joints at the level of the first mobile segment above the fusion, has been found satisfactory. It may also be applied to the management of persisting problems of neck and arm pain following successful anterior cervical fusion.

ix) Synchronous Combined Anterior and Posterior Spinal Fusion, with Internal Fixation

This massive operation has been advocated, in recent years, for the primary treatment of multi-level lumbar disc degeneration and as a salvage procedure following failure of other operations. Good results have been claimed by O'Brien and Kozak (1990) and by Selby and Henderson (1991). Despite its intended purpose even this procedure has failed, sometimes with catastrophic results.

Multi-level degenerative disease of the spine often responds tolerably well to conservative treatment. If surgery is required for its treatment in the lumbar spine, the less radical operation of bilateral foraminal and nerve root canal decompressions, with preservation of the laminal arches, spinous processes and their related ligaments will often give acceptable results (Fig. 9.15).

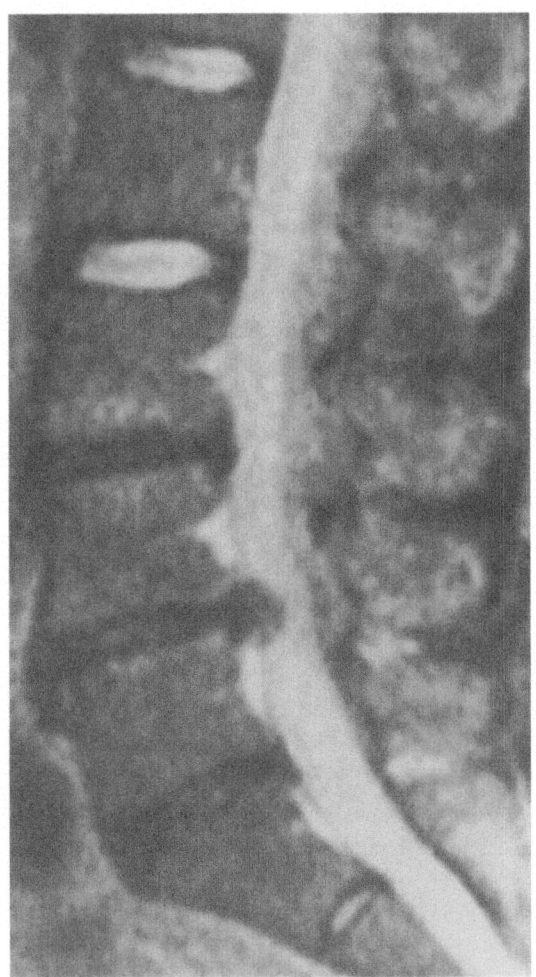

Figure 9.15. A mid-sagittal MR image, T2 weighted sequence, from the lumbar spine of a 24 year old man who presented with recurring episodes of back pain and lumbar scoliosis. He was a sedentary worker. Despite the appearance of a large filling defect related to the dural sac at the L4/5 level, he had no neurological signs on examination. His symptoms subsided with conservative treatment and surgery was not necessary

9.6. Summary

The surgical techniques used in re-exploring the lumbar spine have been described in considerable detail in this chapter. In concluding, attention is focussed on a number of important points:

1. Pay particular attention to the muscles of the back which will be further damaged by the re-exploration operation.
   Release self-retaining retractors every 45 minutes to allow the muscle blood supply to flow for 5 minutes before proceeding with the surgery.
2. Do not leave jagged remnants of laminal bone in the roof of the spinal canal. Preserve the pars interarticularis, leaving smooth laminal margins adjacent to the dural sac. Coat these bony surfaces either with bone wax or with haemostatic agents at the conclusion of the operation.
   Do not leave bony spicules in scar tissue overlying the dura.
3. Pay particular attention to haemostasis during the operation. Avoid electrocoagulation of vessels in the spinal canal as far as possible, relying rather on the use of haemostatic agents such as gelfoam, packed lightly in the paradural gutters at the end of the operation.
4. Use closed suction drainage post-operatively, except in cases where leakage of cerebrospinal fluid may be anticipated.
5. Before embarking on re-explorations of the spinal canal, the surgeon must be familiar with techniques for opening and closing the dural sac or nerve root sheaths. He or she must be aware of the potential danger of cauda equina injury and avoid the use of a strong sucker without the protection of a cotton patty on the sucker tip.
   In treating cauda equina arachnoiditis (p. 213) or in circumstances where multiple rents have occurred in abnormally thin dura in the course of the operation, closure of the dura may not be indicated. Special care must then be exercised in closing the wounds and the patient should be given chemotherapy prophylactically.

9.7. Post-Operative Care

Pain control is often particularly difficult in these patients so that special management with continuous intravenous infusions of Pethidine or Omnopon may be required for a few days. Anticoagulant therapy is advised, particularly after lengthy operations.

Mobilization should start soon after operation and in due course a cautious rehabilitation programme should commence. Warm pool therapy is often useful, though if this is not available, then walking progressive distances is to be recommended. Any vigorous muscular exercise is to be avoided.

Light surgical corsets are often helpful for short-term use.

Medical Aspects in the Management of Spinal Surgical Patients

Bryan P. Galbally, M.B.B.S., F.R.A.C.P.

Surgical procedures on the spinal cord and spinal canal structures are the fifth most commonly performed operations, after biopsies, caesarean section, repair of lacerations in obstetrical patients, hysterectomy, and more common than cholecystectomy, oophorectomy, open reduction of fractures and appendicectomy (National Center for Health Statistics, U.S.A., 1987).

Patients who undergo spinal surgery are usually adults whose pain has been chronic and sometimes disabling. Only a minority of them will suffer acute symptoms requiring spinal surgery on an emergency basis. The majority will have suffered from spinal pain for many months or years and undergone various forms of treatment comprising bed-rest, traction, injections, physical therapy, including chiropractice and osteopathy, acupuncture and varieties of complementary medicine such as homeopathy, naturopathy, aromatherapy, reflexology, herbal medicine, faith healing and special diets, eg macrobiotics; many will have used large doses of different kinds of medication: analgesics, pain-killers, anxiolytics, hypnotics, antidepressants, and non-steroidal anti-inflammatory drugs. It is in the review and assessment of these drugs which are so often taken in combination and in large dosage by patients with chronic spinal pain that the physician has an essential and major role to play in their management. The immediate and beneficial results of spinal surgery may allow drastic modification of the medication regime over several weeks but a number of patients presenting for operation are drug dependant and require special care to moderate the addiction before surgery.

The first 24–48 hours after general anaesthesia, when the patient is receiving intravenous analgesia (usually morphine, pethidine or omnopon) provides the best opportunity to withdraw drugs of dependency. Following the cessation of administration of intravenous narcotics, appropriate drugs are prescribed in moderation, e.g. Voltarol (diclofenac) per rectum, Tylex (codeine and paracetamol), and Aspav (aspirin and papaveretum) orally. The range and dosage of drugs regularly consumed by some patients is often excessive as illustrated in the records of three cases listed in Table 1.

Table 1. Examples of pre-operative daily medication intake in 3 patients at the time of their admission to hospital for repeat spinal surgery

Case 1		Case 2*		Case 3	
Diazepam	50 mg	Diazepam	10 mg	Lorazepam	6 mg
Triazolam	0.375 mg	Nitrazepam	15 mg	Triazolam	1 mg
Thyroxine	150 mcg	Promethazine	20 mg	Paracetamol	4 g
Benzhexol	15 mg	Paracetamol	4 g		
Cyclobenzaprine	30 mg	Aspirin	600 mg		
Metoprolol	300 mg	Dihydrocodeine tartate	300 mg		
Nifedipine	30 mg	Diphenoxylate +	5 mg		
Glyceryl trinitrate		Atropine	50 mcg		
transdermal patch	5 mg	Ranitidine	300 mg		
Beclamethasone aerosol	600 mcg	Hyoscine butylbromide	40 mg		
Aspirin	300 mg	Nabumetone	1 g		
Codeine phosphate	120 mg	Frusemide	80 mg		
Paracetamol	3 g	Potassium chloride	1.2 g		
Dextropropoxyphene	100 mg				
Amitriptyline	200 mg				
Clofibrate	1 g				
Sucralfate	3 g				
Ranitidine	450 mg				
Frusemide	120 mg				
Potassium chloride	3 g				
Diphenoxylate +	5 mg				
Atropine	50 mcg				

* Case 2 developed acute hepatic failure with coma post-operatively on a previous occasion.

All three cases were discharged from hospital following definitive spinal surgery with a markedly reduced intake of drugs.

The patient presenting for spinal surgery may be receiving medication for concomitant pathological conditions: these regimes will require attention and review prior to general anaesthesia and surgery. Conditions such as hypertension, diabetes mellitus, asthma, allergy and hypersensitivity may require further specific investigation and management before operation.

Pre-operative review must include psychological assessment as well as physical examination including dental inspection and other special tests: chest radiography, electrocardiography, haematology, serology and biochemistry profiles. A raised erythrocyte sedimentation rate as a single abnormal finding in an otherwise healthy patient may point to underlying pathology. As an example, an ESR of 40 mm in these circumstances was found to be caused by a uterine infection due to a retained loop which had been in place for several years.

Chronic spinal pain which is severe enough to be disabling is almost always accompanied by psychological disturbances. Many patients have obsessional neuroses and depression reflecting the inevitable stress imposed on the patient's own psyche and the deterioration in lifestyle of the spouse or close family members; these effects may reach others in the near-environment perhaps the family physician, the physiotherapist or osteopath, neighbours and friends, the family nanny or other domestic staff. The result is a network of tangled interpersonal relationships the common thread of which is the patient's response, the ability to cope or otherwise, with chronic disabling spinal pain. The dynamics of the patient's closer interpersonal relationships usually require scrutiny as part of the psychological evaluation. Psychotherapy and/or psychotropic drugs may be indicated.

Practice in North America strongly supports the notion of several days hospitalisation prior to surgery for physical therapy, group therapy and instruction in pre- and post-operative procedures, operative procedures and medico-legal consequences. This approach is not widely accepted in other Western countries. Europeans are less enthusiastic about and certainly less responsive to group therapy and are generally less preoccupied with clinical minutiae and the potential for medico-legal action.

Admission to hospital should be at least one day prior to surgery. However, information must be obtained at least one month earlier with regard to the intake of drugs, in particular certain psychotropics such as monoamine oxidase inhibitors, the contraceptive pill or hormone replacement therapy. These drugs pose threats such as subarachnoid haemorrhage with general anaesthesia and intravenous narcosis or post-operatively of thrombo-embolic manifestations. Also, the intake of alcohol, nicotine and other lifestyle drugs should be restricted to reduce the risks of general anaesthesia.

Unhurried counselling on the major aspects of the patient's individual spinal surgery should be given on admission. Patient care is more satisfactory when the patient has time to become familiar with the hospital environment and with the staff who will be in attendance post-operatively. At this time, the use of special equipment such as the vertical tilting bed, the intravenous infusion pump, the chair with spring-loaded seat, elastic stockings, to enhance venous drainage, and orthoses for use in the neck or other areas of the spine where indicated, may be explained.

However, some patients who have a concomitant illness or a history of complex drug intake may require to be admitted several days prior to surgery. In this time, their general physical condition may be improved, specific treatment given and drug control initiated. Most spinal surgical patients have the opportunity to achieve recovery when their pain is reduced or eliminated and their dependency situation removed as a consequence.

Previously unrecognized concomitant disease discovered following admission to hospital is not uncommon and is cause for concern for the physician: various anaemias (commonly sickle-cell and iron deficiency), carcinomas (lung, bladder and colon), disorders of biochemistry (commonly hyperlipidaemia), hormone secreting tumours (acromegaly and phaeochromocytoma), tuberculosis, neurological disorders, urethral stricture, sexually transmitted diseases including human immuno-deficiency viral infection. Testing for HIV antibodies is desirable in all patients undergoing surgery and requires sensitive counselling both before and after the test. The patient should always be reassured of the strict confidentiality of the test and its result and offered the option of not being informed of the result itself.

Early post-operative complications with spinal surgery relate to malfunction of the gut. Nausea is common with intravenous narcotic medication and a short-lived ileus commonly follows anterior approaches to the thoracic or lumbar spine. Occasionally a more severe ileus occurs requiring naso-gastric drainage, intravenous dextrose and electrolytes and if prolonged, complete parenteral nutrition. If a central venous line is used it should be changed at intervals not exceeding 48 hours. Intensive care is most likely to be required in surgery of the upper cervical spine – here a patient nurse ratio of 1:1 will replace ordinary ward nursing care. Post-operative pain relief is achieved with an intravenous adjustable infusion pump delivering a fixed rate of a suitable narcotic, usually morphine, pethidine or omnopon. Close supervision of the intravenous pump is mandatory noting the patient's respiratory rate and blood pressure at frequent intervals.

Early mobilisation on the day of, or the day after, surgery is facilitated by the use of a vertical tilting bed which places the patient upright and allows him or her to walk freely from the footboard.

Respiratory care, mobilisation and early rehabilitation are supervised by the physical therapist who exercises the patient each day, both morning and afternoon.

Apart from early mobilisation, the risk of post-operative thrombo-embolic manifestations is reduced by the use of heparin injected subcutaneously each day (e.g. Clexane 40 mg, commenced 12 hours prior to surgery) for a week to ten days, and the wearing of above-knee elastic stockings to enhance venous drainage from the lower limbs for at least six weeks after surgery.

A short-lived rise in temperature due to a metabolic response is the norm after spinal surgery. In the presence of significant wound infection on the other hand, the temperature is persistently elevated, the pulse rapid, pain is severe and the patient looks ill.

The management of spinal surgical patients rests on the efforts of a dedicated team under the leadership of the spinal surgeon. Its members include assistant surgeons, fellows-in-training, nurses, physiotherapists and technicians specially trained in the care of patients undergoing spinal surgery together with a physician or physicians who are committed to the aspects of patient care which are briefly outlined above.

References

Adkins, E. W. O.: Lumbo-sacral arthrodesis after laminectomy. J. Bone Joint Surg. *37B*, 208–223 (1955).

Albee, F. H.: Transplantation of a portion of tibia into the spine for Pott's disease. JAMA *57*, 885–886 (1911).

American Academy of Orthopaedic Surgeons Symposium on the Spine, p. 289. St. Louis: C. V. Mosby. 1969.

Armstrong, J. R.: Lumbar disc lesions. Edinburgh: E. and S. Livingstone. 1965.

Aronson, H. A., Dunmore, R. H.: Herniated upper lumbar disc. J. Bone Joint Surg. *45A*, 311–317 (1963).

Arseni, C., Nash, F.: Protrusion of thoracic intervertebral discs. Acta Neurochir. (Wien) *11*, 3–33 (1963).

Assheuer, J.: Neuroradiologist (Köln, Germany). Personal communication (1991).

Beadle, O. A.: The intervertebral disc (Medical Research Council, Special Report Series 161), p. 79. London: His Majesty's Stationery Office. 1931.

Beals, R. K., Hickman, N. W.: Industrial injuries of the back and extremities. J. Bone Joint Surg. 54A, 1593–1611 (1972).

Bickerstaff, E. R.: Neurological examination in clinical practice, 3rd ed. Oxford-London-Edinburgh-Melbourne: Blackwell. 1973.

Blikra, G.: Intradural herniated lumbar disc. J. Neurosurg. *31*, 676–679 (1969).

Bobechko, W. P., Hirsch, C.: Autoimmune response to nucleus pulposus in the rabbit. J. Bone Joint Surg. *47B*, 574–580 (1965).

Bogduk, N., Macintosh, J. E.: The applied anatomy of the thoracolumbar fascia. Spine *9*, 164–170 (1984).

Bohlman, H. H., Cook, S. S.: One-stage decompression and posterolateral interbody fusion for lumbosacral spondyloptosis through a posterior approach. Report of two cases. J. Bone Joint Surg. *64A*, 415–418 (1982).

Bonneville, J. F. (ed.): Focus on Chemonucleolysis, pp. 1–152. Berlin-Heidelberg-New York-Tokyo: Springer. 1986.

Brain, Lord R., Wilkinson, M.: Cervical spondylosis and other disorders of the cervical spine. London: W. Heinemann. 1967.

Brav, E. A., Bruck, S., Fruchter, J. M.: A roentgenologic study of low back and sciatic pain. AJR *48*, 39–46 (1942).

Briggs, H., Krause, K.: The intervertebral foraminotomy for relief of sciatic pain. J. Bone Joint Surg. *27*, 475–478 (1945).

Brown, H. A., Pont, M. E.: Disease of lumbar discs: 10 years of surgical treatment. J. Neurosurg. *20*, 410–417 (1963).

Brown, M. D.: Intradiscal therapy, pp. 1–186. Chicago-London: Year Book Medical Publishers Inc. 1983.

Brown, M. D.: The pathophysiology of disc disease. Orthop. Clin. North Am. *2*, 359–370 (1971).

Buck, J. E.: Direct repair of the bony defect in spondylolisthesis. In: Operative Surgery, 3rd ed., p. 419. London: Butterworths. 1979.

Buck, J. E.: Direct repair of the defect in spondylolisthesis. J. Bone Joint Surg. *52B*,432–437 (1970).

Burton, C. V., Heithoff, K. B., Kirkaldy-Willis, W., Ray, C. D.: Computed tomographic scanning and the lumbar spine, Part II: Clinical considerations. Spine *4*, 356–368 (1979).

Campbell, A. M. G., Phillips, D. G.: Cervical disk lesions with neurological disorder. Brit. Med. J. *2*, 481–485 (1960).

Carson, J., Gumpert, J., Jefferson, A.: Diagnosis and treatment of thoracic intervertebral disc protrusions. J. Neurol. Neurosurg. Psychiatry *34*, 68–77 (1971).

Chari, P. R. (Professor of Orthopaedic Surgery, Hyderabad, India): Personal communication, unpublished.

Charnley, J.: Arthroplasty of the hip. A new operation. Lancet *1*, 1129–1132 (1961).

Chow, S. P., Leong, J. C. Y., Ma, A., Yau, A. C. B. C.: Anterior spinal fusion for deranged lumbar intervertebral disc. Spine *5*, 452–458 (1980).

Cloward, R. B.: Lumbar intervertebral disc surgery. Surgery *32*, 852–857 (1952).

Cloward, R. B.: The treatment of ruptured lumbar intervertebral discs by vertebral body fusion. J. Neurosurg. *10*, 154–168 (1953).

Cloward, R. B.: Multiple ruptured lumbar discs. Ann. Surg. *142*, 190–195 (1955).

Cloward, R. B.: The anterior approach for ruptured cervical discs. J. Neurosurg. *15*, 602–617 (1958).

Cloward, R. B.: Lesions of the intervertebral discs and their treatment by interbody fusion methods. Clin. Orthop. *27*, 51–77 (1963).

Cole, E. S.: Psychiatric aspects of compensable injury. Med. J. Aust. *1*, 93–100 (1970).

Collis, J. S.: Lumbar discography. Springfield, Ill.: Ch. C. Thomas. 1963.

Coventry, M. B., Ghormley, R. K., Kernohan, J. W.: The intervertebral disc: its microscopic anatomy and pathology. J. Bone Joint Surg. *27*, 105–112, 233–247 (1945).

Critchley, E. M. R.: Lumbar spinal stenosis. (Leading article.) Brit. Med. J. *284*, 1588–1589 (1982).

Crock, H. V.: The arterial supply and venous drainage of the bones of the human knee joint. Anat. Rec. *144*, 199–218 (1962).

Crock, H. V.: Post-traumatic erosions of articular cartilage. J. Bone Joint Surg. *64B*, 530–538 (1965).

Crock, H. V.: The blood supply of the lower limb bones in man. Edinburgh-London: E. and S. Livingstone. 1967.

Crock, H. V.: A reappraisal of intervertebral disc lesions. Med. J. Aust. *1*, 983–989 (1970).

Crock, H. V.: Isolated lumbar disc resorption as a cause of nerve root canal stenosis. Clin. Orthop. *115*, 109–115 (1976).

Crock, H. V.: Observations on the management of failed spinal operations. J. Bone Joint Surg. *58B*, 193–199 (1976).

Crock, H. V.: Traumatic disc injury. In: Handbook of clinical neurology (Vinken, P. J., Bruyn, G. W., eds.), pp. 481–511. Amsterdam: North-Holland. 1976.

Crock, H. V.: Surgical management of lumbar disc prolapses. In: Operative surgery, 3rd ed., pp. 404–415. London: Butterworths. 1978.

Crock, H. V.: Anterior lumbar interbody fusion, indications for its use and notes on surgical technique. Clin. Orthop. *165*, 157–163 (1981).

Crock, H. V.: Normal and pathological anatomy of the lumbar spinal nerve root canals. J. Bone Joint Surg. *63B*, 487–490 (1981).

Crock, H. V.: Traitement chirurgical de la calcification du nucleus pulposus du disque intervertébral dorsal et lombaire, chez l'adulte. Revue de chirurgie orthopédique *68*, 171–177 (1982).

Crock, H. V., Crock, M. C.: A technique for decompression of the lumbal spinal canal. Neuro-Orthopaedics *5*, 96–99 (1988).

Crock, H. V., Goldwasser, M.: The fine circulation related to the vertebral end-plates in adult dogs. Spine *9*, 702–706 (1984).

Crock, H. V., Yoshizawa, H.: The blood supply of the vertebral column and spinal cord in man. Wien-New York: Springer. 1977.

Crock, H. V., Yoshizawa, H., Kame, S. K.: Observations on the venous drainage of the human vertebral body. J. Bone Joint Surg. *55B*, 528–533 (1973).

Crockard, H. A.: Anterior approaches to lesions of the upper cervical spine. Clin. Neurosurg. *34*, 389–416 (1988).

Cyriax, J.: The slipped disc. London: Gower Press. 1970.

Dandy, W. E.: Concealed ruptured intervertebral discs: Plea for elimination of contrast media in diagnosis. JAMA *117*, 821–823 (1941).

DeBeyre, J., Delforges, P.: Arthrodèse vertébrale intersomatique. Rev. Chir. Orthop. *45*, 855–894 (1959).

DePalma, A. F., Rothman, R. H.: The intervertebral disc. Philadelphia: W. B. Saunders. 1970.

Dillane, J. B., Fry, J., Kalton, G.: Acute back syndrome – a study from general practice. Brit. Med. J. *2*, 82–84 (1966).

Donisch, E. W., Trapp, W.: The cartilage end plates of the human vertebral column (some considerations of postnatal development). Anat. Rec. *169*, 705–716 (1971).

Doppman, J. L., Di Chiro, G., Ommaya, A. K.: Selective arteriography of the spinal cord. St. Louis: W. H. Green. 1969.

Dreyfus, P. B., Six, B., Dorfmann, H., De Sèze, S.: La hernie discale dorsale. Sem. Hôp. Paris *48*, 3045–3052 (1972).

Dwyer, A. F., Newton, N. C., Sherwood, A. A.: An anterior approach to scoliosis. A preliminary report. Clin. Orthop. *62*, 192–202 (1969).

Dyck, P.: Paraplegia following chemonucleolysis. A case report and discussion of neurotoxicity. Spine *10*, 359–362 (1985).

Dye, E. R.: Kinematics of the human body under crash conditions. Clin. Orthop. *8*, 305–309 (1956).

Ehni, G.: Effects of certain degenerative diseases of the spine, especially spondylosis and disk protrusion, on the neural contents, particularly in the lumbar region. Mayo Clinic Proc. *50*, 327–338 (1975).

Epstein, B.: The spine. New York-London: Lea and Febiger. 1969.

Epstein, J. A., Epstein, B. S., Lavine, L.: Nerve root compression associated with narrowing of the lumbar spinal canal. J. Neurol. Neurosurg. Psychiatry *25*, 165–176 (1962).

Esses, S. I., Sachs, B. L.: Complications of pedicle screw fixation. Paper 64 delivered at the 25th Anniversary Meeting of the Scoliosis Research Society 1991, Minneapolis, Minnesota, USA.

Farfan, H. F., Cossette, J. W., Robertson, G. H., Wells, R. V., Krause, H.: The effects of torsion on the lumbar intervertebral joints: the role of torsion in the production of disc degeneration. J. Bone Joint Surg. *52A*, 468–497 (1970).

Farfan, H. F., Huberdeau, R. M., Dubow, H. I.: Lumbar intervertebral disc degeneration. J. Bone Joint Surg. *54A*, 492–510 (1972).

Ferguson, A. B.: Roentgendiagnostic. Extremities and spine. New York: Hoeber. 1949.

Fineschi, C.: Anatomical anomalies of the lumbar spinal roots. Arch. Putti *2*, 222–236 (1952).

Finneson, B. E.: Low back pain. Philadelphia: J. B. Lippincott. 1973.

Flynn, J. C., Hoque, M. A.: Anterior fusion of the lumbar spine. J. Bone Joint Surg. *61A*, 1143–1150 (1979).

Fraser, R. D.: A wide muscle-splitting approach to the lumbosacral spine. J. Bone Joint Surg. *64B*, 44–46 (1982).

Frederickson, B. E., Baker, D., McHolick, W. J., Yuan, H. A., Lubicky, J. P.: The natural history of spondylolysis and spondylolisthesis. J. Bone Joint Surg. *66A*, 699–707 (1984).

Frederickson, B. E., Baker, D., Murtland, A., Yuan, H. A.: Paper presented at 5th Annual Meeting, North American Spine Society, Monterey, California, August 1990.

Freebody, D., Bendall, R., Taylor, R. D.: Anterior transperitoneal lumbar fusion. J. Bone Joint Surg. *53B,* 617–627 (1971).

Frykholm, R.: Deformities of dural pouches and strictures of dural sheaths in the cervical region producing nerve root compression. A contribution to the aetiology and operative treatment of brachial neuralgia. J. Neurosurg. *4,* 403–413 (1947).

Fujimaki, A., Crock, H. V., Bedbrook, G. M.: The results of 150 anterior lumbar interbody fusion operations performed by two surgeons in Australia. Clin. Orthop. *165,* 164–167 (1982).

Ghosh P. (ed.): The Biology of the intervertebral disc, pp. 1–245. Boca Raton, Florida: CRC Press Inc. 1988. Anniversary meeting of the Scoliosis Research Society, Minneapolis, 1991.

Gill, G. G., Manning, J. C., White, H. L.: Surgical treatment of spondylolisthesis without spine fusion. J. Bone Joint Surg. *37A,* 493–518 (1955).

Gimeno, A.: Arachnoid, neurenteric and other cysts. In: Handbook of clinical neurology: congenital malformations of the spine and spinal cord (Vinken, P. J., Bruyn, G. W., eds.), pp. 393–448. Amsterdam: North-Holland. 1978.

Gonsette, R.: An experimental and clinical assessment of water-soluble contrast medium in neuro-radiology. A new medium Dimer – X. Clin. Radiol. *22,* 44–56 (1971).

Graf, H.: Graf stabilisation system. Lyon, France (1991).

Graham, C. E.: Backache and sciatica. Med. J. Aust. *1,* 5–8 (1974).

Grollmus, J., Perkins, R. K., Russel, W.: Erythrocyte sedimentation rate as a possible indicator of early disc space infection. Neurochirurgia (Stuttg.) *17,* 30–35 (1974).

Gross, D.: Treatment of prolapsed lumbar intervertebral disk. Folia Rheumatologica (Basel) *2,* 1–16 (1965).

Gurdjian, E. S., Webster, J. E., Ostrowski, A. Z., Hardy, W. G., Lindner, D. W., Thomas, L. M.: Herniated lumbar intervertebral discs – an analysis of 1,176 operated cases. J. Trauma *1,* 158–176 (1961).

Hakelius, A., Nilsonne, U., Pernow, B., Zetterquist, S.: The cold sciatic leg. Acta Orthop. Scand. *40,* 614–623 (1969).

Happey, F., Johnson, A. G., Naylor, A., Turner, R. L.: Preliminary observations concerning the fine structure of the intervertebral disc. J. Bone Joint Surg. *46B,* 563–567 (1964).

Hartman, J. T. (Dean, Faculty of Medicine, Texas Tech. University, Lubbock, Texas): Personal Communication, unpublished.

Hasue, M., Ito, R.: Sacral nerve root cyst as a cause of low back pain and sciatica. J. Jap. Orthop. Ass. *46,* 65–72 (1972).

Hasue, M., Kunogi, J., Kikuchi, S.: Imaging methods of the dorsal root ganglion. Diagnostic aids in lumbar spine disease. A preliminary report. Neuro-Orthopaedics *8,* 23–27 (1989).

Helfet, A. J., Gruebel Lee, D. M.: Disorders of the lumbar spine. Philadelphia: J. B. Lippincott. 1978.

Hijikata, S.: Practice of discography. In: Diagnosis of orthopaedic diseases. (Tsuji, H., Takahashi, H., eds), chapter 14, pp. 689–700. Tokyo: Kanehara Shuppan. 1982.

Hijikata, S., Yamagishi, M., Nakayama, T., et al.: Percutaneous disectomy: a new treatment method for lumbar disc herniation. J Toden Hosp. *5,* 5 (1975).

Hirabayashi, K., Satomi, K., Sasaki, T.: Ossification of the posterior longitudinal ligament in the cervical spine. In: The cervical spine. (Serb, H. H., Dunn, E. J., Eismont, F. J., et al., eds.), pp. 678–692. Philadelphia: Lippincott. 1989.

Hirsch, C., Bobechko, W. P.: Auto-immune response to nucleus pulposus in the rabbit. J. Bone Joint Surg. *47B,* 574–580 (1965).

Hirsch, C., Zotterman, Y.: Cervical pain. Proc. Intern. Symp. Wenner-Gren Center, Stockholm, 1971. Oxford: Pergamon Press. 1972.

Hodgson, A. R., Stock, F. E.: Anterior spinal fusion: a preliminary communication of the radical treatment of Pott's disease and Pott's paraplegia. Brit. J. Surg. *44*, 266–275 (1956).

Hooper, J.: Low back pain and manipulation. Med. J. Aust. *1*, 549–551 (1973).

Houdart, R., Djindjian, R., Hurth, M.: Chirurgie des angiomes de la moelle. Neuro-Chirurgie *15*, Suppl. 1 (1969).

Hudgins, W. R.: The predictive value of myelography in the diagnosis of ruptured lumbar discs. J. Neurosurg. *32*, 152–162 (1970).

Hult, L.: The Munk Fors investigation. Acta Orthop. Scand. Suppl. *16*, 1–76 (1954).

Inman, V. T., Saunders, J. B. DeCM: Anatomico-physiological aspects of injuries to the intervertebral disc. J. Bone Joint Surg. *29*, 461–475 (1947).

Jackson, R. K.: The long-term effects of wide laminectomy for lumbar disc excision. J. Bone Joint Surg. *53B*, 609–616 (1971).

Jayson, M.: The lumbar spine and back pain. London: Sector Publishing. 1976.

Jenkins, D. H. R., Weeks, R. D., Yau, A. C. M. C., Du, R. R.: Manual of spinal surgery. London: Butterworths. 1981.

Johnson, R. H.: Cerebro-spinal fluid. In: Scientific foundations of neurology, pp. 281–288. London: W. Heinemann. 1972.

Jones, R. A. C., Thomson, J. L. G.: The narrow lumbar canal. J. Bone Joint Surg. *50B*, 595–605 (1968).

Kellgren, J. H.: Sciatica. Lancet *1*, 561–564 (1941).

Keyes, D. C., Compere, E. L.: The normal and pathological physiology of the nucleus pulposus of the intervertebral disc: an anatomical, clinical and experimental study. J. Bone Joint Surg. *14*, 897–938 (1932).

Kirkaldy-Willis, W. H., Paine, K. W. E., Cauchoix, J., McIvor, G.: Lumbar spinal stenosis. Clin. Orthop. *99*, 30–50 (1974).

Kirkaldy-Willis, W., Hill, R. J.: A more precise diagnosis for low back pain. Spine *4*, 102–109 (1979).

Knutsson, F.: The vacuum phenomenon in intervertebral discs. Acta Radiol. (Stockh.) *23*, 173–179 (1942).

Köhler, A., Zimmer, E. A.: Borderlands of the normal and early pathologic in skeletal roentgenology. New York-London: Grune and Stratton. 1968.

Kramer, J.: Intervertebral disk diseases: causes, diagnosis, treatment and prophylaxis. Stuttgart: G. Thieme. 1981.

Kudelka, P.: Laminectomy in lumbar disc syndrome. Med. J. Aust. *1*, 1120–1122 (1968).

Kulak, R. F., Schultz, A. B., Belytschko, T., Galante, J.: Biomechanical characteristics of vertebral motion segments and intervertebral disc. Orthop. Clin. North Am. *6*, 121–133 (1975).

Lancourt, J. E., Glenn, W. V., jr., Wiltse, L. L.: Multiplanar computerized tomography in the normal spine and in the diagnosis of spinal stenosis: a gross anatomic-computerized tomographic correlation. Spine *4*, 379–390 (1979).

Le Vay, D.: A survey of surgical management of lumbar disc prolapse in the United Kingdom and Eire. Lancet *1*, 1211–1213 (1967).

Lin, P. M., Gill, K.: Lumbar interbody fusion, pp. 1–271. Rockville, Maryland, Royal Tunbridge Wells: Aspen Publishers Inc. 1989.

Lindblom, K.: Diagnostic puncture of intervertebral discs in sciatica. Acta Orthop. Scand. *17*, 231–239 (1948).

Lowther, D. A., Baxter, E.: Isolation of a chondroitin sulphate protein complex from bovine intervertebral discs. Nature (Lond.) *211*, 595–597 (1966).

Lowther, D. A. (Monash University, Melbourne): Personal communication, 1972.

MacCartee, C. C., Griffin, P. P., Byrd, B. E.: Ruptured calcified thoracic disc in a child. J. Bone Joint Surg. *54A*, 1272–1274 (1972).

McKenzie, J. A., Williams, J. F.: The dynamic behaviour of the head and cervical spine during "whiplash". J. Biomech. *4*, 477–490 (1971).

Macnab, I.: Acceleration-extension injuries of the cervical spine. In: American Academy of Orthopaedic Surgeons Symposium on the Spine, p. 16. St. Louis: C. V. Mosby. 1969.

Macnab, I.: Chemonucleolysis. Clin. Neurosurg. *20*, 183–192 (1973).

Macnab, I.: Backache. Baltimore: Williams & Wilkins. 1977.

Macnab, I., McCulloch, J. A., Weiner, D. S., Hugo, E. P., Galway, R. D., Dall, D.: Chemonucleolysis. Can. J. Surg. *14*, 280–289 (1971).

Maroudras, A., Nachemson, A., Stockwell, R. A.: Factors involved in the nutrition of the adult human intervertebral disc. J. Bone Joint Surg. *55A*, 658–659 (1973).

Mathews, J. A.: Epidurography. In: Modern trends in orthopaedics, pp. 148–166. London: Butterworths. 1972.

Matsubara, T., Karube, F., Terashima, I.: Atypical course observed following discography – cases of discitis and disappearing backache. J. Orthop. Surg. (Tokyo) *17*, 124–130 (1966).

Matsuda, H. M., Hirose, T., Shimazu, A., Yoshimura, M., Yamano, Y., Nakajima, K.: Electro-neurophysiological diagnosis by the approach from single nerve root unit in the degenerative spondylolisthesis. Osaka City Med. J. *23*, 155–165 (1977).

Matsuda, H., Hirose, T., Hashimoto, T., Shimazu, A., Yamano, Y., Nakajima, K.: Electro-diagnosis of compression of individual nerve roots of the cauda equina. Intern. Orthop. *2*, 121–131 (1979).

Mayer, H. M., Brock, M.: Percutaneous lumbar disectomy, pp. 1–218. Berlin-Heidelberg-New York: Springer. 1989.

McCulloch, J. A.: Chemonucleolysis. J. Bone Joint Surg. *59B*, 45–52 (1977).

McCulloch, J. A., Macnab, I.: Sciatica and Chymopapain, pp. 1–225. Baltimore-London: Williams and Wilkins. 1983.

McCulloch, J. A.: Principles of micro surgery for lumbar disc disease, pp. 1–307. New York: Raven Press. 1989.

Med. J. Aust. (Editorial): Comments on: Backache and sciatica: a new breakthrough or a new controversy? Med. J. Aust. *1*, 3 (1974).

Mercer, R., Duthie, R. B.: Orthopaedic surgery, 6th ed. London: Edward Arnold. 1964.

Miller, H.: Accident neurosis. Brit. Med. J. *1*, 919–925 (1961).

Mitchell, P. E. G., Hendry, N. G. C., Billewicz, W. Z.: The chemical background of intervertebral disc prolapse. J. Bone Joint Surg. *43B*, 141–151 (1961).

Mixter, W. J., Barr, J. S.: Rupture of the intervertebral disc with involvement of the spinal canal. New Engl. J. Med. *211*, 210–215 (1934).

Moll, J., Wright, T. V.: Measurement of spinal movement. In: The lumbar spine and back pain (Jayson, M., ed.), pp. 93–112. London: Sector Publishing. 1976.

Morgan, F. P., King, T.: Primary vertebral instability as a cause of low back pain. J. Bone Joint Surg. *39B*, 6–22 (1957).

Murphey, F., Simmons, J. H. C., Brunson, B.: Surgical treatment of laterally ruptured cervical disc. Review of 648 cases, 1939–1972. J. Neurosurg. *38*, 679–683 (1973).

Murphey, M. G., Gado, M.: Anterior cervical discectomy without interbody bone graft. J. Neurosurg. *37*, 71–74 (1972).

Nachemson, A.: Mechanical stresses on lumbar disks. In: Current practice in orthopaedic surgery, pp. 208–224. St. Louis: C. V. Mosby. 1966.

Nachemson, A.: Intradiscal measurements of pH in patients with lumbar rhizopathies. Acta Orthop. Scand. *40*, 23–42 (1969).

Nachemson, A. L.: The lumbar spine an orthopaedic challenge. Spine *1*, 59–71 (1976).

Nachemson, A.: Editorial comment. Lumbar discography – where are we today? Spine *14*, 555–557 (1989).

Nachemson, A., Morris, J. M.: In vivo measurements of intradiscal pressure. J. Bone Joint Surg. *46A*, 1077–1092 (1964).

Nashbold, B. S., Hrubec, Z.: Lumbar disc disease: a twenty year follow-up study. St. Louis: C. V. Mosby. 1971.

Naylor, A.: The biophysiological and biochemical aspects of intervertebral disc hernation and degeneration. Ann. Roy. Coll. Surg. Engl. *31*, 91–114 (1962).

Naylor, A.: The late results of laminectomy for lumbar disc prolapse. J. Bone Joint Surg. *56B*, 17–29 (1974).

Naylor, A., Happey, F., Turner, R. L., Shentall, R. D., West, D. C., Richardson, C.: Enzymic and immunological activity in the intervertebral disc. Orthop. Clin. North Am. *6*, 51–58 (1976).

Newman, P. H.: Surgical treatment for derangement of the lumbar spine. J. Bone Joint Surg. *55B*, 7–19 (1973).

Nixon, J. E. (ed.): Spinal stenosis, pp. 1–401. London: Edward Arnold. 1991.

Northfield, D. W. C., Osmond-Clarke, H.: Surgical treatment. In: Cervical spondylosis (Brain, R., Wilkinson, M., eds.), p. 215. London: W. Heinemann. 1967.

O'Connell, J. E. A.: Maternal obstetrical paralysis. Surg. Gynec. Obstet. *79*, 374–382 (1944).

O'Connell, J. E. A.: Protrusions of the lumbar intervertebral discs. A clinical review based on five hundred cases treated by excision of the protrusion. J. Bone Joint Surg. *33B*, 8–30 (1951).

Ohki, K.: Biochemical studies on lumbar disc lesions, changes in the protein-polysaccharide complex. J. Jap. Orthop. Ass. *48*, 567–579 (1974).

Olerud, S., Karlstrom, G., Sjostrom, L.: Transpedicular fixation of thoracolumbar vertebral fractures. In: Clinical orthopaedics and related research, Vol. 227, pp. 44–50. Philadelphia: J. B. Lippincott. 1988.

Olmarker, K.: Spinal nerve root compression, studies from the laboratory of experimental biology, departments of anatomy and orthopaedics, Sahlgren Hospital. University of Goteborg, Sweden. 1990.

Ooi, Y., Mita, F., Satoa, Y.: Myeloscopic study on lumbar spinal canal stenosis with special reference to intermittent claudication. Spine *15*, 544–549 (1990).

Paine, K. W. E., Haung, P. W. H.: Lumbar disc syndrome. J. Neurosurg. *37*, 75–82 (1972).

Palmer, J. J.: Spinal arachnoid cysts. J. Neurosurg. *41*, 728–735 (1974).

Pankovich, A. M., Korngold, L.: A comparison of the antigenic properties of the nucleus pulposus and cartilage protein polysaccharide complexes. J. Immunol. *99*, 431–437 (1967).

Parke, W., Gammel, K., Rothman, R. H.: Arterial vascularization of the cauda equina. J. Bone Joint Surg. *63A*, 53–61 (1981).

Parker, N.: Malingering. Med. J. Aust. *2*, 1308–1311 (1972).

Paulson, S., Sylven, B., Hirsch, C., Snellman, O.: Biophysical and physiological investigations on cartilage and other mesenchymal tissues. The diffusion rate of various substances in normal bovine nucleus pulposus. Biochim. Biophys. Acta (Amst.) *7*, 207–213 (1951).

Peacock, A.: Observations on the post-natal structure of the intervertebral disc in man. J. Anat. (Lond.) *86*, 162–179 (1952).

Peck, F. C., Jr.: A calcified thoracic intervertebral disk with herniation and spinal cord compression in a child. Case report. J. Neurosurg. *14*, 105–109 (1957).

Penning, L.: Functional pathology of the cervical spine. Amsterdam: Excerpta Medica. 1968.

Pennybacker, J. (Oxford University): Personal communication, 1959.

Perot, P. L., Munro, D. D.: Transthoracic removal of mid-line thoracic disc protrusions causing spinal cord compression. J. Neurosurg. *31*, 452–458 (1969).

Postaccini, F.: Lumbar spinal stenosis, pp 1–240. Wien: Springer. Bologna: Aulogaggi. 1989.

Putti, V.: New conceptions in the pathogenesis of sciatic pain. Lancet *2*, 53–60 (1927).

Ransford, A. O., Harries, B. J.: Localized arachnoiditis complicating lumbar disc lesions. J. Bone Joint Surg. *54B*, 656–665 (1972).

330 References

Rathke, F. H., Schlegel, K. F.: Surgery of the spine. In: Atlas of orthopaedic operations (Hackenbroch, M., Witt, A. N., eds.), Vol. 1. Stuttgart: G. Thieme. 1979.

Reynolds, F. C., Katz, S. F.: Herniated lumbar intervertebral disc. In: American Academy of Orthopaedic Surgeons Symposium on the Spine, pp. 84–96. St. Louis: C. V. Mosby. 1969.

Riley, L. H., Robinson, R. A., Johnson, K. A., Walker, A. E.: The results of anterior interbody fusion of the cervical spine. Review of 93 consecutive cases. J. Neurosurg. *30*, 127–133 (1969).

Robinson, R. A., Smith, G. W.: Anterolateral cervical disc removal and interbody fusion for cervical disc syndrome. Bull. Johns Hopkins Hospital *96*, 223–224 (1955).

Robinson, R. A., Walker, A. E., Ferlic, D. C., Wiecking, D. K.: The results of anterior interbody fusion of the cervical spine. J. Bone Joint Surg. *44A*, 1569–1587 (1962).

Rothman, R. H., Simeone, F. A.: The spine, Vol. II. Philadelphia: W. B. Saunders. 1975.

Roy-Camille, R., Lazennec, J. Y., Garreau, C., Saillant, G.: Grade three and grade four L5/S1 spondylolisthesis: Surgical reduction and fixation through a posterior approach about 29 cases. Rachis *3*, 147–158 (1991).

Sacks, S.: Anterior interbody fusion of the lumbar spine. J. Bone Joint Surg. *47B*, 211–233 (1965).

Sarpyener, M. A.: Congenital stricture of the spinal canal. J. Bone Joint Surg. *27*, 70–79 (1945).

Schatzker, J., Pennal, G. F.: Spinal stenosis, a cause of cauda equina compression. J. Bone Joint Surg. *50B*, 606–618 (1968).

Schmorl, G.: Die pathologische Anatomie der Wirbelsäule. Verh. Dtsch. Orthop. Ges. *21*, 3–41 (1926).

Schmorl, G., Junghanns, H.: The human spine in health and disease (translated by Wilk, S. P., Groin, L. S.), p. 38. New York: Grune and Stratton. 1959.

Scott, J. H. S.: The Edinburgh repair of isthmic (Group 2) spondylolysis. J. Bone Joint Surg. *69B*, 491 (1987).

Selby, D. K., Henderson, R. J.: Circumferential (360 degree) spinal fusion. In: The adult spine principles and practice (Frymoyer, J. W., ed.), pp. 1989–2006. New York: Raven Press. 1991.

Simeone, F. A.: The modern treatment of thoracic disc disease. Orthop. Clin. North Am. *2*, 453–462 (1971).

Simpson, J. A.: Electromyography. In: Scientific Foundations of Neurology, pp. 341–356. London: W. Heinemann. 1972.

Smith, B. H.: Clinical spondylosis and its neurological complications. Springfield, Ill.: Ch. C. Thomas. 1968.

Smith, J. W., Serafini-Fracassini, A.: The distribution of the protein polysaccharide complex in the nucleus pulposus matrix in young rabbits. J. Cell. Sci. *3*, 33–40 (1968).

Smith, L., Brown, J. E.: Treatment of lumbar intervertebral disc lesions by direct injection of chymopapain. J. Bone Joint Surg. *49B*, 502–519 (1967).

Sonnabend, D. H., Taylor, T. K. F., Chapman, G. K.: Intervertebral disc calcification syndromes in children. J. Bone Joint Surg. *64B*, 25–31 (1982).

Spangfort, E. V.: The lumbar disc herniation. Acta Orthop. Scand., Suppl. *142*, 1–95 (1972).

Spurling, R. G., Grantham, E. G.: The end results of surgery for ruptured lumbar intervertebral discs. A follow-up study of 327 cases. J. Neurosurg. *6*, 57–64 (1949).

Stauffer, R. N., Coventry, M. B.: Anterior interbody lumbar spine fusion. Analysis of Mayo Clinic series. J. Bone Joint Surg. *54A*, 756–768 (1972).

Stauffer, R. N., Coventry, M. B.: Posterolateral lumbar spine fusion. Analysis of Mayo Clinic series. J. Bone Joint Surg. *54A*, 1195–1204 (1972).

Stevenson, H. G.: Back injury and depression – a medico-legal problem. Med. J. Aust. *1*, 1300–1302 (1970).

Stewart, D. Y.: Current concepts of the "Barré syndrome" or the "posterior cervical sympathetic syndrome". Clin. Orthop. *24*, 40–48 (1962).

Tan, S. B., Kozak, J. A., Graham, J. M.: A modified technique of anterior lumbar fusion with femoral cortical allograft. J. Orthop. Surg. Techn. *5*, 83–93 (1990).

Taylor, T. K. F., Akeson, W. H.: Intervertebral disc prolapse: a review of morphologic and biochemic knowledge concerning the nature of prolapse. Clin. Orthop. *76*, 54–79 (1971).

Torgerson, W. R., Dotter, W. E.: Comparative roentgenographic study of the asymptomatic and symptomatic lumbar spine. J. Bone Joint Surg. *58A*, 850–853 (1976).

Tsuji, H.: Comprehensive atlas of lumbar spine surgery. Mosby year book (1991).

Van Akkerveeken, P. F.: Diagnosis and neuromechanisms: Pain patterns and diagnostic blocks. In: The Lumbar Spine, Chapter 3 (Editorial committee – Weinstein, J. N. and Wiesel, S. W.). W. B. Saunders Company – Harcourt Brace Jovanovich, Inc. 1990.

Venner, R. M., Crock, H. V.: Clinical studies of isolated disc resorption in the lumbar spine. J. Bone Joint Surg. *63B*, 491–494 (1981).

Verbiest, H.: A radicular syndrome from developmental narrowing of the lumbar vertebral canal. J. Bone Joint Surg. *36B*, 230–237 (1954).

Verbiest, H.: Further experience of the pathological influence of a developmental narrowness of the bony lumbar vertebral canal. J. Bone Joint Surg. *37B*, 576–583 (1955).

Verbiest, H.: The lateral approach to the cervical spine. Clin. Neurosurg. *20*, 295–305 (1973).

Verbiest, H.: Neurogenic intermittent claudication. Amsterdam: North-Holland. 1976.

Vogelsang, H.: Intraosseous spinal venography. Amsterdam: Excerpta Medica. 1970.

von Torklus, D., Gehle, W.: The upper cervical spine. London: Butterworths. 1972.

Waddell, G., Kummel, E. G., Lotto, W. N., Graham, J. D., Hall, H., McCulloch, J. A.: Failed lumbar disc surgery and repeat surgery following industrial injuries. J. Bone Joint Surg. *61A*, 201–206 (1979).

Waddell, G., McCulloch, J. A., Kummel, E., Venner, R. M.: Nonorganic physical signs in low-back pain. Spine *5*, 117–125 (1980).

Watkins, M. B.: Postero-lateral bone grafting for fusion of the lumbar and lumbo-sacral spine. J. Bone Joint Surg. *41A*, 388–396 (1959).

Weinstein, P. R., Ehni, G., Wilson, C. B.: Lumbar spondylosis: diagnosis, management and surgical treatment. Chicago: Year Book Medical Publishers. 1977.

White, A. A., Southwick, W. O., Deponte, R. J., Gainor, J. W., Hardy, R.: Relief of pain by anterior cervical spine fusion for spondylosis: report of 65 patients. J. Bone Joint Surg. *55A*, 525–534 (1973).

Williams, P. C.: Reduced lumbosacral joint space: its relation to sciatic irritation. JAMA *99*, 1677–1682 (1932).

Wilson, P. H., MacCarty, W. C.: Discography: its role in the diagnosis of lumbar disc protrusion. J. Neurosurg. *31*, 520–523 (1969).

Wiltberger, B. R.: The dowel intervertebral body fusion as used in lumbar disc surgery. J. Bone Joint Surg. *39A*, 284–292 (1957).

Wiltberger, B. R., Abbott, K. H.: Dowel intervertebral body fusion as used in lumbar disc therapy. J. Int. Coll. Surg. *29*, 204–213 (1958).

Wiltse, L. L.: Spondylolisthesis in children. Clin. Orthop. *21*, 156–163 (1961).

Wiltse, L. L.: The etiology of spondylolisthesis. J. Bone Joint Surg. *44A*, 539–560 (1962).

Wiltse, L. L.: Common problems of the lumbar spine: spondylolisthesis and its treatment. JCE Orthop. *7*, 13–31 (1979).

Wiltse, L. L.: Long term follow up of high grade spondylolisthesis treated by in-situ alar transverse fusions without spinal canal decompression. Video Presentation at 5th Annual Meeting, North American Spine Society, Monterey, California, August 1990.

Wiltse, L. L., Bateman, J. G., Hutchinson, R. H., Nelson, W. E.: The paraspinal sacrospinalis-splitting approach to the lumbar spine. J. Bone Joint Surg. *50A*, 919–926 (1968).

Wiltse, L. L., Hutchinson, R. H.: Surgical treatment of spondylolisthesis. Clin. Orthop. *35*, 116–135 (1964).

Wiltse, L. L., Rocchio, P. D.: Preoperative psychological tests as predictors of success of chemonucleolysis in the treatment of the low-back syndrome. J. Bone Joint Surg. *57A*, 478–483 (1975).

Wiltse, L. L., Widell, E. H., Jr., Jackson, D. W.: Fatigue fracture: the basic lesion in isthmic spondylolisthesis. J. Bone Joint Surg. *57A*, 17–22 (1975).

Wullenweber, R., Brock, M., Hamer, J., Klinger, M., Spoerri, O.: Lumbar disc. Adult hydrocephalus. (Advances in Neurosurgery, Vol. 4.) Berlin-Heidelberg-New York: Springer. 1977.

Yoshizawa, H., O'Brien, J. P., Smith, W. T., Trumper, M.: The neuropathology of intervertebral discs removed for low-back pain. J. Path. *132*, 95–104 (1980).

Zilkens, K. W., Peters, B., Schwanitz, B.: Biochemical markers for an earlier detection of spinal infections. Paper presented to the European Spine Society, Rome, 1991.

Subject Index

Herbert Resch, Emil Beck (eds.)

Arthroscopy of the Shoulder

Diagnosis and Therapy

Translated from the German
by Marie-Louise Antoft and Brigitte Marschall

1992. 125 figs. Approx. 200 pages
Cloth DM 198,-, öS 1386,-
ISBN 3-211-82339-5

Prices are subject to change without notice

This book focuses on arthroscopy of the shoulder joint and the subacromial space. Diagnosis as well as the current therapeutic possibilities are described in explicit detail. The book begins with describing the anatomy of the shoulder joint from an arthroscopic viewpoint. The diagnostic part gives a description of the individual structures in the glenohumeral joint as well as the subacromial space with regard to their pathologic changes and special attention is focused on differentiating between healthy and pathologic structures. The therapeutic part gives a detailed description of the Bankart refixation methods successfully applied by the authors which include a suturing technique, a refixation technique using absorbable tacks and an extraarticular screw fixation technique; furthermore the techniques of subacromial decompression, removal of a calcium deposits and the resection of the lateral end of the clavicle are described in detail. Starting with the indication for arthroscopy and/or arthroscopic therapy, the book then conveys information on positioning, draping, necessary instruments and then goes on the technical realization of the arthroscopic intervention itself, thus it gives all necessary details which are required for arthroscopy of the shoulder.

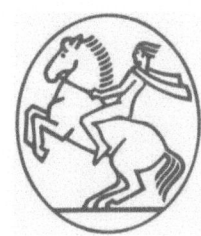

Springer-Verlag Wien New York

Mario Campanacci

Bone and Soft Tissue Tumors

Co-authors of the Soft Tissue Section:
Franco Bertoni and Patrizia Bacchini

Foreword: W. F. Enneking
Translator: Sylvia Notini
Translation from the Italien edition

1990. 881 figs. XI, 1131 pages.
Cloth with slipcase DM 548,-, öS 3.836,-
ISBN 3-211-82186-4

Prices are subject to change without notice

This book systematically treats the tumors of bones and soft tissues. An expert in the fields of pathology and orthopedic surgery, Professor Campanacci describes these tumors in terms of the pathological, clinical, radiographic, and therapeutic points of view. The introductory chapter deals with the classification, frequency, diagnostic tools, biopsies, and therapeutic strategies for these tumors. Following the histological classification, the author describes the primary, secondary, and metastatic tumors, and pseudotumoral lesions in detail.
Bone and Soft Tissue Tumors stems from both Professor Campanacci's 30 years of experience and from the clinical records of 15.000 studied and verified cases of the Instituto Ortopedico Rizzoli, the largest orthopedic clinic in Italy. The book contains illustrations of all varieties of tumors, with special emphasis on those cases which exemplify the typical tumors encountered in daily clinical practice. For the English edition the book has been completely revised and updated. The bibliography has been trimmed down to include only the most significant and recent publications. The addition of uniform subtitles makes this edition more concise and comprehensible.

Jointly published by **Springer-Verlag Wien New York**
and **Aulo Gaggi, Editore, Bologna**

Sole distribution rights: Springer-Verlag Wien New York

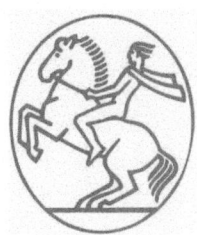

Springer-Verlag Wien New York

The manufacturer's authorised representative in the EU is Springer
Nature Customer Service Centre GmbH, Europaplatz 3, 69115 Heidelberg,
Germany. If you have any concerns regarding our products, please
contact ProductSafety@springernature.com

Printed and bound by CPI Group (UK) Ltd, Croydon, CR0 4YY

29/04/2026
02099553-0003